Praise for *The Truth in Small Doses*

" 'Why have we made so little progress in the war on cancer?' Clifton Leaf asked *Fortune* in 2004. His groundbreaking story went on to describe the failures of researchers and drugmakers alike, and a system so focused on incremental improvements in the treatment of the disease that it could not arrange itself to tackle the roots of a persistent (and still growing) problem. For a decade Leaf has followed the story, and though we are no closer to 'curing' cancer, we can now imagine—thanks to his lucid and fascinating work—what that solution might look like. In Leaf's brilliant new book, he reframes the challenge as one of engineering, not science. As Leaf writes, 'Science determines the limits of the possible. Engineering lets us reach them.' "

—*Fortune*

"According to Leaf, a journalist and cancer survivor, the [1971 National Cancer Act] failed because of the flawed research culture it spawned. In this history of the fight against cancer, he describes how scientists often cannot secure funding for risky research in a culture that rewards competition over collaboration."

—*Scientific American*

"*The Truth in Small Doses* is a detailed, sober myth-busting report."

—Ralph Nader

"As a cancer patient and advocate, I applaud Clifton Leaf for so boldly pulling back the curtain on the 'cancer culture' to reveal why we've made limited progress toward cures. *The Truth in Small Doses*, a book told with the rigor of a brilliant journalist but with the heart of a cancer survivor, is certain to disrupt the conversation on the state of cancer research and inspire new approaches to win this war."

—Kathy Giusti, founder and CEO, Multiple Myeloma Research Foundation and Multiple Myeloma Research Consortium

"Leaf's book serves as a powerful call to action that our current system is too structurally flawed to provide the transformation in cancer care we all seek. . . . The longer format has given Leaf room to explore the wide range of issues in more detail, and several chapters merit reading as stand-alone pieces. . . . Leaf's analysis is clear and accessible to scientists and non-scientists alike, and should probably be read and debated by senior executives at all oncology-focused drug companies."

—Pharmagellan.com

"In this brave and important book, Clifton Leaf explains the state of cancer research today, traces the battles we have won and lost in the war on cancer, and most importantly shows the ways in which doctors, researchers, and even patients might improve what we are doing to combat this disease. Leaf's own path—from cancer patient to journalist to author—is an inspiring story itself, and his book will benefit both patient and doctor alike. *The Truth in Small Doses* will be the most important 'discovery' in cancer this year."

—David B. Agus, M.D., author of *The End of Illness*

"In this lucid, convincing, and gripping book, Clifton Leaf lays out, in heart-breaking detail, why our well-intentioned war on cancer has produced such dispiriting results. Leaf's command of the science is masterful, his passion is palpable, and his critique of a broken research system is utterly convincing. But, like the best advocacy journalism, *The Truth in Small Doses* is ultimately inspiring, pointing the way toward a more hopeful future. It is a landmark achievement."

—Jason Tanz, executive editor of *WIRED*

"It matters because: We've been at war with cancer since 1971, and despite endless promises, are not much closer to truly winning that battle. In this refreshingly impassioned volume, Leaf explains why while offering a path forward. . . . Perfect for: Anyone curious about the history of medicine, as well as the fraught intersection of pharmacology, public policy, and the corporate world."

—TheAtlanticWire.com

"Beautifully written, with the twists, turns, and suspense of a great novel, *The Truth in Small Doses* tells the tale of the great individual successes and collective failure of both government and the pharmaceutical industry to impact the increasing number of cancer diagnoses and deaths in the U.S. But Clifton Leaf offers more than a history of our national cancer effort: He provides a vision and a roadmap for a creative and bold national cancer strategy."

—Frank M. Torti, MD, MPH, Dean, University of Connecticut School of Medicine; former director, Wake Forest Comprehensive Cancer Center; and former acting commissioner of the FDA

"An important evaluative study meriting serious public discussion."

—*Kirkus Reviews*

"[An] eye-opening look at why the U.S. is losing the war on cancer . . . *The Emperor of All Maladies* got Americans talking about the stalled battle against cancer. Leaf's book keeps the conversation on track."

—*Booklist*

"Through flowing prose Leaf delivers, alongside facts and data, stories on personalities involved in research, the fascinating process of solving an unusual and highly deadly cancer in Africa, and the heartbreaking realities of cancer treatment in children today. Leaf's extensively investigated treatise will resonate with researchers and patients frustrated by the bureaucratic woes he delineates. Public policy makers, grant reviewers, and pharmaceutical researchers alike must consider Leaf's indictment and proposed solutions."

—*Publishers Weekly*

"[*The Truth in Small Doses*] is the book you love so much that you write about it not simply to fill a hungry page with words but because of a genuine conviction that people need to read this thing. . . . A fiercely written book on a fiercely urgent subject is too hard to resist."

—TheAtlanticWire.com

"A fascinating resource for anyone interested in understanding more about the biological mechanisms of cancer and curious about the history, politics, and ethics of the current cancer culture."

—HuffingtonPost.com

"Provocative . . . his prescription is dead on."

—*New York Post*

The
Truth
in Small
Doses

Why We're Losing the War on Cancer—
and How to Win It

Clifton Leaf

Simon & Schuster

New York   London   Toronto   Sydney   New Delhi

Simon & Schuster Paperbacks
A Division of Simon & Schuster, Inc.
1230 Avenue of the Americas
New York, NY 10020

First Simon & Schuster trade paperback edition August 2014

SIMON & SCHUSTER PAPERBACKS and colophon are registered trademarks of Simon & Schuster, Inc.

For information about special discounts for bulk purchases, please contact Simon & Schuster Special Sales at 1-866-506-1949 or business@simonandschuster.com.

The Simon & Schuster Speakers Bureau can bring authors to your live event. For more information or to book an event contact the Simon & Schuster Speakers Bureau at 1-866-248-3049 or visit our website at www.simonspeakers.com.

Designed by Ruth Lee-Mui

Manufactured in the United States of America

10   9   8   7   6   5   4   3   2   1

Library of Congress Cataloging-in-Publication Data
  Leaf, Clifton.
  The truth in small doses : why we're losing the war on cancer—and how to win it / Clifton Leaf.
     p. ; cm.
  Includes bibliographical references and index.
  I. Title.
  [DNLM: 1. Neoplasms—drug therapy—Popular Works. 2. Antineoplastic Agents—economics—Popular Works. 3. Drug Discovery—history—Popular Works. 4. History, 20th Century—Popular Works. 5. Neoplasms—mortality—Popular Works. QZ 201]
  RC271.C5
  616.99'4061—dc23
                                                            2013005817

ISBN 978-1-4767-3998-4
ISBN 978-1-4767-3999-1 (pbk)
ISBN 978-1-4767-4000-3 (ebook)

For Alicia and Sofia, the loves of my life.

Contents

Part Four: The Way Forward

How Did We Get Here?

Two years before I came to believe that we were losing the "war on cancer," I had concluded that we were on the brink of victory. The notion had spun out of an extraordinary conversation I'd had in February 2002 with Daniel Vasella, then the chief executive officer of the Swiss pharmaceutical firm Novartis. He was in New York for the World Economic Forum, the annual gathering of business titans, statesmen, movie stars, and savants traditionally held in Davos, a resort town tucked high in the Swiss Alps. But this particular winter, the first after 9/11, the gathering had moved to midtown Manhattan, and the forty-eight-year-old Vasella had settled into the lobby bar at the St. Regis Hotel for a string of interviews with the business press.

I was reluctant to join the line. It was late in the day, and I was sure I was in for a lengthy pitch on some revolutionary age-spot cream then in clinical trials, or a rundown of the company's ever-expanding portfolio of medicines. I was then an editor at *Fortune* and oversaw the magazine's investing coverage, among other things, so such conversations were common. But this time the phrase *drug pipeline* was not uttered once. Nor was *revenue stream*. Nor *share price*. Vasella hardly mentioned his company at all.

Instead, he spoke about the anguish caused by endemic malaria, the soaring cost of prescription drugs, and the preventable diseases still plaguing half the world. His industry, he said with surprising candor, had not done enough to address these crises. He spoke of the challenges of innovation in a big corporation and of dismantling the walls of ancient corporate fiefdoms. (Vasella had helped engineer, in 1996, the merger of two century-old Swiss chemical companies, Sandoz and Ciba-Geigy, and had become CEO of the newly formed Novartis.)

As the conversation continued in the dim light of the hotel bar, the subjects grew more personal and raw, and dotted lines between our histories emerged. Vasella spoke of his older sister Ursula's battle with Hodgkin's disease, a cancer of the lymph system, and of watching her waste away during a grueling three-year fight. Vasella was ten at the time of her death; she was eighteen.

I too had struggled with Hodgkin's (at age fifteen), but had survived thanks to a unique chemotherapy regimen that had been pioneered at the National Cancer Institute (NCI) a decade or so prior to my diagnosis in 1978. The discovery had, unfortunately, come a few years too late to save young Ursula.

An uncannier connection was Vasella's work in the late 1980s. In his first managerial job at a pharmaceutical company, he was responsible for an obscure injectable drug, somatostatin, that was shown to relieve some of the worst symptoms of carcinoid syndrome, a rare intestinal cancer. My mother had been one of the few people in the world to rely on the drug, which had alleviated some of the daily diarrhea and near-constant skin flushing that made her disease so debilitating. Like Vasella's sister, she would eventually succumb to her cancer, in 1995.

Vasella had been surrounded by illness and tragedy as a child. At the age of five, his asthma grew so severe during the summer months that his parents sent him to live on a farm in the mountains, away from the family. When he was eight, a bout with tuberculosis, followed by meningitis, forced him to spend a full year in a hospital and sanatorium. Five years later his father, a history professor, died of complications from surgery. Then a second sister died as well, from a car accident.

Vasella related only a tiny portion of this story as we sat with our Scotches in the hotel bar.

He had gone to medical school, received his degree, and practiced medicine in Bern, Switzerland, before giving it up for a junior marketing position at Sandoz. Six years later he was in the corner office. Among the chief executives of major drug companies, Vasella was the only physician, the only one who had ever taken care of patients.

A few journalists would later venture that it was this clinically trained eye that helped him see the vast potential of the leukemia drug called Gleevec, which many oncologists were then hailing as a genuine breakthrough and as a model for cancer therapy in the generation to come. Others involved in the drug's development would give Vasella far less credit. I knew none of this at the time.

What I did know, what I could hear in our first conversation, was how Vasella spoke of the drug, which had been approved by the Food and Drug Administration just nine months earlier. He spoke the way a first-time parent speaks about his child's first recital.

Gleevec worked, he explained, in a radically new way: by homing in on a "mutant" protein found in the white blood cells of patients with an uncommon form of leukemia. This aberrant protein, created as the result of a genetic glitch, relayed instructions that sent those white blood cells into a continual replicative loop. They divided and divided until eventually they crowded out every other type of cell in the blood, and the patient died. Novartis's remarkable molecule blocked that protein from passing along its deadly message. And it was so precisely aimed that, even as it shut down the mutants, it spared the healthy cells around them. (Traditional chemotherapy, by contrast, is a sledgehammer: it decimates many normal cells as it strikes the malignant.)

Gleevec, said Vasella, had established the principle of *targeted* cancer therapy. Now it was only a matter of time until scientists designed molecules to disable the wayward signaling mechanisms central to every cancer.

As dramatic and exciting as the story line was, I failed to grasp its significance. Over the next few months, Vasella and I spoke again and again, but little about cancer. Our sprawling conversations focused on the challenges of running an enormous global company, the unyielding pressure from Wall Street, and the unexpected crises of confidence that leaders face—subjects closer to *Fortune's* editorial focus. (He and I turned the interviews into an essay for the magazine, entitled "Temptation Is All Around Us," in which Vasella thoughtfully, and forthrightly, bared some of his driving fears and desires.)

As for the revolution then going on in cancer therapy, I did not think about it again until another drug company CEO, Sam Waksal, was in the news. Waksal had founded, with his brother Harlan, a small biotech company called ImClone, which also had a targeted cancer medicine in development.

Sam Waksal was the anti-Vasella—a showman and socialite famous for hosting lavish, celebrity-brimming parties at his "art-filled SoHo loft," as New York's gossip pages put it. In 2001, he made tens of millions of dollars cashing in ImClone stock, which had soared on rumors of the imminent approval of the company's cancer agent. Like Gleevec, this new molecule was designed to interrupt the growth signaling of a specific protein.

ImClone's experimental agent, soon to be known as Erbitux, operated by way of a different mechanism: a biological one. Unlike traditional chemistry-based drugs, Erbitux was an antibody, one cultivated in the living factories of cultured cells. Conceived by a well-respected cancer researcher at Houston's MD Anderson Cancer Center, the molecule had been in the making for some twenty years. And by late 2001, at long last, it looked as if the agent would be approved by the Food and Drug Administration.

Although results from the initial trials with the antibody were nowhere near as dramatic as those for Gleevec, Erbitux's quarry was more plentiful—a protein receptor found in excess on cells in roughly a third of all cancers. Its "market," therefore, was potentially huge. That was why giant Bristol-Myers Squibb had invested a head-shaking $2 billion in ImClone earlier in the year, and why several Wall Street analysts were predicting that Erbitux would become a billion–dollar-a-year medicine. ImClone's antibody, proclaimed the brokerage firm UBS Warburg as early as January 2001, "represents a significant market opportunity, with an overall target population of well over 400,000 patients and blockbuster sales potential." Morgan Stanley Dean Witter chimed in, "In our view, ImClone is poised to become one of the next commercial success stories in biotechnology." Erbitux was to be Gleevec writ large.

But there was a snag. As 2001 drew to a close, reviewers at the FDA refused even to evaluate ImClone's antibody for licensing, citing critical problems with the way the company had set up its clinical trials and analyzed its data, among other complaints. Sam Waksal tried to dump shares of ImClone stock before the bad news came to light, passed along the confidential information to family members (who also sold stock), misrepresented the FDA's objections to public shareholders, and got caught. The style doyenne Martha Stewart also sold shares after getting advance warning. She and Waksal would both go to jail.

Every nugget from the story was savored in the press. My own magazine published nearly a dozen articles on the subject over a two-year stretch. The name ImClone became an eponym of corporate scandal like Enron, WorldCom, and so many others. Yet this story was different from the others. Waksal's white-collar crimes had a cost, it seemed, that went well beyond shareholder loss. They had left a good drug, a lifesaving drug, in the lurch.

Had ImClone's top management not botched the Erbitux clinical trials, then papered over the problems, then outright lied, the medicine might have been in cancer patients in *months*. It would now take years.

That was the sad coda to so many ImClone stories in the media. And that, oddly enough, was what made me think we were winning the war on cancer.

There was a narrative that connected the sober, truth-telling Dan Vasella with the double-talking New York social climber Sam Waksal. ImClone, the company that couldn't shoot straight, and Novartis, the one that couldn't miss, were aiming at the same surprising scientific bull's-eye.

So were dozens of other companies. And at least according to the

FDA, a few were hitting it. In May 2003, the US drug agency approved two highly touted cancer medicines: Iressa, from the European pharmaceutical company AstraZeneca, and Velcade, from a small biotech firm based in Cambridge, Massachusetts. Both were of the new genus of sophisticated drugs that zoomed in on specific antigens, enzymes, or receptors to interrupt an improper growth command or gum up a cellular mechanism that had gone dangerously awry. Iressa was going after the same high-stakes target as Erbitux.

A few weeks later, more than twenty thousand cancer doctors gathered in Chicago for the annual meeting of the American Society of Clinical Oncology (ASCO), the world's leading guild for cancer physicians. There, too, the major headlines focused on the new breed of inhibitors— notably, an antibody called Avastin, which was designed to squeeze the life out of tumors by robbing them of their blood supply. Indeed, when researchers announced the results of a new clinical trial testing Avastin in patients with advanced colon and rectal cancers, the packed hall at the McCormick Place Convention Center erupted in applause.

I had followed these developments not as a cancer patient whose life depended on knowing what new treatments offered hope, nor as a doctor who understood the context of these gains and the desperate need of those whom they cared for, nor as a science writer who studied the vagaries of the drug-discovery process and the nuances of these agents' biological mechanisms. I had followed these apparent milestones—I am embarrassed to admit—with the detached eye of a business editor. The pharmaceutical industry had long boasted of the progress it was making in the war on cancer. Here was proof, it seemed.

Even the medicine that Sam Waksal had hawked—and nearly destroyed through his carelessness—had come back from the brink of irrelevance. The evidence dangled from ImClone's suddenly lofty stock price. Between June 12, 2002, when Waksal was arrested for insider trading, and June 10, 2003, when he was sentenced to more than seven years in prison, ImClone's share price had soared 364 percent. (The Standard & Poor's 500 stock index had dropped by 3 percent over the same period.) Erbitux, the firm's only major drug, was still months away from approval. But reports from various clinical trials had been promising. It now seemed as if both the oncology experts and investors might be right after all: The antibody *worked*. Many were betting on that, at any rate.

It was a great story—and, frankly, an upbeat one in an era beset by scandal. So in the fall of 2003, I set out to report on the scientific revolution that was transforming cancer medicine. The thesis was not original. (*Fortune*'s longtime rival *BusinessWeek* had done a fine cover story on the subject a few months earlier, focusing on Erbitux.) I had promised myself to look more broadly, if possible, to see how the long war on cancer was being won on multiple levels, not just with a new fleet of drugs.

Right from the start, however, I was confused. The numbers did not add up. For years, even before drugs such as Gleevec and Erbitux came on the market, US health officials were saying that the death rate from cancer had steadily been dropping. But in the simplest terms—in raw numbers—more people in the United States were dying of cancer each year. Officials used a death rate that adjusted for both the rising population and its changing age demographics. But even with such filters in place, the rate had barely budged since 1971, when President Nixon signed the National Cancer Act, launching what became known as the war on cancer. Nor had the rate dipped much from its 1950 level.

Nor did it look as if the vaunted new cancer medicines, the targeted agents, would be able to make much of a dent. The more data I read from completed clinical trials, difficult as they were to read and comprehend, the more I wondered if the new therapies did any good at all. I was missing something, obviously. Cancer officials had been talking of declining death rates for years. Every few weeks, it seemed, came reports of a new clinical advance.

I kept looking. The nation was spending far more to study cancer, and exponentially more to treat it, than we had a decade or two earlier. Official patient survival rates had crept up a little, but even these figures were suspect, as I would discover later.

In an unexpected way, the cancer story was unfolding like so many of the sordid business sagas that had appeared in *Fortune* and *BusinessWeek* and the *Wall Street Journal* over the previous few years. There was a profound disconnect between the rhetoric of top management and the numbers. NCI officials and leading oncologists were talking about "steady progress" and "turned corners" and "breakthroughs," but the statistics told a far more depressing tale.

I began to get that old Wall Street feeling: Could we be *losing* the war on cancer?

Over the next few months of reporting I came to believe the answer was yes. I wrote a cover story for *Fortune* in March 2004 that made that sad argument. The analysis was based on more than just the numbers. Interviews with scores of scientists and doctors, regulators, and other warriors in the cancer arena had painted a disturbing picture. Their often candid testimony described what I called a dysfunctional "cancer culture"—

a groupthink that pushes tens of thousands of physicians and scientists toward the goal of finding the tiniest improvements in treatment rather than genuine breakthroughs; that fosters isolated (and redundant) prob-lem solving instead of cooperation; and rewards academic achievement and publication over all else.

At each step along the way from basic science to patient bedside, investigators rely on models that are consistently lousy at predicting success—to the point where hundreds of cancer drugs are thrust into the pipeline, and many are approved by the FDA, even though their proven "activity" has little to do with curing cancer.

Each participant in the system did the proverbial best he or she could. Everyone involved wanted to contribute. But the way the system worked day in and day out seemed almost designed to keep progress at bay—to discourage substantive collaborations, to prevent the timely sharing of data, to slow the rate at which new laboratory discoveries could be devel-oped into viable therapies. As Andy Grove, longtime CEO of microchip maker Intel, cancer survivor, and philanthropist, described it to me in early 2004, "It's like a Greek tragedy."

The letters poured in, as they always did after a provocative *Fortune* cover. I had anticipated a spirited defense from cancer doctors, but in-stead I got dozens of invitations.

Researchers, medical oncologists, cancer center directors, and patient advocates wrote with requests to continue the conversation. Some said, with surprising amiability, that I had gotten some things dead wrong; most wanted to tell me more—to share with me their own frustrations with a broken system. Patients and, harder to bear, the parents of children with cancer wrote me of their panic and despair—and, often, "in spite of what some *Fortune* reporter had written," of their resolute, unshakable hope. One man told of the high school sweetheart he had married and lost to the disease, though he still refused to believe she was gone; a father e-mailed to see if there was anything, *anything at all,* that could fend off his daughter's far-gone lymphoma.

My wife and I read the letters, one by one, and cried. She was seven months pregnant with our first child when the story came out. I was then an executive editor at the magazine—a business magazine, I reminded myself. One that published stories about Walmart and IBM; that opined about corporate strategy and investment opportunities. It was not the time to continue my inquiry into the war on cancer. I had never written a "science" article other than this one. I nearly failed high school biology, and for good reason. I wasn't qualified to write about any of this.

And yet I couldn't stop myself. There was still a story I wanted to tell. It was the one prompted by a question that went unanswered in interview after interview. If the efforts to win the fight against cancer were paralyzed by a dysfunctional cancer culture, how did we get here?

Those five words—*How did we get here?*—became the focus of my life for the next nine years. They are, indeed, the core of this book.

Cancer scientists speak eloquently about the need to study the biological mechanisms of cancer, to understand its genetic roots. Only with such comprehension, say many, can we figure out ways to stop the disease. The same can be said for the culture of cancer science: we need to know how it became the way it is before we can fix it.

The forces in this culture—some dramatic, others subtle, a few nearly imperceptible—have evolved over decades, if not centuries. Trying to single them out is like trying to point to the rainstorm that carved a canyon. But that is the thing about cultures: they form in such slow motion that the process is often ignored until the ground has been thoroughly redrawn.

I have tried nonetheless. Over the past nine years, I have spoken with well over a thousand people involved in the cancer fight around the world—oncologists, geneticists, pharmacologists and drug designers, university professors, officials at the NCI and the FDA, surgeons and radiologists, statisticians, politicians, big-company executives and start-up entrepreneurs, foundation leaders, cancer nurses, veteran advocates, care-takers, and, most of all, patients. Some of the conversations have been formal interviews; many more have been chats over coffee in the hallway of a conference center, or long-running e-mail exchanges.

In the process of reporting and writing this book, I have changed as well, beginning the journey as a business editor and ending, in some ways, as a proponent of reform. I served for three years on the national board of directors for Susan G. Komen for the Cure not as a journalist, but as an advocate for Komen's tens of thousands of volunteers and for millions of people with breast cancer. I served as a grants reviewer, and on various advisory boards and committees, not as a reporter, but rather as a participant, panelist, or member. My experiences in these roles have shaped my perspective.

In all this time I have emerged certain of only *one* conclusion: this is a story without any villains. Unlike in so many aspects of American business, personal greed has played little part in the failure of the na-tional cancer enterprise. Some readers may find that assertion difficult to believe—or may find it naïve of me to make it—but after nine years of wandering in this realm I am confident of this claim.

That said, plenty of heroes appear in the pages that follow, and through their stories—tales of lessons learned and lost, and of Herculean struggles waged for decades—this book's argument is made. In Part One, I have tried to give a complete assessment of the growing cancer burden, one now carried by millions of people, but which is barely reflected in the statistics health officials use in reporting progress in the cancer war. Part Two shows why the scientific strategy we have chosen cannot suc-ceed in lessening the terrifying human cost of cancer, and offers the only viable path to achieving that goal, which in my view is to interrupt the disease process in its earliest stages of development. (As chapter 7 makes clear, the barriers to this approach are hardly insignificant. We have little choice, though, but to attack these challenges head-on.)

Part Three is the story of the dysfunctional cancer culture itself. It begins with a wrong turn at a critical juncture in history: the start of the modern cancer effort in 1971. Chapter 8 tells the surprising tale of what happened in the legislative wrangling over the National Cancer Act—and how that act of Congress, instead of hastening a "cure," set in place (or reinforced) many of the barriers to success we face today.

No doubt many will assume that the biggest of these barriers involves money. Nearly every cancer scientist and advocate, after all, contends that our failure to make significant headway against the disease is due to a lack of sufficient funding, and politicians and stewards of the national cancer program have long agreed. Chapter 9 punctures that myth. Money is at the core of many of the failings in the modern cancer effort. The greatest of these problems stem, however, not from a lack of money, but rather from the way it is spent. This chapter, along with the next three, make that clear.

Chapter 10 reveals the career and financial incentives (and academic traditions) that push investigators to think narrowly and impede collaboration. Chapter 11 bares the mind-set that limits risk-taking in cancer drug development and all but ensures that treatment will improve in the slowest, most incremental fashion; while chapter 12 shows how thin the line between risk-taking and recklessness can be, and why we sometimes have to be willing to approach that line to save lives. Chapter 13 explains why so much of the raw data generated in the modern high-tech research effort never translates into clinical knowledge, and why even a tiny investment in low-tech infrastructure might change that.

What may be surprising to many readers is how well-known these systemic failures are to the cancer community—not only to rank-and-file researchers and oncologists, but also to those in positions of leadership in science, medicine, industry, and, yes, government. One official report after the next has cataloged the problems and promised reform. Still, little of substance is ever done to change them.

Part of the reason, indeed, may be due to the cancer culture itself. In this realm, there is little incentive for investigators to look to the past—to search for wisdom in the pages of ancient, musty journals, to follow up on the fledgling insights, or experimental teases, of scientists who came earlier. The result is that much of what is learned in one generation is forgotten in the next.

Among these myriad bits of lost wisdom, one stands out: It is the story, told in chapter 14, of a one-eyed, Irish surgeon named Denis Burkitt, who taught the world how powerful true scientific collaboration can be. Far-flung investigators, working together, unraveled a cancer mystery that no single scientist would ever have solved on his own. The tale in this chapter took place half a century and half a world away, but its lesson remains as essential today as ever.

Part Four, notably, is the shortest section of the book. It contains but one chapter ("Matterhorn"), where I have tried to lay out a way forward in our century-old cancer crusade. It may seem to some that a three-hundred-page history of how and why we have failed in the war on cancer ought to be balanced by more than a single, brief chapter for the proposed solution. There may seem to be something cowardly in spending so much time dissecting a broken system without also offering a litany of concrete "fixes." Over the past several years, I have felt that way many times myself.

But then, as will have been made clear by then, I hope, the route to victory in the cancer war is not as complex as it might seem. It does not require another act of Congress—a thousand-page bill forming new committees, oversight boards, and complicated mandates. Nor does it necessarily take a huge influx of taxpayer money to create a system that encourages researchers to think in novel ways, to share ideas more freely, and to take more entrepreneurial leaps in their scientific exploration. What is needed to reach this goal is a different sort of political will: a fierce public commitment to undo the incentives, rules, and daily practices that don't work. Many of them are so entrenched that it will take an army of citizen–scientists and warrior patients to remove them. It will take even more public will to pursue an authentic "war" on cancer, one that honestly lays out the mission and follows a coordinated plan to achieve it.

Mustering a nation's will is no easy aim. Summoning it depends first on telling the truth about the cancer burden today, and what the future holds as the American population continues to expand and age. Admittedly, some people will have a difficult time accepting such a blunt message. Grateful survivors may reflect upon their own victories and conclude that the effort is not failing at all.

Each rescued life, certainly, is a victory over cancer that ought to be celebrated. But the fact that there are millions of cancer survivors does not validate our approach in the anticancer campaign—any more than a growing number of soldiers returning from the front suggests a war is being won. All it really means is that more people have been sent into battle.

Others may contend that reporting on the lack of progress made against cancer steals precious hope from those who need it most. With each life saved, with each *report* of success, they say, comes renewed hope for those newly diagnosed, and for their loved ones.

I do not dispute the raw power of hope. I have felt it myself, believed in its magic to help me through my own bout with cancer long ago. I have seen my mother rely on it, wield it, call it forth in the darkest hours of her own fight. None of us, perhaps, could live without it.

But for hope to be more than mere wishing, it needs vision; it needs a commitment of will; it needs a clear perspective on where we are and where we need to go.

And for that, it helps to know how we got here.

Part One

The Burden

Chapter 1

Counting

J oe Hin Tjio couldn't believe his eyes. Staring down at the jumble of filaments on the glass slide, he counted again. And again. And again until he was sure.

Few lights were on at the Institute of Genetics, a low-slung, redbrick building on the outskirts of Lund. Beyond Tjio's first-floor window was only darkness. This was the Skåne region of southern Sweden, where the ground was swept flat and the winter night made the landscape colder and emptier still. It was 2:00 a.m., three days before Christmas 1955. For Tjio, a thirty-six-year-old visiting professor, that meant prime laboratory time.

He was a strange fellow—moody, defensive, prone to emotional outbursts. Effortlessly, he could turn an offhand comment from a colleague into a personal slight. The most minor of disagreements could evolve into a long-lasting feud. His Swedish coworkers, for the most part, shrugged off the behavior, attributing Tjio's hypersensitivity to the traumas he had suffered as a young man.

Born in Java in 1919, in what was then the Dutch East Indies, to

Chinese parents, Tjio (pronounced *CHEE-oh*) was a Peranakan, the name given to second-, third-, and later-generation Chinese Indonesians, who often spoke a patois of Malay and Chinese. The word translated to "local-born" or "descendant"—though it was hard to imagine Tjio descending from anywhere. He was a rootless amalgam: a Dutch-educated Chinese Indonesian, employed in Basque-speaking Spain, on sabbattical in Sweden, married to a woman from Iceland. He could move fluidly between French, English, German, and Dutch, languages he'd learned at the severe colonial schools where he'd spent his youth. He spoke Japanese as well, though for him that language conjured up bitterness and anger.

Tjio had just turned twenty-two years old when the Second World War stormed into the Indonesian archipelago. The Japanese Imperial Forces invaded much of Southeast Asia, and Tjio, along with thousands of others, was sent to a squalid, bamboo-fenced internment camp, where he was imprisoned for three years and tortured by the guards. Even the war's end offered little respite, as Indonesian authorities accused Tjio of being a Communist and detained him—until he'd at last managed to get on board a Red Cross boat for "displaced persons" bound for Holland.

He had studied plant breeding before the war, hoping to create a strain of potato resistant to disease. And after a brief study in Holland, he had landed a job at a Spanish university in the northern city of Zaragoza.

Now, Tjio was, once again, a world away from anything that could be called home. He had come to Lund to work in the laboratory of an accomplished geneticist named Albert Levan. And here in the dead of night, in the euphoria of discovery, the emotional, itinerant cell biologist from nowhere in particular had no one with whom to share his extraordinary news.

Again and again Tjio counted the tiny bended strands. They were human chromosomes, taken from the embryonic cells of an unformed lung. Thanks to a bit of chemical manipulation, he had managed to "freeze" the chromosomes in the midst of cell division—a point at which the cell's DNA was held in tightly wound, compacted coils. Ordinarily, this particular stage of the division, known as metaphase, was fleeting. But the young scientist had treated the slide with colchicine, a deadly poison found in the stem and seeds of the disarmingly beautiful autumn crocus. The poison had stopped mitosis in its tracks. Now, the wiry strands—each one a unique packet of genes—were dense enough to be seen with a light microscope. It was a marvel.

Twenty-three pairs of chromosomes. Forty-six in all. Clear as could be.

If he'd made no mistake in the preparation of the slide—and mistakes, he knew, were easy to make in this delicate art—the finding was startling. More than that, it was momentous. The textbooks would have to be re-written.

Theophilus Shickel Painter had shown, in 1921, that human cells had two roughly matching sets of twenty-four chromosomes, for a total of forty-eight. (The sole exception to the rule being the germ cells, sperm and egg, each of which had only one set.) Painter, a zoologist who'd spent most of his career at the University of Texas, had been a pioneer in mammalian chromosome studies, or cytogenetics, as the discipline was starting to be known. A careful scientist, ever attentive to detail, he was an authority in the field.

If Tjio was right, that meant Painter was wrong—humans had two *fewer* chromosomes than previously believed.

Tjio, aware of the historic nature of the moment, snapped a few photographs through the microscope. On the bottom left-hand side of one of these photomicrographs, he inscribed, *Human cell with 46 chromosomes observed 1955 on December 22nd at 2.00 a.m.* He annotated a second photo in French. In the coming days, he would ceremoniously give these mementos to friends.

It took until late January, however, for him and Levan, his laboratory boss, to do the backup experiments required to make their case to the world. By then they'd inspected the nuclear DNA of cultured cells from four separate embryos, making 261 counts in all. In nearly every case, they could clearly make out forty-six strands. The researchers prepared an article and submitted it to the Swedish journal *Hereditas,* which published the piece in its next issue.

In what would be the biggest professional battle of Tjio's long career, he argued bitterly with Levan over who would be "first author" on the paper—an honor that, then, typically went to the lab chief. Tjio tearfully threatened to destroy all the work he'd done if his name wasn't listed first, daring his boss to reproduce it. Levan eventually conceded.

There was no hint of this Sturm und Drang in the title of the article that ran in the April *Hereditas*, nor even of the provocative conclusion inside. But within months of the publication of "The Chromosome Number of Man," it became clear that an earthquake of sorts had occurred. The ground of human cytogenetics had cracked. What was for more than three decades considered by scientists around the world to be "normal" (forty-eight chromosomes) wasn't normal at all. Several labs quickly reproduced the results of the Swedish group, and the revised number was *re*set in stone. In less than a year, the established wisdom changed.

More remarkable, however, was that a fair number of chromosome researchers (even some in Lund) had already come to the same conclusion—but had kept quiet. After the *Hereditas* article was published, several researchers wrote Tjio and Levan to confess that they, too, had spied only forty-six chromosomes in their cell preparations, but had thrown out the results because they were in conflict with established knowledge. Photographic evidence of the true number had, in fact, been published long before. A black-and-white photo of the human karyotype (the complement of chromosomes divided in matched pairs) in a widely read textbook of the day, by the eminent British geneticist Cyril Darlington, clearly showed forty-six chromosomes. The photo caption, however, read forty-eight.

The belief was so powerful, so set in the culture of biological research, that at least one respected scientist continued to find phantom chromosomes in normal human cells even after several labs had verified the correct number. Masuo Kodani, writing in the prestigious journal *Science* shortly after Tjio and Levan's paper, acknowledged that forty-six chromosomes were certainly "possible" in man, but claimed there were other acceptable totals, too. Kodani reported that he'd found forty-eight of the gene-carrying strands in a full third of the Japanese men he had studied. In one case, he'd found forty-seven strands. Kodani, to put it kindly, had been confused. Chromosome counts in normal, healthy human beings— or in any other species, for that matter—do not vary from one individual to the next. (A critical exception comes with cancer, a hallmark of which is a change in the chromosomal counts of cells. Such change, called aneuploidy, is often dramatic.)

By year's end, if there were additional doubts or confusion about the "new" number, they were unlikely to be published in a serious academic journal. Just like that, scientific *truth* had changed. The sun didn't revolve around the earth. The earth wasn't flat. And human cells carried twenty-three—not twenty-four—pairs of chromosomes.

In the long, twisting history of science, the chromosome upheaval of 1956 barely registers. High school science teachers don't teach it. It is not standard fare in biology textbooks. Among the great frame-shifts in human knowledge—from Newton's gravity to Planck's quantum and Pauling's chemical bond—Joe Hin Tjio's late-night discovery has gotten the attention of a footnote.

But this minirevolution in science ought to stand out in part for its pedestrian nature: Chromosome researchers before Tjio and Levan didn't need their eyes *opened* to anything. They just needed to trust themselves enough to believe what they'd already seen.

Over a period of at least thirty years, many scientists—people trained to challenge conventions, to mistrust their own ingrained biases, to sharpen their instinct of skepticism—refused to question a finding that they had suspected was wrong. They'd accepted as incontrovertible fact something contrary to their own investigation and experience.

The question is, why? Why had so many scientists abandoned science when confronted with dogma?

This is the question that hovers over cancer research today. For the past several decades, reports of shining advances in cancer biology and treatment have streamed into newspapers, magazines, and television sets the world over. But during that time, there has been only minor change in the prospects for most people with active disease: survival numbers have barely improved; new cases keep mounting; death counts continue to rise.

Cancer doctors *see* this in their own clinics, despite offering their patients the newest, smartest drugs and treatment options in the oncology arsenal. Many of these same physicians, however, will tell you that they believe significant progress is being made in the war against cancer—for that is the story they've been hearing and reading, too. But that is not because they have witnessed it themselves.

The mythology extends from outrageously rosy assessments of the drug pipeline to the distortion of critical cancer statistics. And the cultural imperative to believe that we are winning is so powerful that when someone openly questions our progress, he risks a public shunning.

That is what happened to John Bailar.

I had spoken to the man twice, at length over the phone, before he agreed to an interview in person. We met at his office at the National Academy of Sciences building in Washington, not far from the White House.

John C. Bailar III is six feet four inches tall with a barrel chest. His thick, white hair shoots straight up from the top of his head like a forest of birch trees. His voice is a resonant baritone. Physically, he is something of a giant—which made his tentativeness at our meeting all the more surprising. Something about the man suggested vulnerability. His gait was careful, his words and tone measured.

Some of this aura of caution, no doubt, was the product of his academic heritage. Bailar was not merely trained to be a research scientist; he was genetically engineered to be one. His mother taught mathematics. His father—John Jr.—winner of the Priestley Medal, chemistry's highest honor shy of the Nobel, was an acknowledged pioneer in inorganic chemistry and author of a classic textbook. And both of Bailar's grandfathers had been professors: his mother's father taught economics at Purdue; his father's father taught chemistry at a small Colorado college.

As for John Bailar III, there seemed to be the briefest hope of reprieve from a life of scholarly analysis and serial publication. After getting an undergraduate degree in chemistry, he enrolled at Yale to become a physician. But then, with his MD in hand and a two-year hospital stint completed, Bailar decided to trade the clinic once and for all for a career in research. He was back in the family business.

The realm that called to him was known as biometry (or biostatistics), and it intersected all of the academic fields he had come to love—bringing a detached, mathematical analysis to human biology, medicine, and epidemiology. Bailar, who would go on to earn a PhD in statistics from American University, found in the National Cancer Institute the perfect place to practice his new art.

He soon emerged as a star on the institute's lush, woody campus in Bethesda, Maryland, heading up the NCI's demography section. He then took charge of the government's Third National Cancer Survey, conducted from 1969 through 1971. If Joe Hin Tjio was the consummate outsider, John Christian Bailar III was an unquestioned member of the club. The bullet points on his résumé said it all: editor in chief of the *Journal of the National Cancer Institute* for six years, statistical consultant to the *New England Journal of Medicine* for eleven years, lecturer in biostatistics at Harvard's School of Public Health for seven. By 1986, the fifty-three-year-old researcher was a respected leader in his field.

Then he publicly questioned our progress in the fight against cancer.

His doubts had been building for at least a decade, since shortly after President Nixon declared a national "war on cancer" in 1971. "Sometime during the 1970s, I began to have increasing questions about the effectiveness of the cancer research program as a whole," Bailar told me in 2004. "When I left the NCI in 1980, I thought that it was best not to say much, at least for a while."

By 1986, however, he felt as if he could not wait any longer. With Elaine Smith, an epidemiologist at the University of Iowa Medical Center, Bailar wrote a piece that May for the *New England Journal of Medicine* entitled "Progress Against Cancer?"

The headline, a sheepish fraction of a question, belied the devastating argument that would follow. Measuring cancer incidence and death in the United States back to the year 1950, Bailar and Smith found "no evidence that some 35 years of intense and growing efforts to improve the treatment of cancer have had much overall effect on the most fundamental measure of clinical outcome—death." The odds of dying from cancer had *increased* in the previous decades, not decreased. For instance, in 1962, there were 151 cancer deaths for every 100,000 Americans; by 1982, there were close to 189—a gain of 25 percent. Taking into account changes in the age of the US population (Americans had gotten older, on the whole, in the intervening years), the jump in the cancer death rate was more modest, climbing just under 9 percent in the previous two decades. But *up* 9 percent was *up*. As Bailar and Smith pointed out in an accompanying table, 155,000 more people in the United States died of cancer in 1982 than in 1962. The only conclusion they could draw was that the war on cancer "must be judged a qualified failure. Results have not been what they were intended and expected to be."

At the time, officials at the National Cancer Institute were busy talking up their goal of slashing the cancer death rate in half by the year 2000. Lawmakers in Congress had just boosted NCI appropriations to new heights (and overridden a veto by President Reagan to do so). And Bailar and Smith were now saying the cancer effort had been misfocused from the start.

The major problem, they said, was a blind focus on trying to cure cancer, rather than trying to prevent it. Prevention meant more than just getting people to quit smoking (though that was critical). It included everything from studying the role of diet in cancer to identifying and eliminating cancer-causing chemicals in the environment. It meant doing a much better job of analyzing risk factors, understanding with far greater precision *who* was getting cancer, and researching new ways to detect the disease in its earliest, most curable stages. Prevention even extended to treatment in some respects—including the prospect of using drugs to halt or reverse the early cellular abnormalities that, if unchecked, were likely to progress to malignancy and metastasis.

This strategy was the same one, after all, that had, since the 1950s, sharply reduced death from heart disease and stroke, then the leading and third-leading killers, respectively, in the country. Prevention by way of vaccines had all but eliminated polio and other once-devastating infections. Prevention by way of seat belts and speed limits had even reduced deaths from car accidents.

Bailar and Smith never proposed that research on treatment be stopped altogether. What was needed, Bailar later explained, was "a substantial realignment of the balance between treatment and prevention, and in an age of limited resources this may well mean curtailing efforts focused on therapy."

Published just as the giant annual meeting of oncologists was convening, the article brought a swift and hammerlike response. It fell most heavily upon the study's senior author—someone who should have known better. The president of the American Society of Clinical Oncology (ASCO), the powerful professional organization of cancer doctors, called Bailar "the great naysayer of our time." Others angrily questioned his motives, or his intelligence, or derided his use of "old data."

It was as if the man had never been a member of the science fraternity. Critics snapped that the experienced statistician had flubbed the statistical analysis, and several leaders in the field implied that he was too dim-witted to comprehend the "molecular revolution" then occurring in cancer medicine. Perhaps the angriest response came from the NCI director himself, Vincent T. DeVita Jr., the scientist who had led the discovery of the first successful drug therapy for Hodgkin's disease and one of the most respected figures in cancer medicine. DeVita called Bailar's paper "reprehensible," irresponsible, and misleading and claimed the statistician had "departed with reality." Bailar, who had only years earlier been a trusted part of the NCI fold, was now, in the eyes of some cancer leaders, "that son of a bitch." (This, according to Bailar, was how he'd been described at a meeting of the National Cancer Advisory Board in the wake of the *New England Journal* article.)

Bailar wasn't just offended by the reaction, he was shaken. He couldn't believe that his colleagues were attacking him personally. As he saw it, he had told the truth, which was his job as a scientist, and people treated him like an infidel . . . or a traitor.

The blowback from the cancer community came in stages, Bailar recalled: "First was absolute rage. 'How could anybody say these terrible things?' they wondered. A few weeks later came a second reaction from my colleagues and fellow epidemiologists saying, essentially, 'Everybody knows that.' Well, it was clear that everybody *didn't* know that."

Not long after the article was published, Bailar was approached by an elderly physician at a cancer meeting in Minneapolis. The doctor told him, gratefully, "that he'd been treating patients throughout his career and he didn't understand why they weren't doing any better than they were years before. Then he read my paper and saw that this was a general problem—not just his own. This man had read the newspapers like everybody else and thought there was lots of progress."

Eleven years later Bailar and a second colleague, Heather Gornik, published a follow-up study in the *New England Journal,* entitled "Cancer Undefeated," arguing that little had been done to lessen the burden of the disease. They built their case upon cancerdom's own official statistics. But as before, other researchers dismissed the findings, lacing into Bailar for his "defeatism," "underlying bias," and "cavalier attitude" toward those lives that *had* been saved in the anticancer effort. One prominent scientist, who chaired the government-appointed National Cancer Advisory Board, told a journalist that Bailar had "gone beyond the data in order to dramatize the issues" and suggested the scientist had "taken liberties with data to get the attention of the media."

Such personal attacks aside, however, the feeling in research circles overall wasn't that Bailar had botched the statistical analysis. It was that, in the words of one NCI official, he "was trying to predict the future simply by looking at the past." And scientific discovery was changing cancer treatment so dramatically that mortality trends of the past were irrelevant. Bailar's problem, said many, was that he didn't get it: *he didn't get the science.*

At long last, Bailar's critics claimed, biologists and geneticists were beginning to comprehend what the cancer process looked like—not merely at the cellular level, but on the infinitesimal scale of molecules within the cell: the (mostly) protein messengers that wriggled and jostled and signaled each other from beyond the cell membrane, across the cytoplasm, to the nuclear crypts of DNA, and back. This mystical dance of molecules was, in reality, an ancient and well-regulated system for communication—the means by which a healthy cell took its cues for when to grow, divide, and die. Except in a cancer cell, that is.

With cancer, the signaling goes terribly wrong. Decades of study and billions of dollars in research grants were now paying off, many argued, for scientists were beginning to see precisely how these communications pathways—those inside the transformed cell as well as outside—were going awry: how they were telling the cell to replicate with abandon, ignoring all instructions to stop; how they told the renegade to recruit new blood vessels, sucking up vital oxygen and nutrients at the expense of neighboring cells and tissues; how they told the malignant renegade to pack up from one site in the body and migrate to another, where it did not belong.

The implications of this hard-won knowledge were undeniable. With a detailed "route map" of cancer signaling now in hand, research scientists were confident that they could soon construct their own molecular barricades at key junctions along the way. Drug developers, the thinking went, could design chemical compounds (or even man–made antibodies) that would insert themselves between the faulty proteins and their cellular "receptors," thereby interrupting the conspiratorial whispers between them. It was a bit like blocking an electrical signal by sliding a piece of rubber between two live copper wires.

This was, at long last, a "rational," targeted approach to cancer interdiction—a far cry from the brutal systemic therapies that had largely defined cancer treatment to that point, an approach that even many oncologists derided as "slash and burn." Genuine cures were on the horizon. The excitement was palpable.

Bailar had felt it, too. He "got" the science. The spate of discoveries being reported, often breathlessly, in the medical literature were marvels to him as well. But then, he had heard such revelatory talk before. New treatment paradigms had come and gone since 1956, the year Bailar had joined the NCI as a field investigator. The argument that somehow *this time was different* was "similar in tone and rhetoric to those of decades past about chemotherapy, tumor virology, immunology, and other approaches," he and Gornik wrote in responding to critics. "In our view, prudence requires a skeptical view of the tacit assumption that marvelous new treatments for cancer are just waiting to be discovered."

A significant number of researchers and oncologists who were treating cancer patients day to day had seen firsthand what Bailar's data had spelled out. But almost no one said anything in support. At the huge annual gatherings of cancer scientists, in the prominent medical journals, nobody spoke up: Bailar the Naysayer was left to swing in the wind.

His career was not over—but it had changed. From then on, he continued to do epidemiological research, publishing analyses on such things as asbestos risk, smoking, Gulf War syndrome, and air-quality issues in Canada. But he wrote little more about the nation's progress in the war on cancer. There were only so many times he could tell the truth, it seemed, before people stopped believing him altogether.

In all the criticism of Bailar's conclusions about the cancer war, no one had questioned the data underlying them. The raw mortality figures he had cited were familiar to health officials and cancer researchers everywhere. They were the US government's own numbers, published annually by the National Center for Health Statistics (which, like the NCI, was an arm of the sprawling Public Health Service). Since long before the first of Bailar's *New England Journal* studies was published in 1986, cancer deaths had been piling up at rates significantly faster than the growth in population.

This was the same dismal trend, indeed, that had led Congress to pass the National Cancer Act—the legislation that began America's war on cancer in 1971. The slew of touted drugs and discoveries that had come since had not lessened the crisis—that much Bailar's blunt-edged data had shown. Yet the same progression of drugs and discoveries had convinced many of the nation's top scientists and doctors that the war on this disease was being won. As with the case of human chromosomes, the best and brightest had chosen to believe and repeat the textbook line—not what, in many cases, they had seen and counted and measured with their own eyes.

Yet what was most surprising, perhaps, about the whole Bailar affair was not his sobering message, nor even its wholesale rejection by the cancer community. Rather, it was that it had all happened before. Three-quarters of a century before John Bailar's public challenge, another statistician had offered a starkly similar warning.

Frederick Ludwig Hoffman was a wisp of a man, five feet seven inches tall and wiry thin. His receding blond hair was combed back; his high, wide forehead funneled to a mere point of a chin. The face was a cone, with prominent lines in his brow that looked as if they'd been carved by a palette knife. It was not that the man looked old or even tired for his forty-eight years. He looked merely as though he had lived. His eyes, large and serious and hollowed into the underside of his brow, seemed almost haunted. He bore an uncanny resemblance to Vincent van Gogh, who had been born not long before him only a few hundred miles from Hoffman's hometown of Varel, in East Friesland, a stretch of Germany carved around the North Sea.

Hoffman had run away from those salt-marsh lowlands at the age of nineteen. Throughout his miserable youth he had failed at everything he had tried. His mother had berated him incessantly, brutally, as a lazy good-for-nothing. His father had died of tuberculosis years before, leaving behind a lonely ten–year-old boy who would grow weak and rheumatic into his teenage years. The young Hoffman had balanced on the edge of suicide—until the gift of a steamer ticket to America saved him.

When his ship docked at New York Harbor in November 1884, he had twenty marks (less than $5) in his pocket. He weighed only one hundred pounds. It was mere accident that immigration authorities did not suspect him of tuberculosis and send him straight back across the Atlantic.

Or maybe it was something else—a sign, perhaps, that his luck had changed. From the moment Hoffman stepped off the boat, it seemed his fortunes improved. Opposite to his every experience in Germany, the young immigrant excelled at whatever odd job he took, with each new clerkship or sales position or bill-collecting post leading to another. None of that quite explained how, on March 26, 1913, some three decades after sailing penniless from home, he came to be addressing the membership of the New Jersey Academy of Medicine.

Dressed in a high wingtip collar and Windsor knot, his beard and mustache trimmed to perfection, he looked like a person of stature and accomplishment. Which he was, to an extent. Hoffman had, by then, published 250 tracts and treatises on matters of public health, part of what would be more than 1,200 papers and books he produced during his lifetime. Yet, such prolific output aside, he was an unusual choice to deliver a medical speech to a society of physicians. That was because

Hoffman wasn't a doctor at all. He was an actuary. For a life insurance company in Newark.

The health care research he had done focused not on organs and cells, but on *numbers*—vital statistics, actuarial tables, census reports, claims records. Hoffman, the in–house statistician for the Prudential Insurance Company of America, had until then published an odd sprawl of studies that ranged from the prescient (drawing a link between "inorganic dust" and lung disease in coal miners) to the obscure (the underestimated dangers of railroad crossings) to the outrageous. He had caused a stir, in 1896, by asserting that the sharp health disparity between whites and blacks in late-nineteenth-century America was due to what he termed a "constitutional weakness" in the latter. (W. E. B. Du Bois had been one of several scholars to debunk the ridiculous assertion and challenge the data behind it; years later, Hoffman would largely reverse the position, contending instead that factors of environment rather than race accounted for any measurable health differences between blacks and whites.) Now he stood before a sober audience of doctors for a talk titled "The Menace of Cancer."

Recorded by physicians in Egypt three thousand years before Christ, named by Hippocrates, found in bones from pre-Columbian Peru and Neolithic Europe, noted in writings of ancient India and Mesopotamia, preserved in the fossil record of prehistory, cancer had left its mark on man for so long and in so many places that it was almost pointless to point to a beginning. But, said Hoffman, this scourge had been awakened now into a kind of fury. New cases of cancer were surging by the thousands every year. All of a sudden, an ancient malady had become a monumental new threat.

The actuary summed up his warning in a single, heavily accented sentence:

It must be admitted that there are many perplexing problems in the analysis of cancer mortality which seem to contradict this conclusion, but as regards myself, I am not in doubt but that apparent increase in the cancer death rate, practically from year to year and from decade to decade, and for nearly every civilized country in the world, is not apparent, but real.

At the time, few if any practicing physicians thought cancer to be a significant public health issue. The disease was feared, but as a specter, as a monster under the bed. The chance of dying from cancer was remote, most medical practitioners believed, especially when compared with ubiquitous killers such as pneumonia, influenza, and tuberculosis.

Nevertheless, the man at the podium had seen something no one else had seen. And that was because he had done something no one else had done, at least with any precision: *he had counted.* Prudential's methodical actuary had gone through his company's own life insurance payouts for the previous year and had discovered that two words kept recurring in the ledgers: *malignant neoplasm.* Cancer.

A shocking number of deaths, primarily to policyowners forty-five or older, were due to cancer. During the first decade of the twentieth century, roughly one in every twelve deaths in men in that age cohort was the result of the disease; for women of that age, the figure was close to one in six. That made cancer, in Prudential's experience, the leading cause of death for middle-aged and older women and the third-leading cause for men.

From there, Hoffman began scouring statistical data from dozens of other sources, from state health boards to hospitals. He found that cancer deaths nationally were increasing at an alarming rate. Hoffman told his audience what had happened in just the short span of a decade: For males twenty-five and older, the annual cancer death rate in the United States had jumped some 30 percent between the years 1901 and 1911; for females, rates had risen by nearly a quarter.* And the older the age group, the more dramatic the jumps. For men age fifty-five to sixty-four, for example, cancer death rates had climbed a stunning 39 percent between 1901 and 1911; for women the increase was 27 percent.

But Hoffman's most glaring statistic was still to come. Unlike the others, this one was not a rate: it was a big, round number—and one that everyone in the auditorium could understand. By his calculation some

---

*When Hoffman made statistical corrections for differences in population age during the two periods, the percentage leaps were nearly identical to those cited: just over 30 percent for men and 22 percent for women.

seventy-five thousand Americans would die of cancer in 1913 alone, a number that was significantly higher than the government's estimate. And the death toll was climbing fast.

The actuary's speech drew a flurry of attention in the medical community—so much that when Hoffman redelivered it six weeks later at the American Gynecological Society's annual gathering in Washington, DC, the *New York Times* sent a man to report on it. But even so, Hoffman's conclusion that cancer was becoming a genuine and deepening problem for the nation was hard for many to accept.

The first question skeptics raised was whether Americans were really dying more from cancer . . . or *less* from other diseases, and particularly from tuberculosis. As terrifying as the threat of TB was in 1913, public health measures since the turn of the century had contained its spread (decades before the discovery of antibiotics even) so that that rate of death had fallen by a quarter since 1900. There were similar drops in mortality from diarrheal diseases, scarlet fever, and other childhood infections. Women were also less likely than at the turn of the century to die during childbirth. When all of these advances were taken together, the skeptics said, Americans who might otherwise have perished young were now living long enough to die of cancer. (Hoffman had, however, made such adjustments for the aging population in his calculations.)

Beyond the aging issue were other reasons for doubt. Cancer, for instance, was better understood than it had been in the past, meaning that physicians were more likely to diagnose it. How was one to know whether cancer rates were truly rising or whether pathologists were doing a better job of identifying it as the cause of death?

A third complaint, by contrast, was that cancer remained so *poorly* understood that medical workers ascribed whatever ailment they could not diagnose to this family of diseases. Who knew how many mysterious infections or chronic conditions were written off as cancers?

Finally came an argument that had little to do with Hoffman's data: even if his dire warnings were true, people could not be trusted with the knowledge that cancer was on the rise. The American Medical Association called it "cancer phobia." The mere "specter" that any mole or wart could be diagnosed as cancerous, said the AMA, was "capable of shattering even a normal mentality." It might even drive some to run away from the doctor rather than seek help.

There was a measure of truth to all of these complaints—but together, they did not change the fact that Hoffman's cancer findings were essentially correct. What they did prove to the actuary, however, was that he would have to do a better job of making his case.

Convincing the world that numbers currently so small could mean something so enormous in the coming decades, he knew, would require a statistical investigation unlike any other. Hoffman got to work. He devoted the next two years to compiling a survey of cancer prevalence and death so thorough that when the Prudential Insurance Company published Hoffman's findings in May 1915, it was obvious even to skeptics that his claims were valid.

At 826 dense pages, *The Mortality from Cancer Throughout the World* was the most comprehensive global census of a single disease ever done. Hoffman had sifted through data from not only the Prudential, but also from the Mutual Life Insurance Company of New York, the Washington Life Insurance Company, the Gresham Life Assurance Society, Clergy Mutual, Northwestern Mutual Life, and some two dozen other American companies. Outside of the United States, he had studied figures from the Scottish Widows' Fund, the Gotha and Germania companies of Germany, the Austrian Phoenix, and many others, compiling them into 121 neat tables of raw fatality counts, causes of death, and percentages. He had pored over the records of institutions ranging from the Frankfurt Medical Society to Britain's Imperial Cancer Research Fund and dissected scores of articles in the medical literature. He'd canvassed officials in state after state, city after city, in twenty-four countries, compiling records from Tasmania, Australia, to Lima, Peru (an additional 378 statistical tables). In the end, he had arrived at a lamentable truth nearly identical to his findings two years earlier.

There were now more than eighty thousand deaths from cancer a year in the United States, and the pace was increasing by a blistering 2.5 percent each year. "If the present rate of increase continues unchecked," Hoffman exclaimed, "the annual cancer mortality in the continental United States will soon exceed 100,000!"

But the cancer menace wasn't just a problem for the United States. Combining the returns for the United Kingdom, Norway, Holland, Austria, and a half dozen other countries, Hoffman found that the death rate from cancer had doubled in just thirty years. The trend had climbed mountains and crossed oceans; it had transcended language and culture and race. The plague was universal.

The change in death rates was not the only thing the statistician had uncovered in his survey. He also found more evidence to support the connection of "chronic irritation" from smoking with the rise in cancers of the mouth and throat. "The relation of smoking to cancer of the buccal [oral] cavity," he wrote, "is apparently so well established as not to admit of even a question of doubt." (By 1931, he would draw an unequivocal link between smoking and lung cancer—a connection it would take the surgeon general an additional three decades to accept.)

Nor did Hoffman neglect the future financial cost of this subterranean epidemic. By the end of 1914, 40,204,119 life insurance policies were in force in the United States. "It is for this reason," Hoffman noted, "that life insurance companies are directly interested in the nationwide effort to control a disease, which has not inappropriately been described as a scourge."

As the Prudential man saw it nearly a century ago, the nation—and indeed the world—was about to assume the biggest casualty risk in history, and it was unaware. Dangerously so. No reserves had been set up to cover this cancer burden. It was a disaster in the making.

Hoffman was right. What a lone actuary in Newark saw reflected in his ordinary insurance tables is what we now see reflected in history.

In 1913, the year Hoffman issued his meticulous warning to the New Jersey Academy of Medicine, cancer was the eighth leading cause of death in the United States—behind accidents, diarrheal disease, stroke, nephritis, pneumonia/influenza, tuberculosis, and heart disease. A year later it rose to sixth. A decade later it was fourth. Three years after that, third.

By 1927, cancer was killing some 145,000 Americans a year. Even so, it took another decade, until 1937, for the nation to awaken to the crisis. Early in the year, Henry Luce's *Fortune* magazine published a cover story entitled "Cancer: The Great Darkness," which highlighted the soaring mortality numbers and asked why, when so many American lives were being lost, so little money and effort was being spent on cancer research. Quickly, similar articles followed in two other magazines owned by Luce, *Life* and *Time*. The trio of articles prompted tens of thousands of Americans to write their congressmen and senators demanding action—with one historian later calling this response to the cancer threat a "spontaneous national referendum."

It took just weeks for a spate of cancer-battling resolutions to sweep through various congressional committees. "The people," as Thomas Parran Jr., Franklin Delano Roosevelt's surgeon general, would later reflect, had "accepted the idea that a disease which takes a sweeping toll of lives each year from the productive ages of our population; a disease which knows no state or county boundaries; a disease which is so costly in its diagnosis and treatment that but few of its victims can pay the costs unaided—is a public health problem."

Still, the dilemma that Hoffman had faced when he announced his startling findings a quarter century earlier remained. So little was known about the disease—how seemingly normal cells transformed into lawless hordes, how they infiltrated faraway organs, escaped the vigilant sentries of the immune system, survived in tissues devoid even of oxygen—that it was hard to know how to proceed. So Congress did what it does well: it requisitioned a sparkling new research center in which to figure out such mysteries.

America's first assault on cancer began in 1937 with the construction of a $750,000 "National Cancer Institute" on a stretch of donated land called Tree Tops, in Bethesda, Maryland. Ninety-six senators—the entire membership of the Senate—signed the bill that year to create the center, making it the first time in history that a measure had been "sponsored" by the full slate of either legislative chamber. And *that,* said one senator, was testament enough to the government's "grim determination to stamp out a disease that was threatening every home in America." The following year cancer would claim the number two rank among America's killers, overtaking every other cause of death except for heart disease, a spot it still claims today.

Figure 1

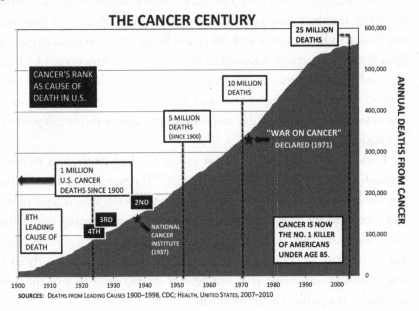

THE CANCER CENTURY

SOURCES: DEATHS FROM LEADING CAUSES 1900–1998, CDC; HEALTH, UNITED STATES, 2007–2010

And so it went for the three and a half decades that followed. Until 1971, when the National Cancer Act was signed into law and a new "war" against the cancer menace was declared by President Nixon.

And so it has gone for the four decades since. Americans continue to die from the illness at a startling rate. The rise in annual deaths is not quite as steep as it was in the early part of the last century, when the Prudential insurance man raised his alarm, but the mountain is already so high that any direction other than down is alarming: the latest war on the disease has not lowered the burden.

If anything, the toll's relentless rise looks more singular and dramatic now because so many other plagues of old and middle age are in retreat. Consider the progress made against heart disease: the number of yearly fatalities for every hundred thousand Americans—what researchers call the "crude death rate"—fell 47 percent between 1970 (the year before the cancer war began) and 2010 (the latest figures available in January 2013).

But even this remarkable drop merely hints at the scope of the turn-around. To grasp the drama, one has to look at the raw numbers. From 1970 to 2010, America's population swelled by more than 100 million. Its residents aged and fattened. Yet there were 138,000 *fewer* deaths from heart disease in 2010 than in 1970.

Figure 2

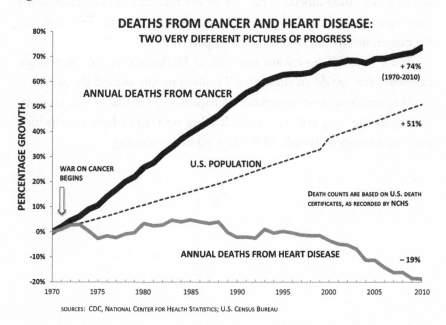

The United States now has tens of millions of additional beating hearts racing to catch commuter trains and airplanes, thumping their way through traffic jams and long office meetings—but fewer of them are breaking down each year.

Nor is this seeming miracle an outlier. The crude rate of death from stroke—then the country's number three killer—has been more than cut in half since the Nixon era, which translates into 78,000 fewer deaths per year. The death rate from influenza and pneumonia has dropped by over 40 percent (equating to 13,000 fewer deaths a year); liver disease, by more than a third.

The pattern holds, strikingly, for causes of death that have nothing to do with chronic illness—from fire-related fatalities to accidental drownings to deadly strikes of lightning. Even to car accidents. America's highways now carry 140 million more vehicles than roads did in 1970. Freeways across the country snarl with congestion. *Road rage* has not so quietly entered the lexicon. And still there were 19,000 fewer motor-vehicle-related fatalities in 2010 than in 1970.

The tale can be summed up in a single syllogism: Over the past four decades, the crude mortality rate for all the myriad causes of death *apart* from cancer, considered together, has dropped 24 percent. The same rate for cancer, meanwhile, has climbed 14 percent.

Some 580,000 Americans now fall to Hoffman's menace in a single calendar year—as do an additional 7 million people around the globe.

No great insight or observation is required to see that we are far from victory in the long war on cancer. It takes no leap of logic to conclude that our strategy is flawed. All it takes is a little counting.

Chapter 2

The Truth in Small Doses

If the rising toll from cancer is plain to see, if the hard numbers from death registers seem an unshakable reality, there is another way to count them. The method is so firmly established, and so commonly used by health care researchers and policymakers, that few remember anymore that it's a statistical sleight of hand. But that it is—and one powerful enough to transform nearly six hundred thousand annual deaths into a victory-in–progress.

To see its magic at work, one has only to read the lead commentary in the November 15, 2007, issue of *Cancer,* the venerable journal published by the American Cancer Society. Here, a group of top epidemiologists and statisticians from the National Cancer Institute and other institutions shared what seemed to be exciting news: "Overall cancer death rates *decreased* by 2.1% per year from 2002 through 2004, nearly twice the annual decrease of 1.1% per year from 1993 through 2002."

The study prompted the American Cancer Society to say in a separate report, "Death rates are declining in measurable, inspiring numbers." The

NCI, meanwhile, announced the findings on its own website, under the banner:

ANNUAL REPORT TO THE NATION FINDS
CANCER DEATH RATE DECLINE DOUBLING

Hundreds of news outlets across the United States ran with the story, with most echoing the "doubling" theme.

"Cancer Death Rates Dropping Fast," blared the *Washington Post*, running a story by the Associated Press. "The news has never been better in the war on cancer," echoed the on–air reporter for the *CBS Evening News*—with anchor Katie Couric, a celebrated anticancer campaigner in her own right, remarking that the study was "the clearest sign yet that all the research, new treatments, and plain old nagging are having a dramatic effect in reducing cancer deaths in this country."

Leaders of the cancer effort, from public officials and cancer center directors to famous oncologists, embraced the news as if it were an exclamation point on a sentence they'd read long ago. The cancer "death rate" had been declining for a decade and a half; every epidemiologist *knew* that after all.

Over the next few years, several additional studies would reinforce the 2007 findings. The cancer death rate was seen to be falling so precipitously that a few experts were now openly predicting an end to the plague in the coming few decades.

Andrew von Eschenbach, NCI director from 2002 to 2005, had famously pledged early in his term to "eliminate suffering and death due to cancer by the year 2015"—a goal he had repeated so many times it had become a part of the NCI's mission statement. At the time, much of the cancer community snickered at the presumption. The numbers arriving in an American Cancer Society report in January 2013, however, made the prospect almost conceivable. Between the years 1990 and 2009, the death rate for the disease was reported to have dropped 20 percent, an achievement the ACS hailed as a "milestone." Almost twenty years of steady declines in cancer death rates, boasted a charity press release, "translates to almost 1.2 million deaths from cancer that were avoided."

Only a cynic, it seemed, could not have been elated by the finding. Yet, for anyone who had been following the raw numbers coming from the National Center for Health Statistics (NCHS), the US government's chief collector of mortality data, the wave of celebratory reports must have caused some cognitive dissonance. There were 567,628 deaths from cancer in 2009, some 62,000 more than there were in 1990. How was it possible that an *additional 62,000 cancer deaths per year* could translate into a celebration? (Sixty-two thousand deaths is more than US losses from the entire Vietnam War.) How could anyone have scanned the rising toll from cancer, decade after decade, and concluded that the "news had never been better"?

Herein lies one of the fundamental misconceptions of the cancer war. Unraveling it requires a relearning of words and concepts that most people assume they understand. Cancer accounting, in this respect, is much like financial accounting, where terms that mean one thing to corporate executives and Wall Street analysts are often construed as something else by the lay investor. In the same way that "profits" and "cash flow" and "risk" have been redefined by thousands of companies over the past few decades, so the familiar notions of "death" and "counting" have been reinterpreted in the realm of cancer research.

The annual death toll is what statisticians call a *crude* measure. It has yet to be refined, shaped, or processed. It is simply what it is: a tally of death certificates. When that raw number is viewed in relation to a given population, the statistic is referred to as a crude death rate, which is traditionally presented per every 100,000 people in the group being studied.

There is nothing exotic about the concept. The "rate," in this case, is a simple exercise of division (the number of cancer deaths in a calendar year)/(the number of individuals in the population). Many of us rely daily on some form of crude rate—every time, for instance, we eye the calories per serving on the back of a cereal box or size up prices per gallon at the gas pump. Such rates are as ubiquitous as they are straightforward.

And in the case of cancer or any other ailment, crude rates offer the best gauge of the burden of disease in a given year.

In 2009, for example, the crude death rate for cancer in the United States was 184.9 per 100,000 people, a figure that does not seem particularly immense until one considers that a nation of 307 million (the population of the United States that year) has 3,070 "slices" of 100,000 people. Multiplying 184.9 times 3,070 yields an annual death toll of 567,643—just about what the actual death count was that year (567,628).

In 1990, 505,322 cancer deaths were recorded in the United States, a nation then of 248.7 million people—which works out to 203.2 deaths per every 100,000 residents.

So the crude rate did, in fact, go down over these nineteen years (from 203.2 to 184.9), which is good news. Yet, this encouraging 9 percent decline is *less than half* the drop reported by the NCI for the same period. The difference translates to tens of thousands of lives each year.

Go back to the start of the modern cancer war, and the disconnect becomes far more dramatic. Per the figures posted by the NCHS, the 2009 crude rate of death is up 14 percent from its level in 1970 (even with the recent drop). Leaders of the national cancer effort, however, maintain that the death rate actually *fell* 13 percent over the same period.

The divide between these versions of history, it's worth noting, has nothing to do with the underlying number of dead. And no one is lying. The confusion stems from the term *death rate* itself. This first meaning gap begins here.

When talking about the progress made against cancer or other illnesses, officials seldom mention crude rates. They instead refer to a statistic called an "age-adjusted" or "standardized" rate. Adjusting a crude rate lets a researcher filter out a factor that would otherwise trip up many epidemiological investigations: namely, the *age* of the population being studied.

There is good reason for this filter: advancing age is such an enormous and obvious "risk factor" for the development of cancer (just as it is for nearly every other major illness) that its shadow often hides any other factor. The median age of cancer incidence, for example, is sixty-six—meaning that half of all cases are diagnosed in people over that age and half under it. That means that any region with an older population is likely to have a higher rate of cancer incidence and death than one with younger residents, simply on the basis of age distribution alone.

Figure 3

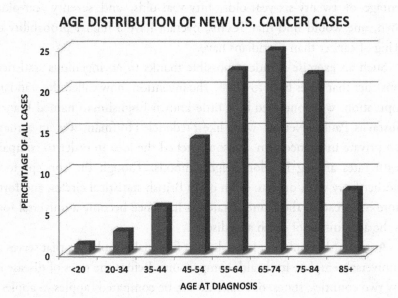

AGE DISTRIBUTION OF NEW U.S. CANCER CASES

SOURCE: Howlader et al. 2012, *NCI SEER CSR 1975–2009*, table 1.10.

To see how powerful the age effect can be, one has only to compare cancer mortality in the states of Florida and Texas. In 2009, the Sunshine State recorded some 41,000 deaths from the disease—far more than might have been expected from a population of just under 19 million. (The crude death rate was 217, well above the national average.) Texas, by comparison, with some 6 million more residents than Florida, had nearly 5,300 fewer cancer deaths during the year. On the basis of such raw mortality figures, one might suspect that Florida is a hotbed of carcinogens, or, alternatively, that hardscrabble Texas has been overrun by nonsmoking, yoga-practicing vegans.

Neither is true. Florida's excess cancer mortality is tied simply and ir-revocably to its oceans of retirees. More than 17 percent of state residents, according to the 2010 census, are sixty-five or older (by far the highest share in the United States), compared with just 10 percent for Texas (the nation's third-lowest).

But what if one were to pretend, somehow, that both states have an equal proportion of residents at each specific age—the exact same per-centage of twenty-six-year-olds, fifty-year-olds, and seventy-year-olds? Then, one would find that Texans, overall, have a higher probability of dying of cancer than Floridians have.

Such an exercise is indeed possible thanks to an ingenious statistical construct that dates back to 1844. The invention, now called the standard population, was conceived by a little-known Englishman named Francis Gustavus Paulus Neison, who, like Frederick Hoffman, was an actuary at a private insurance firm. Neison hatched the idea in order to compare death rates among London neighborhoods. Though the concept took another forty years or so to catch on in British statistical circles, and forty more to spread to the United States, it has since become a universal tool in the accounting of death and disease.

A standard population is, in short, a fictional population that serves as a universal template for health comparisons. Before the rates of disease in any two counties, states, or countries can be compared "apples to apples," Neison contended, their actual age distributions have to be made identi-cal. The simplest way to do this, he proposed, is to realign the age break-down of *every* subpopulation in the country (or in the world) so that they match the imaginary one's.

To say that the standard is imaginary is not to suggest that it is drawn from thin air. It generally mirrors the actual population in a given census year: the current US standard, for example, faithfully copies the age pyra-mid reported in the 2000 census. (Prior to that, the template was based on the 1970 breakdown, though many researchers still clung to the 1940 model, or to another one entirely.)

But unlike a real population, this population is frozen in time, a statis-tical Neverland in which no one gets older or dies. None move in or out. Whatever flux the broader world might experience, the distribution of ages here remains in suspended animation for thirty years or longer—that is, until a new template assumes its place.

Whatever the standard chosen, to calculate an age-adjusted death rate for cancer, for instance, a researcher first has to measure the actual (or crude) cancer death rate for every age group in the region (i.e., those four years old and under, five through nine, up to eighty-five and over). Each of these *age-specific* rates is then "adjusted" by a percentage factor that reflects the group's fixed share in the standard population. Adding up the lot results in an overall age-adjusted rate for that area.

The exercise has merit. Eliminating the variable of age makes it possible to see important disparities that would surely be missed by looking at crude rates or counts alone. Thanks to Neison's clever device, for example, it is plain to see that African–Americans have a shockingly higher risk of death, matched age to age, than white Americans across a spectrum of cancers. (This has been the case for decades.) Or that, since roughly the 1960s, white men in Montana have experienced unusually high rates of death from prostate cancer compared with white men in most other states. Or that women in Spain and Japan have a dramatically lower risk of dying from cancer than American women do.

Why these patterns are true—are the differences due primarily to diet, lifestyle, environment, genetic makeup, access to care, something else?—are mysteries that standardizing alone cannot solve. But this method has at least allowed once-unseen differences between groups to emerge into plain sight.

Given how eye-opening it can be to compare age-adjusted rates among different populations at the same time, it might seem no great leap to use the method for comparing the *same* population at different times. Here, though, is where more confusion arises.

The aim of the first is to unearth often subtle variances in risk that would otherwise be obscured. The point of the second, ostensibly, is to assess progress over time. (This is clearly what the American Cancer Society implied it was doing in reporting the drop in the US cancer death rate from 1990 to 2009. The message was that the US cancer burden had not only gone down, but gone down dramatically.)

In the case of the first, Neison's clever game is played by—and generally *for*—epidemiologists, who know all along that it is a statistical construct. A useful fiction. In the case of the second, though, only a tiny fraction of people realize that such is the case.

Of the millions of people who heard the cancer establishment's upbeat message, few were aware that the "death rates" in question had little to do with the *actual* frequency of cancer death in the actual US population during those years. Most people assumed the rates were, well . . . real.

Such assumptions are hardwired into human nature. We are primed to read any rate or number as a true measure. This instinct is especially true when it comes to data on injury and death. War casualty figures, the published reports of tsunamis and hurricanes and plane crashes, all recount the number of wounded (injured) and dead. Murders are reported as a simple toll—or as a crude rate, say, for every 10,000 residents in the city or state. When the World Health Organization or CDC offer situation updates on the spread of an infectious disease, such as the H1N1 "swine flu" pandemic of 2009, they tell of the number of those infected and killed. Of the thousands of reports filed on the events of September 11, no one ever thought to age-adjust the victims.

Standardized rates are different. They are not measures of *burden*—of how many people have gotten a disease or died from it during a given period—they are rather gauges of risk. And even risk, in this context, does not mean what the average person thinks it means. What is being evaluated is not absolute risk, but rather the comparative risk of two or more populations aligned to the same mythical age standard. Change the standard, and—poof!—the measure of risk changes with it.

For a glimpse of the extraordinary and inherent malleability of such rates, consider the following published rates for lung cancer deaths among US women in 1990 (Table 1). Even when the same standard population year is used (see shaded area of table), the "value" implied by any age-adjusted rate can change based on something as minor as how many age groups (five-year breakdowns or ten–year breakdowns, for example) are used in the calculation, or even on whether or not one uses rounded population numbers.

Table 1

When Age-Adjusting Keeps Adjusting . . .

Age-Adjusted Death Rate from Lung Cancer in 1990 for Females (All Ages)—
as Reported in Various Official Government Sources

	Published rate (per 100,000 people)	Standard population year cited	Number of actual deaths undercounted*	% below actual count*
Health, United States, 1998	26.2	1940	16,731	33.4%
Health, United States, 2000	25.6	1940	17,496	34.9%
Health, United States, 2002	37.1	2000	2,833	5.7%
SEER Cancer Statistics Review, 1975–2005	36.8	2000	3,216	6.4%
SEER Cancer Statistics Review, 1973–1993	31.6	1970	9,846	19.6%

*Compared with the raw number reported in 1990. Estimate of undercounting is calculated by multiplying age-adjusted rate by 1,275. (On April 1, 1990, there were approximately 127,500,000 female residents in the United States, or 1,275 "segments" of 100,000 each.) This figure is then subtracted from the confirmed number of female lung cancer fatalities that year (50,136), based on death certificates.

SOURCES: National Center for Health Statistics, *HUS 1998*, p. 235, table 41; *HUS 2000*, p. 195, table 40; *HUS 2002*, p. 151, table 40; Ries et al. 2005, *SEER 1975–2005*, p. 8, table XV-6; Ries et al. 1996, *SEER 1973–1993*, p. 6, table XV-6. For complete source information, see List of References.

If nonexperts are unaware of the distinction between crude rates and their standardized counterparts, it is perhaps surprising how many experts are as well. Alas, the tendency among veteran researchers and policymakers to conflate age-adjusted rates with the true burden of disease is so common that the National Center for Health Statistics has issued one caveat after another telling people not to do so. Warns one of the agency's instructional guides:

The age-adjusted death rate does not reflect the mortality risk of a "real" population. The average risk of mortality of a real population is represented by the crude death rate. The numerical value of an age-adjusted death rate depends on the standard used and, therefore, is not meaningful by itself.

Cautions another:

It is very important to realize that the age-adjusted death rate (ADR) is an artificial measure whose absolute value has no intrinsic meaning. The ADR is useful for comparison purposes only, not to measure absolute magnitude. (To compare absolute magnitude, crude rates are used.)

If nothing else, this mouthful of a term—*age-adjusted death rate*—ought to signal its own modest warning, suggesting that the meaning may not be quite so obvious. But then, much of the time, the ungainly modifier is dropped like a dinner jacket, and by the time the news is passed along to the public, *death rate* has often settled into *deaths.* As a result, millions of people miss the enormous hypothetical that follows each report of victory in the war on cancer. Even the experts breeze by this elephant of an "if":

Yes, cancer deaths have been falling . . . but only *if* the United States is a living wax museum where each inhabitant's age is fixed for eternity. Only *if* real life is a still life.

It isn't, of course. The country's population grew from 1990 to 2009—not only much bigger (adding 58 million residents), but older, too. The nation's median age jumped by nearly four years, to 36.7.

Moreover, it aged in a nonobvious way. America, it turned out, began to bulge in the midriff, like a caricature of a prosperous middle-aged burgher. Over this brief span of time, for instance, the cohort of 45-to-64-year-olds surged by more than 33 million people—increasing its representation in the overall population by 7.3 percentage points as the proportions of younger groups, in turn, declined.

This is exactly what real populations do—they swell and shrink in often sweeping ways. America in 2009 looked no more like the 2000 standard than a distant cousin, and it resembled even less the America of 1990. The cohort of 45-to-64-year-olds in 2009 accounted for nearly 26 percent of the US population, far above the share reserved in the 2000 template (22 percent), and in 1990 (19 percent). And by 2020, this crop of baby boomers will constitute a still larger share of the country.

The point is important. For here, in this group of middle-aged

Americans, can be found more than a third of all new cancer cases and more than a quarter of all deaths. Each year, the disease kills more people in this otherwise vital age group than the next three leading causes of death (heart disease, accidents, and chronic lower respiratory disease) combined.

So if for no other reason than the group's surging numbers, there were more cancer fatalities in 2009 among 45-to-64-year-olds—some twenty-three thousand more, in fact—than there had been nineteen years earlier. The group's share of overall cancer mortality, moreover, had gone *up*, not down since 1990. Yet by the time the raw mortality figures for 2009 emerged from the standardization model, most of these additional deaths had vanished from the accounting. Scaled out of the age-distribution model, they simply did not exist. Gone were thousands of people, relegated to a statistical potter's field.

By the NCI's accounting, the "death rate" for this ample slice of the population fell an incredible 31 percent over the period.

As great as the undercounting has been, the more profound concern is not what has already happened, but what will.

A demographic storm is coming to the United States. According to the Census Bureau, the number of Americans age sixty-five through eighty-four will soar in the coming decades. And as high as the actual cancer death rates are in the great swath of middle age (where much of the boomer generation now sits), they are over three times higher in the age group above.

Already, according to the 2010 census, nearly 35 million people between the ages of sixty-five and eighty-four reside in the United States. By 2025, this age group is projected to number 57 million, representing roughly 16 percent of the nation.

The shift in the population pyramid will be as consequential for America as it is colossal. Legions of social scientists and think-tankers have already spun one scary scenario after the next on the fates of Social Security and Medicare. But the sheer scale of the country's expanding cancer burden has yet to be recognized by those entrusted with measuring it. Nor is this fast-rising burden likely to be acknowledged in the NCI's annual progress reports anytime soon. After all, in the *official* playbook, the proportion of people age sixty-five through eighty-four stands at a mere 11 percent . . . and that figure is not due for a revision until 2030.*

Eventually, of course, the cancer leadership's own assessment will have to catch up with reality. America's aging population cannot be filtered out of the question "How many people are dying of cancer?" It is not a confounding artifact in the cancer burden. It is the main driver.

Cancer death rates aren't the only statistics that convey a misleading picture of progress. So do the numbers for patient survival. Here, too, the cancer community's official measure paints over the experiences of millions of patients and their families. Here, too, making sense of the numbers requires relearning a concept most people think they understand.

The confusion centers on the statistic commonly called the survival rate. According to the most recent data from the National Cancer Institute, some 67 percent of new patients are expected to "survive." As with the age-adjusted death rate, however, the cancer world's definition of survival tows behind it a string of asterisks. The actual statistic, compiled by researchers at the NCI's surveillance and epidemiology arm—a program called SEER—gauges something more limited: the percentage of cancer patients who are still alive *five years after their diagnosis.*

This "observed survival rate," then, is rejiggered slightly so that it can be seen in relation to those in the general population (of the same age, sex, and race) who would ordinarily live that long. The aim is to filter out

---

*Each time the standard population is changed, an immense volume of statistical data from numerous federal and state agencies must be recalculated along with it. So, by convention, the switch to a new standard happens only once every thirty years. Prior to switching to the 2000-year standard population in 1999, the National Cancer Institute SEER program computed cancer incidence and mortality data with the 1970 standard, even as other federal and state agencies clung to a standard based on the 1940 US population. The National Center for Health Statistics, the government's central collector of vital statistics, primarily used the 1940 standard for more than half a century (from 1943 to 1999), though some data were computed with other standards as well.

deaths from causes other than cancer, and in this case, the adjustment makes sense. If an eighty-year-old man dies three years after being diagnosed with early-stage prostate cancer, one should not assume that cancer was the cause. In many older men, the disease is so slow-growing as to be a nonfactor.

Reflecting both this broader context as well as the limited time horizon, the statistic is officially termed the *five-year relative survival rate*. But whether the full name is used or not, the measure leaves out a critical piece of information: it gives no clue as to how many survivors are free of their disease. Included in this percentage are tens of thousands of patients who will be battling their cancers to the five-year mark and beyond, who will spend the first half decade of their ordeal enduring one toxic treatment protocol after the next.

Unmentioned in the tally of survivors is how many are likely to relapse after the five-year benchmark or succumb to metastases later on. The overall survival rate in breast cancer, for example, declines another five percentage points between five years after diagnosis and ten. In kidney cancer and leukemia, the drop-off in survival soon after the five-year mark is steeper. Nonetheless, in official recordkeeping, a patient who dies after a grueling six-year fight with breast cancer is placed in the "survived" category. (By such accounting, the late Elizabeth Edwards is considered a treatment success.)

The National Center for Health Statistics, trying to correct the common misperception, says the measure is properly "used to estimate the proportion of cancer patients *potentially curable*." When authorities in the cancer war speak of gains in patient survival, though, they rarely hint at how tentative the official assessment is. It is like an infantry commander declaring that a key hill has been taken, without mentioning the enemy troops massing nearby, who may take it back the next day.

To be sure, any statistical measure has its limitations. Whatever the flaws of the official survival rate, it does make clear that a greater share of patients today are living at least five years with their cancers compared with the mid-1970s. The most recent rate (available in January 2013) is some 19 percentage points higher than the rate in the late 1970s—an achievement that the American Association for Cancer Research told

Congress is "a direct result of our national commitment to funding cancer research, screening, and treatment programs at the NCI, NIH, and other agencies across the federal government."

So where's the catch? Though more cancer patients are living longer today—and even, in some cases, beating their diseases outright—only a small portion of that improvement has derived from advances in *cancer treatment,* or at least from any medicine that has come to the clinic during the past quarter century. Despite the seemingly endless procession of discoveries in the lab, despite the spate of reported "wonder drugs," the deadliest malignancies are still nearly as deadly in 2013 as they were at the start of the cancer war (see Figure 4). Fewer than a fifth of Americans diagnosed today with a cancer of the lung, pancreas, liver, or esophagus are expected to live five years. Likewise, cancers of the stomach, brain, and ovary largely remain the killers they were at the start of the cancer war.

Figure 4

DEADLY AS EVER

This year, hundreds of thousands of people in the U.S. will be diagnosed with a cancer in which the five-year survival rate is less than 50 percent.

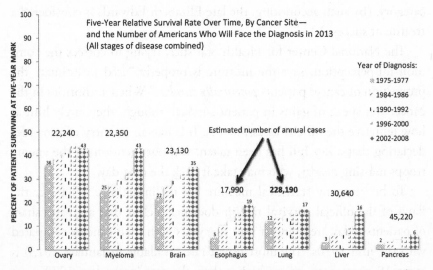

SOURCES: Siegel et al. 2013, *Cancer Statistics, 2013,* table 12. Howlader et al. 2012, table 1.4, cite slightly lower patient survival rates for the period 2002–2008.

As oncologists point out, even modest improvements in the survival rates for such cancers are hardly negligible to the patients who are now living longer. "We're making incremental—first base, second base—gains in the major solid tumors," Gwen Fyfe, a physician and former Genentech executive involved in cancer drug development, told me years ago. "If you're looking for a cure, that's disappointing. On the other hand, if you are a physician taking care of patients, these are steps which translate into real patient benefit—getting to go to your child's graduation, having Christmas, having an anniversary. Those are things that make a big difference in people's lives."

But even in the case of a common malignancy such as breast cancer, where overall five-year survival rates now approach 90 percent and which many oncologists now consider a treatment success story, the bulk of the improvement since the 1970s has not derived from "breakthrough" drugs and other research advances; rather, as will be made clear in chapter 6, the change is due mostly to the fact that we are now catching a greater share of cases in earlier stages, when tumors are far easier to remove and treat. Indeed, to the extent that progress has been made in improving patient survival, it is due less to the things on which Americans spend many billions of dollars a year (cancer research and treatment) than to what we have long given short shrift (early detection).

To understand how this could be possible, it helps to examine the official survival rate through a different prism—the "stage at diagnosis," or how far the malignancy has advanced at the point at which it is detected (Figure 5). With some notable exceptions, patients diagnosed today with a localized (early-stage) cancer have an excellent chance of living at least five years. That's great news, certainly—but such was the case in the 1970s as well. And sadly, the same parallel can be seen for those diagnosed with an advanced stage of cancer: Outcomes for most patients have improved little over the decades.

There is one critical difference between now and then, however. It is scale. In 2013 alone, some half a million Americans will be told they have a cancer in which the overall survival rate is less than 50 percent. That is far larger than the number who faced such a diagnosis in 1971.

Figure 5

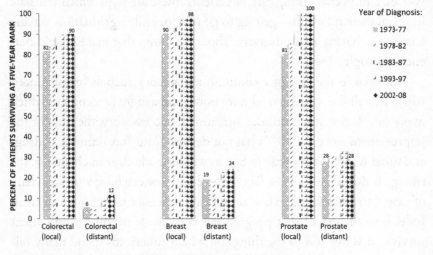

TWO REALITIES

Even four decades ago, most patients with early-stage disease lived at least five years. But patients with metastatic cancer still face nearly the same dire odds they did at the start of the cancer war.

Local — Early stage; cancer has not spread from initial site at diagnosis.
Distant — Advanced stage; cancer has already spread to other sites in body.

Year of Diagnosis:
- 1973-77
- 1978-82
- 1983-87
- 1993-97
- 2002-08

PERCENT OF PATIENTS SURVIVING AT FIVE-YEAR MARK

Colorectal (local), Colorectal (distant), Breast (local), Breast (distant), Prostate (local), Prostate (distant)

SOURCES: *Cancer Statistics* for years 1986, 1992, 2008, and 2013 *CA Cancer J Clin* (American Cancer Society)

The distorted, or incomplete, accounting of our progress is not the fault of a single individual, or two, or ten. There is no conspiracy at work, nor even perhaps the intention to deceive. Rather, the distortion has been spread through academic training and long-standing practice. It has been woven into the cancer culture itself. That diffusion is what makes it so credible, and so troubling. The ease with which the concrete is transformed into the amorphous, at which flesh and blood withers into the abstract, is the ease of convention. Cancer's data keepers and crunchers are not deliberately misleading us. They are simply performing the same adjustments that others have done before them. Their formulas are trusted and venerable—even logical within their own cramped universes of meaning.

Some researchers privately acknowledge that the official gauges of cancer progress do not reflect the reality of the growing cancer burden.

But as with those who counted the correct number of human chromosomes (and then disregarded it), almost no one has publicly questioned the way cancer mortality and survival are assessed. Instead, the cancer world draws further into its paradox—into the cultural koan that seems as if it could have been lifted from young Alice's Wonderland: We see only what we measure, and we measure only what has been measured before.

The thinking guides research that goes well beyond the assessments of mortality and survival, well beyond the calculations of either risk or burden. So deeply embedded is this cultural doctrine that it seems to drive the development, testing, and even regulatory approval of cancer medicines. The oncology world's strange traditions of measurement turned dozens of failed agents into "wonder drugs"—into "breakthrough" discoveries. And no one seems to acknowledge that they don't work. Or hardly anyone, that is.

At first glance, the April 2003 edition of the *Journal of Clinical Oncology* was nothing out of the ordinary. The *JCO* is the official journal of the American Society of Clinical Oncology, which in turn, is the official guild for some twenty-seven thousand practicing cancer doctors. In the hierarchy of cancer journals, *JCO* ranks way up at the top. As such, reports of the most exciting and highest-impact clinical trials are often published here first. But as with any medical journal, the vast majority of its contributions tend toward the workaday. In medicine, lightning bolts do not strike often.

The April 2003 issue carried three dozen articles reporting on various stages of clinical trials, potential prognostic tools for cancer, long-term outcome studies, and even an investigation of the role of faith for patients in making decisions about their care. (The authors concluded that faith in God was important—but ranked second after faith in one's oncologist.) Chances are that few busy cancer doctors made it to the thirty-first article in the issue, "End Points and United States Food and Drug Administration Approval of Oncology Drugs." But the article contained probably the most important finding *JCO* had published in years.

When a pharmaceutical company believes it might have an effective drug compound and wants to test the molecule in humans, it files for what is called a New Drug Application, or NDA. That gets the long journey to approval rolling. The FDA, which oversees the process, requires a tremendous amount of evidence to support any drug approval, which means that the developer (known in the endless jargon of the industry as the *sponsor*) has to send in reams of data, covering not only every patient in every human trial, but nearly every preclinical study as well. The agency's reviewers pore over the information and present a recommendation to an advisory committee, which, after a public hearing, gives either a yea or nay. The FDA then makes the final decision on whether to approve the drug for sale.

In theory at least, a compound is given the okay if it meets two criteria. First, the sponsor has to demonstrate in clinical trials that the drug is safe, or reasonably so in the context of its intended use. An antibaldness drug, for example, would be expected to have no major side effects. When the aim is to treat cancer, on the other hand, FDA regulators often give a passing grade to brutally toxic chemicals. (The vast majority of cancer medicines in use today are poisons, essentially. Their job is to kill cells.)

The second hurdle for any investigational drug is to prove that it does something useful. Federal regulators generally do not approve an agent unless it is shown to be *more* effective in treating a condition than the "standard therapy" (the one already on the market). But again, depending on the disease, the spectrum of judgment can be wide. For new would-be cancer drugs, the bar for "efficacy," as the FDA calls it, can be low.

What the three authors of the prosaically worded "End Point" study did was to show exactly *how* low. They went back nearly thirteen years from November 2002 (to January 1990) and examined each of the seventy-one occasions when the FDA told a company it was okay to market a cancer drug. Then the authors recorded the stated reason for approval: Did the new drug improve patient survival compared with existing therapy? Was it better tolerated? Did it lessen nausea?

The results were shocking: 75 percent of the permissions were granted for a reason *other* than that the drugs helped patients live longer. It is the kind of sentence you have to say out loud, slowly, for the meaning to seep in: three-quarters of the cancer medicines approved over the period did no more to keep people alive than the older, cheaper treatments did. These were the rare compounds that made it through more than a decade's worth of animal and human testing, with each drug, on average, costing hundreds of millions of dollars to develop. In some cases, patients or their health insurers had to pay as much as $20,000 per month for these new medicines.

Telling as the statistic was, it was also remarkable who told it. The study's senior author was Richard Pazdur, a former practicing medical oncologist at MD Anderson Cancer Center, in Houston, who was then, as now, the FDA's chief regulator of cancer drugs. Pazdur has been the agency's "cancer czar" since April 1999, when he gave up not only his flourishing clinical practice, but also a tenured professorship at the University of Texas to go to Washington.

"The overwhelming reason why oncology drugs do not get approved in the United States, is the failure to demonstrate efficacy," Pazdur sums up. "To put it in [blunter] words: It's the efficacy, stupid." The vaunted new cancer drugs are simply not keeping people alive.

To understand how paralyzed the cancer research effort is, however, it is important to know why—if not for prolonging lives—the myriad agents in the Pazdur study *were* approved. In half of the cases (50.7 percent), the primary reason was something called "partial tumor response rate."

That sounds reasonable enough, but it represents a regulatory contortion that stretches and twists the sinews of reason. The definition captures it best: a partial tumor response is "a 50% decrease from baseline in the sum of the cross-products of all bidimensionally measurable tumors lasting at least 1 month." In plain English, it means that a patient's tumors shrank . . . for at least one month. So, 50.7 percent of the FDA's cancer drug approvals from 1990 through 2002 were based on the fact that the drugs in question shrank tumors for at least a month.

The problem is, shrinking tumors has little to do with curing patients of cancer. In 90 percent of cases, it is not the initial tumor that kills people but rather the process of metastasis. Aggressive cells break off from the primary tumor site—*even when the sum of its cross-products is being shrunk by at least 50 percent from the baseline*—and these tough, destructive cells spread to the bones or the brain, to the liver or lungs, or to some other vital area of the body.

It happens too often in breast cancer, even when the entire tumor is seemingly removed; and even when the nearby lymph nodes are negative. It happens in cancers of the ovary, the stomach, the head and neck. Metastasis—the thing that makes cancer *cancer*—is what kills.

End of story? Well, not quite. As it turns out, the seventy-one FDA approvals during the Pazdur study fell short in another surprising way: there weren't seventy-one drugs to begin with.

On the list, for example, was the well-prescribed chemotherapy agent Taxol (known generically as paclitaxel). This one drug accounted for *six* of the approvals reported in the study. Moreover, seven other cancer medicines in the Pazdur study were each approved for sale by the FDA, and then reapproved, and then *re*-reapproved during the thirteen–year period the authors examined. An additional seven compounds each had two official go-aheads from the drug agency—revealing yet another Alice-in–Wonderland truth about the cancer world: in FDA math, seventy-one drug approvals adds up to just forty-five actual drugs.

How could that be? The answer has to do with the intricate rules of US drug regulation. Even when officials permit a new medicine to be sold in American pharmacies, they set limits as to how, and to whom, it can be marketed. This limit is the drug's "indication," or, in pharma-speak, "the label." Legally, a medicine can be sold to treat only a specified condition, such as ovarian cancer or multiple myeloma. And the label's limits can be quite limited. Taxol, for instance, was first approved in 1992 for the treatment of advanced, metastatic ovarian cancer—but only for patients who had already been given (and failed to respond to) the conventional and highly toxic therapy of the time. In 1994, the FDA gave Bristol-Myers Squibb its blessing to market Taxol as a breast cancer medicine—but again, only for patients whose disease had not responded to standard chemotherapies. Another approval came in 1997 for the treatment of Kaposi's sarcoma, a rare cancer that strikes those with severely weakened immune systems, such as people with AIDS. One more permission (1998) followed for the early treatment of ovarian cancer; a fifth (1998), for non–small-cell lung cancer; and a sixth (1999) for early-stage breast cancer. Six approvals in all—one lone drug.

Once supplemental approvals for the same compound are put aside, the number of cancer drugs that actually prolonged the lives of patients drops considerably. From January 1990 through November 2002, the world's laboratories produced just twelve drugs that showed they could extend the lives of *any* group of cancer patients even by weeks or months. Nonetheless, during this same period, the media managed to find cancer breakthroughs everywhere; that phrase, *cancer breakthrough,* appeared in 691 published articles. The celebratory headlines, which continue to this day, did not come from thin air. The "news" that prompted them was often plucked from the newsletters and press releases of cancer centers, research hospitals, and universities, or from articles published in the major medical journals, or from high-profile presentations at scientific conferences.

Each tiny improvement in clinical treatment or biological understanding went through a kind of grade inflation as it passed from one source to the next: An experimental finding, no matter how minor, became a "Discovery." A discovery morphed into a "Breakthrough." A tweak to a treatment protocol, even if it did not improve the longevity of patients, became an "Advance."

The optimistic announcements played into the desperate need for hope, and in turn, the desperation pushed both researchers and reporters to hype each laboratory finding even more. The cycle proved virtuous for raising money for cancer research, which fueled the cycle all the more. And the result was that the disconnect between the public's impression of progress and actual progress grew.

It grew and grew—until only the strange math of the cancer culture could bridge the gap:

691 breakthroughs = 71 cancer drug approvals = 45 drugs = 12 drugs that barely extended patient lives.

The cover of *Public Affairs Pamphlet No. 286* carried an illustration of a father, a mother, and a child leaving a clinic together. Their faces were obscured in charcoal hash marks, their bodies off-balance as they descended the steps at the clinic's front door. They were holding hands.

"When a Family Faces Cancer," published in 1959 by the Public Affairs Committee in cooperation with the American Cancer Society, was a lively read, as public health pamphlets went. The text began:

After an eternity of waiting, Allen Todd saw his family doctor coming down the hospital corridor. He stood up, but couldn't speak a word.

Dr. Nielsen led him to a chair, seated himself, and said, "She's doing fine, Allen. They've just put her in the recovery room. In an hour or so you can see her."

"Did you—was it—a complete hysterectomy?"

"Yes."

"Cancer?"

"It *was*. The surgeon got it all, he thinks. He'll be down here in a moment."

"Cancer." Allen looked stricken. "Don't tell Kate, please. She couldn't stand it."

The soap opera continues for another page and a half—at which point the aim of the pamphlet becomes clear. It answers the torturous question that confronted every family hit with cancer: "How much truth can a patient face?"

Some patients, when told, are so overwhelmed they might give up the struggle, the booklet explains. Others become rash and suicidal. Yet to tell the person nothing of his or her malignancy risks having the family member resist or refuse urgently needed treatment, such as surgery.

In the end, the pamphlet's author makes the only appropriate resolution to this dilemma clear: "What the patient is told about his illness is for the doctor to decide." And the doctor's best approach is to offer "truth in small doses."

Here, in these four words, lies the heart of the cancer culture.

Chapter 3

A War of Attrition

On a Sunday in July 2004, at four o'clock in the morning, four-year-old Brian Quinlan awoke from a deep sleep and cried harder than he ever had in his life.

"That must have been some nightmare," thought Brian's mother, Nancy, as she came into his room and sat on the edge of his bed. She stroked the boy's back, murmuring that everything was okay, and when that didn't work, she cradled him in her arms. No matter what she tried, she could not console him.

Nancy felt her son's forehead. It was clammy, but just barely. Brian rubbed his tummy and managed to say, in between wails, the word *hurt*. No wonder his tummy hurt, Nancy thought. He'd been crying for twenty minutes.

Nancy Quinlan was hardly the excitable type. Even with her older son, Brendan, she had been relaxed as a mom—a quality that served her equally well in her other role, as a federal prosecutor. Nancy had spent fourteen years with the US attorney's office in the Southern District of Florida, much of that as a senior prosecutor. Generally, she was methodical in her thinking: Crimes had their perpetrators; mysteries had their explanations. When a little boy woke from a dead sleep at four in the morning, crying as all get-out, it meant he was scared, uncomfortable, or in pain.

The problem didn't appear to be the first. So she called her pediatrician and left her phone number with the answering service. When the doctor called back, he groggily told her to take the child to the emergency room. Nancy had anticipated as much.

Within twenty minutes, they were in a noisy hospital triage room in West Palm Beach, Florida. A resident came and pushed his fingertips into Brian's appendix.

No appendicitis.

Probably constipation, said the doctor. He gave the child a laxative in a suppository and sent the Quinlans home. It was past daybreak now, and just as the doctor had predicted, Brian was back to his old, cheerful self. So that was that, Nancy thought.

And then it happened again.

Two weeks later, Brian woke in the middle of the night, wailing in agony. This time, it seemed, Brian's stomach was swollen—but not dramatically so. His forehead was warm, as it had been on and off for a couple of days. These were hardly symptoms worth getting nervous about. Nevertheless, Nancy coaxed her tired son out of bed and they returned to the same ER. The doctor on the graveyard shift X-rayed Brian, checked him for a rare bowel disorder called intussusception, and this time tried an enema. Again, Brian felt better immediately.

A few days later, Nancy brought her son to a local gastroenterologist for a follow-up. The doctor offered a matter-of-fact explanation for Brian's bizarre nighttime behavior: "Constipation . . . with 'psychological withholding.' Come back in thirty days." The diagnosis was almost comically mild, Nancy thought. She would have been relieved, certainly, but for one small problem: she didn't believe it. She *knew* her son. And "psychological withholding," well, it wasn't Brian. Except for the rare sniffle, he'd never been sick. The boy never wanted to rest, sit down, sleep. He was one of those kids—an ever-grinning, leap-out-of-bed, perpetual-motion machine.

Like his brother, Brendan, Brian was a natural-born athlete. Most kids had to learn to hit a baseball off a plastic tee in the backyard. Both Brian and Brendan could pound line drives off their dad's pitches by the time they were three. By age four, Brian had discovered a still greater love in swimming; he had an even more natural grace in the water than on land.

The Quinlans' one-story ranch house was a few blocks from the Intracoastal Waterway, and just beyond that, the ocean sand. In the tiny backyard, dwarfing the family's cement-block home, was a pool. Brian seemed to be constantly at its edge, poised to leap in with his knees tucked under his arms. The chlorine and sun had made his hair flaxen and shiny. His eyes were bluer than the water—"turquoise," his mom called them. In his long, baggy swim trunks, agile and confident, oblivious of the weather, Brian was the quintessential surfer dude—at age four.

He was like Mom in that regard. Nancy Quinlan, tanned, green–eyed, and blond, still kept her surfboard in the garage. She was certified as a scuba diver, though it had been a long time since she'd been out on the reefs. Her other job had consumed most of her attention for the past several months. Nancy had been at the helm of a major government drug case. She'd coordinated a long interagency investigation, gotten a federal judge to approve dozens of wiretaps, and served as chief prosecutor at trial, sending twenty-seven defendants to jail. "Investigators recovered a lot of cocaine and cash and guns," she later recalled. "A *lot* of guns."

Her strength in the case had come from being prepared, not ferocious. (She hated the cliché of the tough federal prosecutor. "You don't have to be tough," she'd say. "The statutes are tough enough. You just have to be thorough.") It was that need for thoroughness, to bury the doubt that nagged her, that pushed her to get the names of two experts in pediatric gastroenterology.

She made an appointment to see one of them after Labor Day, two hours away at the University of Miami. She gathered all the X-rays and physician reports from the local hospital and stuck them in the backseat of her car. Then, ten days before the appointment in Miami, Brian awoke in agony in the middle of a Sunday night. It was an unwritten law of nature, it seemed, that medical emergencies had to happen on Sundays, or in the middle of the night, or as it was in this case—*both*. Now, in the fullest expression of that unwritten law, a Category 4 hurricane was pounding several islands in the Caribbean with 145-mile-an-hour winds. The storm was bearing straight for the Florida coast.

Nancy thought for a moment. In a minute she was in Brian's room, lifting the sixty-pound child into her arms and rushing him to the car. Her husband, Patrick, a lawyer with the county attorney's office, would have to stay home from work to watch Brendan, Nancy thought. If they waited to see if Brian's symptoms resolved themselves, and Brian got worse, the boy could end up back in the same ER in West Palm Beach. Nancy wasn't going to let that happen. She was going to take her son to see the specialist in Miami. She'd wait outside his house if necessary.

It wasn't until she was an hour down the interstate, with the sun rising and the radio updating forecasts on the approaching storm, that Nancy began to have second thoughts about continuing to Miami. Brian's pain was getting worse. He was now moaning in the backseat. She saw a sign for Hollywood Boulevard and took the exit. She was now only minutes from Joe DiMaggio Children's Hospital, where Dr. Mario Tano worked. Tano was the *other* pediatric gastroenterologist on Nancy's list.

Once more, she and her son waited in the triage room. Brian was wheeled to an X-ray table. Again, the films showed that his bowel was impacted. It was as if she and her son were trapped in the movie *Groundhog Day,* Nancy thought. The same pattern was unfolding for a third time. In her head, she could hear the one-word diagnosis coming from the doctor's mouth: *constipation.* This doctor, however, seemed different from the green, eyelid-drooping interns the Quinlans had seen before.

And this time, Brian wasn't merely in pain, he was also pale and limp. His torso was angled forward, just perceptibly, and he had the tiniest trouble walking. He looked, as Nancy would later tell the doctor, "floppy."

In the least frantic voice she could summon, Nancy begged the ER doctor to call Dr. Tano at home and ask if he might come in. Two hours later, the Quinlans were sitting with Tano in his office at Joe DiMaggio Children's hospital. Then something remarkable happened. The doctor asked Nancy to talk. He wanted her to tell him everything she could about Brian and the events of the past month.

She began the story from the beginning, detailing each symptom and test and change in mood and what Brian had eaten for dinner the evening before. Tano nodded his head as he placed his enormous hands all over Brian's neck, arms, chest, abdomen. It looked as if an old, blind man were trying to find his way from Brian's head to his toes. As Nancy continued her narrative, her voice began to crack. She could feel a score of emotions bubbling inside. Someone was at last taking her concerns seriously, she thought. A doctor actually seemed to believe that a mother could know her son.

"He just listened to everything," Nancy later recalled. "What I was seeing in Brian, what was different about Brian, what was worrying me."

She spoke for twenty minutes, and when she could think of nothing else to add, Dr. Tano said simply, "We will figure out what's wrong with your son."

When she first heard the report, four days later, Nancy was relieved. The words did not quite have the ring of "psychological withholding," but they didn't seem all that frightening either.

Dr. Tano had asked an infectious disease specialist at the hospital to take a look at Brian. The boy's blood counts had been within the normal range, but just to be safe, the specialist wanted to take some MRI images of Brian's spine and pelvis. Now, she was reporting to Nancy and Patrick Quinlan what the radiologist had "noticed" on the films: "diffuse infiltrate of the bone marrow." For whatever reason, Nancy assumed that the words meant that Brian had an infection, a mild bacterial invasion that could be quashed by antibiotics.

The specialist, then, gently explained that the finding was consistent with leukemia. There was a brief moment as the meaning gelled in Nancy's mind. And then, she says, "it was like someone had thrown a fire extinguisher in my face. I couldn't breathe."

It was four long days of waiting before a bone marrow biopsy could be performed. That was the test that would either confirm the doctor's guess or give the Quinlans a reprieve. First came Hurricane Frances, which shut down much of the hospital from Friday through Sunday. Then came Monday, which in its own measure of agony was also Labor Day, a day on which only emergency medical procedures were done. Finding out whether their son had cancer didn't qualify as an emergency.

The Quinlans had entered cancer's otherworldly realm even before they knew they were there. In the four days of wait, Patrick had scouted out a hospital computer and had researched everything he could about leukemia on the Internet. He had read several research papers. He and Nancy had called everyone they knew in the medical profession. Nancy had spent an hour on the phone with a colleague whose young daughter had been diagnosed with leukemia long ago.

The bottom line was terrifying: the disease was rapidly fatal if left unchecked. It killed by infiltrating and corrupting the warm marrow of life itself. Leukemia, in short, was a cancer of the blood.

For all its mystery, cancer is an illness that comes with ready-made images. Just hearing the word is enough to prompt a cascade of mental snapshots: mysterious lumps, rapacious tumors, misshapen moles.

Imagining what cancer is, indeed, is far too easy. It is too easy to picture internal organs under attack by a raging brigade of cells; to see, in the mind's eye, the peaceful space of a liver or lung being swarmed by an unruly mob. Cancer might well be a continuing enigma to scientists, but to the rest of mankind it is as familiar as an Arctic polar bear or a Tahitian sunset—an image seen, perhaps, only in mental postcards, but recognizable nonetheless.

That said, few people are able to picture a cancer of the blood. The internal gallery of snapshots offers not so much as a hint as to how such a thing might work. And there is that obvious conceptual barrier—the notion of blood as a coursing red river. A *liquid*. How could there be cancer of a liquid? As it turns out, though, that traditional idea of blood isn't quite right. Much of what makes up blood is a watery serum (called plasma), laced with assorted protein bits, sugars, fatty acids, electrolytes, and waste. But also within is teeming life—tens of trillions of individual cells, coursing lap after lap throughout the body. That is the first image to overcome: Blood is not an inanimate sauce. It is a bodily tissue composed of cells—any one of which can be set upon a malignant course.

Picturing that is not enough, however. An equal challenge is to reconcile the idea of this living, pullulating stream with another widely held notion—that cancer is a disease of fast-growing tumors. Where, after all, are these fixed masses in the mad rush of blood? Do they protrude from the walls of veins like boulders in the path of white-water rapids?

The answer to these questions holds what is likely to be the disease's biggest surprise: Though the expanding tumor is the most familiar aspect of cancer (the word *neoplasm* means "new growth"), cancer is not merely an illness of rapid cell growth.* Fundamentally, it is a disease of subversion. Cancer is a subversion of rules, the corruption of an organism's cohesion and structural order. When a single cell begins to exploit its biological machinery to promote its own survival and proliferation above all else—stealing resources from its neighbors, failing to perform its normal duties, ignoring the greater good of the organism—cancer has begun. When the instigator of this rebellion is a type of blood cell known as a leukocyte (or white blood cell), the cancer is called leukemia.

Even that, however, is just a shorthand explanation. To understand leukemia, one has to take yet another conceptual leap and consider its opposite—that is to say, the *normal* way in which white blood cells (and all other blood cells) develop and die.

Laid end to end, the blood vessels of an adult human being would stretch an estimated sixty thousand miles or more—well over twice the circumference of the earth. The circuit travels to every square millimeter of the body, in an obstacle course that ranges from thick, pulsing arteries to serpentine canals five times narrower than the thinnest of human hairs. Many capillaries are so narrow that the most common white blood cells have to sputter and contort to squeeze through them. Yet more extraordinary than the marvels of circulation is the way in which all of these myriad passages are populated—and continuously repopulated—with cells.

The challenge is that blood cells, by and large, do not live long. Virtually all of the 30 trillion or so blood cells circulating in the human body are erythrocytes (red blood cells), the scarlet-hued, jelly-doughnut-shaped bundles that ferry oxygen. On average they survive for 120 days. That

---

*Cells in a healthy human embryo grow at an even faster rate.

brief span is an eternity compared with the existence of various white blood cells, whose life spans range from mere hours to a couple of weeks. (Exceptions to the rule include plasma cells and classes of lymphocytes called memory B cells and T cells, which can live for decades.) Platelets, tiny blood-clotting elements that break off from large cells called mega-karyocytes, typically last for just over a week before being degraded.

The result is that on any given day, up to a *trillion* blood cells of various types die and are replaced—a marvelous feat of recycling. To protect itself against a limitless range of pathogens and foreign molecules, for example, the body relies upon a diverse army of leukocytes, a dozen or so different divisions (or "lineages") of immune cells, each with its own role in defense. Various types of these white blood cells, for instance, release little bomblets of toxin to kill invaders such as bacteria and parasites; others attach themselves to their targets and swallow them whole; still others rush en masse to a site of trauma or infection in a kind of protective scrum called inflammation.

Reinforcing and replacing all of these warriors is no minor task, and the limits of space make the job nearly impossible. Blood cells, after all, grow in the marrow, in the soft inner core of bones—a nest too cramped to have a lifetime's worth of backups ready and waiting. Nature has conjured up an ingenious solution by producing every type of blood cell (white, red, and platelets, too) from a single class of progenitors known as stem cells.

When one of these rare matriarchs divide, the first of its two twin daughters remains a stem cell, thereby ensuring that the supply never runs out. The second, meanwhile, can develop into any kind of blood cell, depending on the need. Going through a stepwise process called differentiation, the daughter matures from a roundish blob known as a blast to the ultimate functional cell she is to become.

Such efficient adaptations come with their own unsolved mysteries, as does every other aspect of *hematopoiesis*, the technical term for the making of blood cells. This process is almost too complex to fathom. Information about which types of reinforcements are required (and where) is continually passed along from one cell to another through a great multitude of signaling molecules whose rapid-fire communications somehow preserve the order. As new cells make their way from the marrow, where the blood's elements are made, to the bloodstream, the balance of old dying cells and the newly born is forever recalibrated on the most sensitive of scales. To effect the ideal balance, in fact, tens of billions of perfectly healthy white blood cells are routinely instructed to self-destruct, a process called apoptosis.

Almost all of the time, in almost everyone, in almost all of the trillions upon trillions of cell lives, deaths, and regenerations, these multiple layers of protection work. Once in a rare while they do not. Something happens that collapses this finely tuned network onto itself. Pristine order devolves into turmoil. The entire system breaks down in a matter of weeks or months. And it starts with the tiniest of changes made to a *single cell.* Cancer's subversion begins when the DNA within a lone cell is damaged, removed, rearranged, or overproduced in precisely the wrong ways.

In the case of acute leukemia, that cell is a blast, the early-stage precursor to a mature white blood cell. It is a baby of sorts. An odd and random collusion of genetic injuries keeps that one cell "stuck" in mid-metamorphosis, preventing it from becoming a fully functional granulocyte or lymphocyte.

Additional mutations send the blast (or more likely, one of her descendants) deeper into malignancy. With each cell division, the transformed cell passes along to each newly minted "clone" the same tiny section (or sections) of garbled DNA that allows the first to outsurvive and outcompete her neighbors. Fail-safes fail at every turn. Self-destruct signals are ignored. Cancer is biology's version of Murphy's Law: everything that can go wrong does.

Even in this framework of anarchy, though, acute leukemia stands out. The renegade blast and its progeny reproduce so quickly that they soon take over the cozy spaces of the bone marrow—crowding out not only other white blood cells of every stage, but also red blood cells and the megakaryocytes that spore off wound-healing platelets by the thousands. Eventually, the leukemic cells push their way through the borders of the marrow and into the peripheral blood.

The scenario now enters a critical phase: with fewer new red blood cells being made to replace their dying cousins, tissues throughout the body begin to suffer. Every human cell needs the oxygen that erythrocytes ferry. Without it, muscles and joints ache in cellular hunger. Exhaustion sets in.

Along with anemia and fatigue comes bruising and bleeding. If the leukemic cycle isn't stopped, blood vessels and organs soon begin to hemorrhage. The biological breakdown, likewise, continues on a third path, as one predatory infection after another takes hold. For even though leukemia is a disease of "too many white cells," the immature cells produced are not up to the task of fending off the body's relentless attackers—viruses, bacteria, fungi, parasites. Instead, the increasing numbers of leukemic blasts keep other critical lines of white blood cells from being formed. Without them, there is little hope of a comprehensive defense.

Protecting the body is a communal job. It requires the coordination of dozens of cell types and molecular helpers. Leukemia upends that cooperation. The cancer kills, in sum, by subverting the most essential aspect of hematopoiesis: its perfect, incomprehensible sense of balance. Leukemia is the cruel opposite of normal.

And as recently as the 1960s, nine of every ten children diagnosed with acute forms of the disease died this way: starved of oxygen, hemorrhaging from eyes, the mouth, and internal organs, ravaged by infection.

That was what the Quinlans, sitting in the family room at Joe DiMaggio Children's Hospital, were beginning to learn. Patrick had found only scattered bits of information online, clipped explanations and medicalese. In his research, though, one fact stood out. In 2003, around 3,600 Americans, two-thirds of whom were children, were diagnosed with acute lymphocytic leukemia, a disease best known by its initials: ALL. (To confuse matters, the same cancer is variously called acute lymphoblastic leukemia, acute leukemia, or childhood leukemia.) An additional 10,500 Americans that year were told they had AML, or acute myeloid leukemia (sometimes called acute myelogenous leukemia). Only a fraction of these patients were children.

As the word *acute* suggested, both versions are aggressive and quick moving. The distinction between them lies in the type of white blood cell that is transformed: in ALL, the malignancy begins in a lymphoid cell (a future lymphocyte); in AML, the renegades are of a type called myeloid (would-be granulocytes).

But what Patrick cared about wasn't cell lineage. It was the odds. As best he could tell, the survival rate for children with ALL nationwide, lumping all stages and subtypes together, was an estimated 85 percent, roughly eighty-five out of every hundred kids diagnosed with the disease were likely to live for at least five years. The survival rate for kids with AML was around 50 percent.

The night before Brian's bone-marrow biopsy, Patrick Quinlan found himself in the strange position of *hoping* his son had a specific type of leukemia. In his heart he somehow knew his son had cancer. Now, he desperately prayed that it was the right kind—the lesser of evils. Patrick called up one of his oldest friends. "We've lost a couple ones along the way here," Patrick told him, as if psyching himself up in a football huddle. "We've got to win this one. This game we *have* to win. We have to win the ALL versus AML matchup."

On Tuesday morning, just after nine, a doctor at last put a thick needle into Brian's hip and aspirated some marrow. By one in the afternoon, the Quinlans heard the report. It was what now passed for good news—ALL. They'd gotten what they'd prayed for.

A chemotherapy nurse walking down the hall stopped in front of Nancy, who was resting with her head in her hands. "Are you getting all the information you need?" the nurse kindly asked. In fact, they had no idea what the treatment would be like or even where Brian would go to get it. Patrick had learned in his Internet research that the cure rates for ALL were best at St. Jude Children's Research Hospital in Memphis, where many of the pioneering studies in the disease had been done. One more name that had stuck out in Patrick's investigation was Ching-Hon Pui, the St. Jude clinician who had emerged as the foremost expert in the field.

But how on earth, Nancy asked the nurse, would they get Brian treated there? And if they managed it, where would they stay? How long would they need to be at the hospital? What would they do with their son Brendan, who was in the third grade?

The nurse reassured her that the answers would come in time, then disappeared down the hall. Minutes later, when she reappeared, she was waving for Nancy to come with her: "Dr. Pui's on the phone."

The moment after Nancy hung up the phone, she ran to her husband, shouting, "We're going to Graceland. We're going to Graceland." Pui had agreed to admit Brian onto an ongoing clinical study—but only if they got to Memphis that same night. ALL was an exceptionally aggressive disease. Treatment had to begin right away.

The last flight of the evening departed from West Palm Beach at 6:30 p.m. It was then two o'clock and they were a good hour away from home on the interstate. Hurricane Frances had laid havoc to most of the roads in the area. The Quinlans' car, slammed by three days of nonstop wind and rain, refused to start.

Thirty minutes passed before the engine turned over. Patrick floored the accelerator the whole way home. And then, as the Quinlans pulled into their driveway, they saw something bizarre: several of their neighbors were standing on the lawn, holding open suitcases and flashlights. The power was out across the neighborhood. Although it was just past four o'clock, the Quinlans' home was pitch-black. Within seconds, Nancy and Patrick were racing through their blackened house, emptying closets and bureaus into the suitcases as their friends hovered nearby with flashlights. The Quinlans would have made the plane with only minutes to spare— but, as it turned out, the flight was delayed.

It was nearly midnight when the four Quinlans stood at the baggage claim in the Memphis airport, watching the carousel go around and around. Suitcases were rolling by but the Quinlans had no idea which ones were theirs—none of the bags, after all, belonged to them. They grabbed nearly every piece of luggage as it rounded the belt, looking for some sign of familiarity. In the strangeness of the scene, Nancy and Patrick and the two boys broke into laughter. It wasn't just the luggage. The entire scenario was so hard to believe. Just four days earlier, Brian was an unstoppable four-year-old swimming sensation with an odd case of night constipation. Now he was one of those kids you hear about—the friend of a friend's kid who's got leukemia.

It would have been impossible for the Quinlans to have imagined the speed with which their lives would change. In less than two hours, an IV would be in Brian's arm, blood would be drawn, and pictures of his bones taken with sound waves. Within four hours, his white blood cells would be analyzed down to the molecular level; the DNA inside the deranged blast cells would be scanned for key mutations that could offer either hope or gloom. By morning Brian would be assigned to a treatment protocol based on this analysis. That day he would start an unthinkably complex and brutal drug treatment—and if all went perfectly well, continue it for three straight years without a single week of rest.

As dawn broke on Wednesday, September 8, 2004, Nancy knelt at the foot of her child's hospital bed and started crying. She wasn't sad, she would later explain. She was grateful. Simply, overwhelmingly grateful.

Over the next several months, Nancy would remain grateful. For the expert hands of the chemo nurses. For Shawn, the twentysomething St. Jude patient liaison, who cleverly, reassuringly showed Brian how to swallow the gargantuan capsules that composed part of his chemotherapy, an achievement that made every day to come that much easier. Nancy would remain ever so grateful for Dr. Pui and his animated confidence.

There were rare moments when the renowned oncologist could speak with a certainty that bordered on brusque. But never with children in the leukemia ward. With them, his patience was unending. Older kids poked and chased him; younger ones tugged at his long, white smock. Brian took to the doctor right away. Pui brought Nancy an unexpected calm when they spoke. There was nothing about the disease, or the potential effects from treating it, that the man did not seem to know.

Nancy was thankful for St. Jude. For its cartoon murals and low-hanging ceilings—a framing designed for a child's playhouse rather than a hospital. She was thankful for the red wheelbarrows strewn across the reception area. The people at St. Jude had answers for everything—where the family would stay, where Brian's older brother, Brendan, would go to school, what all of it would cost (nothing more than their insurance would cover). She was thankful for the "friends of friends" in Memphis who had adopted them upon first meeting, welcoming the Quinlans into their homes and lives as if they were long-lost family. Over the next three years, there would be an abundance of care and comfort, of kindness bestowed from friends and strangers. Nancy would be deeply thankful for all of it.

But on the morning of September 8, it was a single fact that made her weep in relief. That was the one Patrick had learned in his frantic computer research at Joe DiMaggio Children's Hospital: the statistic that said her son would likely survive.

In 1963, the five-year survival rate for children diagnosed with acute lymphocytic leukemia—a disease that accounted for three in ten childhood cancers overall—was around 14 percent. By 2004, some 87 percent of young ALL patients across the United States lived at least five years, with the overwhelming majority beating their disease outright. At St. Jude, by all accounts, a child's chances were even better. Recent studies suggested that the five-year survival rate there had climbed to just over 90 percent.

It was a breathtaking transformation. Acute lymphocytic leukemia was a horror-movie villain come to life—and the heroes of the cancer war had found a way to stop it. That was the reason Nancy Quinlan dropped to her knees in thanks.

Talk to just about any leader in the cancer fight about what progress has been achieved and he or she is almost certain to bring up the near-triumph over acute lymphocytic leukemia and other childhood malignancies. Indeed, as with ALL, stunning advances have occurred over the past several decades in the five-year survival rates for Hodgkin's disease, Wilms' tumor, neuroblastoma, Ewing's sarcoma, and several other cancers common to young people—making the turnabout in childhood cancers the greatest success story in the long war on cancer.

To be sure, roughly a fifth of children who get cancer still end up dying from it. Cancer remains the biggest disease killer of children in the United States, killing more kids between the ages of one and fifteen each year than heart disease, influenza, pneumonia, suicide, bronchitis, meningitis, anemia, septicemia, diabetes, measles, hepatitis, HIV, and appendicitis combined. But had death rates never dropped over the years from 1975 to 2006, as Malcolm Smith and colleagues at the NCI recently calculated, the death toll would have included an additional thirty-eight thousand children and teenagers.

By any measure, the transformation in childhood cancers has been remarkable. Yet hovering over these lifesaving achievements is a sobering and uncomfortable truth. To voice it is to challenge the most fundamental assumption of the decades-old cancer war: that the route to victory is finding the "cure" (or cures) for cancer.

It is not. Indeed, even if the five-year survival rate for all pediatric malignancies were to reach 100 percent tomorrow, even in the improbable event that prognoses for every type and stage of the disease were to experience the miraculous turnaround we have seen with ALL, we would still be far from victory in the war on cancer.

The reason can be seen in yet another statistic regarding childhood cancers: 12,060. That was the estimated number of new cases of pediatric cancer in the year 2012. The annual count has jumped by more than 40 percent since 2000, even as the general population in this age group has inched up less than 3 percent over the same period. The leapfrogging tallies of new cases from year to year have, obviously, nothing to do with an aging America. (Correcting for differences in population size and age, the NCI says the incidence of childhood cancers has risen by 0.6 percent a year between 1975 and 2006.) No one quite knows why the rate of new cases has been growing so fast, though theories include everything from exposure to infectious agents to the increasing birth weight of babies. But in the national cancer effort, not enough emphasis has been placed on finding out.

The central aim of the cancer war is to keep patients with cancer alive longer—that mandate can never be sacrificed. But remarkably little effort is aimed at preventing people from getting cancer in the first place; a mere 7 percent of the NCI budget in 2010 was devoted to "cancer prevention and control," by the agency's own assessment. "I'm not saying that we should quit looking for cures," says John Bailar, the former NCI statistician who first warned about our failing cancer war more than a quarter century ago. "But I think it's a bad, bad mistake to assume that this focus on treatment will eventually be effective" if we do nothing to reduce the number of new cancers. We will only find ourselves deeper in this war of attrition, with each new year bringing a growing number of patients to the front lines. And in the case of childhood cancers, the battle is more fierce and lasting than many people know.

On the night that four-year-old Brian Quinlan first lay in a hospital bed at St. Jude, his so-called blast count was just 26 percent—a figure, happily, that was low for children diagnosed with ALL. His white blood count was only mildly elevated. His central nervous system was free of disease. No leukemic cells were in his spleen or his liver. The so-called lineage of his leukemic cells, pre-B cell, offered the best prognosis. They also had a telltale molecular aberration called TEL-AML1, which augured well. He had responded early and dramatically to the fierce remission–induction treatment, which was the best-known predictor of long-term success. He was the right age. He was a strong and healthy kid.

And still, he would have to endure three years of grueling, nonstop chemotherapy—treatment that would change every facet of his young life, consisting of drugs that would sharply raise his risk for heart problems, stroke, and a secondary cancer in adulthood. Pediatric cancer survivors have a sixfold greater risk of getting a second malignancy than untreated children have of getting a first.

The transformation in survival rates for pediatric malignancies is our greatest triumph in the war on cancer. Yet the cost of that victory is growing, not lessening, as more American families pay the price each year.

Alarming as is the increase in childhood cancer incidence, the number of adult diagnoses in the United States each year dwarfs the scale of new pediatric cases. That number has soared 158 percent from 1971 to 2012, a rate of growth that is three times that of the population as a whole.

In 2013, an estimated 1,660,290 Americans are expected to be diagnosed with an invasive cancer. That does not include more than a million annual cases of nonmelanoma skin cancers. (Tumor registries do not keep track of such lesions, which are mostly slow-growing and generally do not metastasize.) Nor do the government figures include most of the in situ tumors that are discovered, more than sixty thousand of which are found in women's breasts each year. The Latin term means "in its place," which reflects that these pockets of abnormally growing cells have remained in the spot where they formed. There is heated debate within the research community as to whether such neoplasms are truly malignant or *prema-lignant*, and about what sort of long-term danger they might pose.

Figure 6

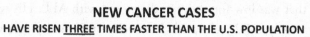

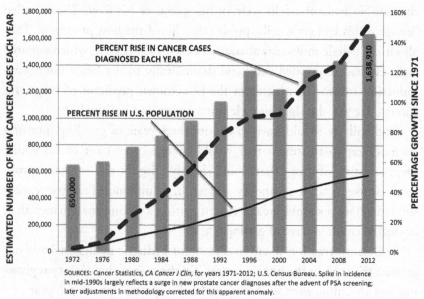

NEW CANCER CASES
HAVE RISEN <u>THREE</u> TIMES FASTER THAN THE U.S. POPULATION

SOURCES: Cancer Statistics, *CA Cancer J Clin*, for years 1971-2012; U.S. Census Bureau. Spike in incidence in mid-1990s largely reflects a surge in new prostate cancer diagnoses after the advent of PSA screening; later adjustments in methodology corrected for this apparent anomaly.

But no matter what is, or is not, figured into the official tally, the overall cancer burden—the number of people getting the disease, enduring treatment, and facing the often lifelong effects of that treatment—is clearly soaring. So, too, is the already enormous cost burden of cancer. Americans spent some $103 billion a year on cancer treatment in 2010, a national bill that has climbed more than 80 percent in just the previous nine years. (Even adjusting for both inflation and the increase in US population, cancer health expenditures grew by a staggering 37 percent between 2001 and 2010.)

Cancer patients spend more than 10 million days in hospitals a year, and untold more hours in outpatient clinics and doctor's offices. Even for those with health insurance, the cost is frequently devastating: copays and out-of-pockets accumulate relentlessly; sick days vanish in a flash, wages are lost—a combination that wipes out the savings of tens of thousands of families each year.

But treatment creates the greatest burden of all. Some of the 1.6 million cancers diagnosed each year are products of unintentional over-diagnosis (an issue that will be discussed in chapter 6). In accounting for this aspect of the disease burden, though, it matters little whether the cancer is "real" and aggressive or not: nearly everyone is treated as if that were the case.

For some, that means radical surgery and morbid rearrangement of their body. For some patients, treatment means a jumble of caustic therapies, heaped upon one another in complicated protocols, or strung out in what seems a never-ending succession. For others, it is urgent and unexpected—a parade of blood transfusions, antibiotic infusions, and marrow transplants. In some cases, the cocktail of chemical poisons in the IV drip damages the heart or muddles the mind; or the targeted radiation inadvertently sears the delicate tissue of the lungs. Or the toxic combination triggers a second cancer, and the process begins all over again.

Cancer treatment can feel like an exhausting board game come to life, a route in which every other square requires a new blood test, scan, or X-ray, where the path is stalled by interminable waiting-room waits, insurance forms, and unanswered questions. For many patients, there is little difference between treatment and disease. Pain from one melds into pain from the other; fear of the cancer is subsumed, at times, by the immediate dread of a brutal drug or procedure. They are the two faces of the same ordeal. That is cancer for hundreds of thousands of new patients each year.

Nor, for many people, does the emotional trauma end with the final round of treatment. The diagnosis continues to tow behind it the nag of uncertainty, whispering anew with each swollen gland, fever, or malaise. Even when the cancer is truly gone, even when the scans are clean, it can seem that the "cure" is held in an escrow of medical testing and follow-up.

Quantifying such costs, putting precise numbers or percentages next to this litany, is impossible—in no small part because the National Cancer Institute has collected only scattershot data on this. The costs, paid by patients and devoted caregivers, are measured in lives, in traumatized families, in missed opportunities, in lost employment, not just in dollars. While these costs remain largely unaccounted, they do not go away, and the more they grow, the further we are from victory in the war on cancer.

By Week 84 of Brian Quinlan's treatment at St. Jude, he was feeling well. Brian had been allowed to take swimming lessons over the summer, and he was now in the pool, home in Florida, much of the day. "He's got a really beautiful freestyle and he's learning to breathe to the side," said Nancy, as we spoke on the phone. "We're just working on his endurance."

In the middle of her comment, another call beeped in. "That was St. Jude's," she said flatly. "They're going to increase his medicine because his counts are too high. His white counts. They want to keep them in a certain range weekly, and his have been a little bit too high. So they might increase the 6-MP he gets every night." If Nancy was worried, she did not let on. Such changes had become routine.

The 6-MP wasn't nearly as bad as the other drugs. When Brian would take vincristine and dexamethasone together, he would get unbelievable tremors. "He would sit in my lap and shake. Those are the wild rides, because the vincristine makes you feel terrible and you've got the leg pain and all that, and the dex affects your mood and your appetite enormously," said his dad.

Twice daily, Brian took a prophylactic antibiotic, Septra or Bactrim, which made his stools turn a pond-silt green. Every Thursday, he got a shot of methotrexate in the leg, except for the last Thursday of the month, on which he was given vincristine. That one, said Patrick, was "wicked."

During the intense phase of treatment called consolidation, Brian received the methotrexate in enormous dosages. The drug, on its own, would have slaughtered his white blood cells to near extinction. So every six hours, Patrick or Nancy had to "rescue" Brian by injecting a drug called leucovorin (essentially, folic acid) directly into his Hickman port, an IV dock embedded in his chest.

In Brian's first few months of treatment, Nancy was alone in Memphis on a high-dose methotrexate day. She had managed the four o'clock and ten o'clock rescue injections of leucovorin, but was afraid that she would fall sleep and miss the next scheduled injection. "She had a number of people calling her at four o'clock in the morning because she was panicked about not getting the medicine to him in time," Patrick once told me. "And it is nerve-racking. There's a lot at stake in the leucovorin rescue. The doctors have you convinced that it has to be right to the exact minute or else there is danger."

There was danger in all of it. The Quinlans had rushed Brian to the hospital eight times in the previous year because of infections. In ALL, even a mild infection can kill. Their six-year-old boy could not swim in the ocean or pet a dog.

"It's funny how normal changes—your view of what normal is," Patrick said. "Brian woke up two days ago and he walked into the bathroom and he started throwing up in the toilet. And he threw up for about ten minutes and then he walked out and lay on the couch and watched a little TV. And Nancy started to give him medicine to calm his stomach and he threw that up. And he went over to the toilet and threw up again.

"And later in the day, I was remembering the morning and thinking, 'We almost treated it like it was run–of-the-mill.' I was feeling guilty that I didn't do more to try and comfort him. And then I came home and told him.

"I actually thought about it, stupidly enough, on the basketball court. Because I had hurt myself. Part of me wanted to come out of the game. And then I thought about Brian. I thought, 'Gosh, he was such a hero this morning. I should have said more to him this morning about how much of a hero he is.'"

Chapter 4

The Soldier

When my father proposed to my mother, she was barely nineteen. He was twenty-four, a lieutenant at a US army Nike-missile base in Reading, Massachusetts; she was in college.

They had met two years before, when both were counselors at summer camp: he at a boys' camp; she at the girls' camp across the lake. At an evening social, my mother had asked my father to find a boy to dance with her younger sister. My father grabbed one of his frightened charges by the ears and dragged him over. My father danced with my mother and fell in love. It was likely, even then, that her cancer was under way.

The first time she felt anything was wrong was a few summers later; she and my father were camping. She doubled over in pain at what she thought were cramps. Days later, a surgeon found a large tumor in her small intestine and removed several feet of the organ. The cancer had metastasized to nearby lymph nodes, and those came out as well. The doctor gave her six weeks to live.

My mother did not die in six weeks, however. Nor in six months. When the tumor recurred in her liver, a second round of doctors gave her another estimate of time remaining: it wasn't promising. She had a rare form of cancer in which carcinoid tumors formed in her digestive tract. Releasing huge doses of the neurotransmitter serotonin into the bloodstream, the tumors created a constellation of symptoms in her body—skin flushing, palpitations, diarrhea—known as carcinoid syndrome. Her heart and lungs would, in time, deteriorate; the coughing jags would turn her stomach. Still, my mother survived.

She loved to travel—far more than my father did. With great pride she set out to climb the steps of the abbey at Mont Saint-Michel in Normandy. When she got to the top, my father was exhausted. He had held her, half carried her, the whole way. She threw up after most of the meals in France. (My father blamed the richness of the food and saved the thick leather menus as if to rewrite the memories.)

Years later, she would be tethered to an oxygen tank, rolling from one room to the next, a green plastic cannula in her tiny nose. She was beautiful even then. My father made her feel more so. They still traveled. They went to the opera, both of them dressed to the nines. He bought a hospital bed that made it easier for my mother to sleep upright; she could no longer lie flat without choking. He bought two of the beds, pushed them together, and slept at the same incline. He had an electric stairway built into the house so that my mother could go upstairs and down at will. Once every so often I would see him, by then in his fifties, carrying her. Their embrace, precarious on the narrow steps, made them look like newlyweds.

My mother was brilliant, pugnacious, and brave. My father was big. That was the word that always came to mind when I thought of him. Six foot one and barrel-chested, he could summon a booming voice that could startle anyone. When two of my school friends were over for dinner one evening, my father suddenly pounded the table with his fist and shouted, "Damnit, Louise . . . I love you!" My friends did not know whether to laugh or cower.

My father had always been big with gestures and kindnesses, generous with hugs and handshakes. He had always been big with people—voted Big Man on Campus at Washington University; named head of the

Intrafraternity Council. When the St. Louis country club hosting the annual fraternity dance refused to allow a black fraternity in, my father refused to hold it there. In the end, the club backed down. The dance was integrated for the first time.

After the army, he went to law school on the GI Bill, aced the bar exam, became a litigator, started his own firm, ran for trustee of our small town—one of only two times I had ever known him to lose anything. My father had green combs embossed with VOTE FOR MARTY LEAF.

The other time was when my mother died, drifting off to death on Friday the thirteenth, January 1995. She was fifty-seven years old.

It was sixteen years earlier, though, when my father loomed largest of all. At least to me. He was waiting—keeping vigil—in a hospital room at New York's Columbia-Presbyterian hospital. This time, though, it was not my mother in the bed. It was me.

Some ten months before then, at the age of fifteen, I had been diagnosed with an advanced stage of Hodgkin's disease. The cancer had overtaken the lymph nodes in my lungs and neck, destroyed my spleen, ventured into my abdomen.

After each round of chemotherapy, my father had been there, holding my forehead as I retched into the night, wiping my face with a cool cloth. The clinic waiting rooms at the National Cancer Institute were as cold as fever chills. I never knew why they kept the rooms so icy. My father's big hands were perpetual ovens. I was embarrassed to cradle my hands in them. I did anyway.

To stave off the nausea, my father—the attorney for our small hometown—had conjured up sandwich bags of marijuana to smoke. Somehow, he had charmed the nurses into finding us an empty room in the government's sprawling cancer hospital. Jauntily, he showed me how to smoke, trying to get me to smile. He never told me where he got the pot—or where he had learned to roll a joint. I was too sullen, too adolescent, to admit to being impressed.

On the night my father sat beside me at Columbia-Presbyterian hospital, though, all of this had passed. By then I had completed three months of chemotherapy. Then a month of daily radiation therapy,

4,000 rads in all—a punch equivalent to getting twenty thousand chest X-rays a day, five days a week, for four weeks. Then three more months of chemotherapy. My parents had enrolled me in an NCI clinical trial, testing a strategy that the doctors called Ping Pong. The aim had been to see if alternating drug therapy with radiation was more effective than doing just one or the other. I was due for the final Pong—a second month of radiation—but had gotten too sick to continue.

The combination therapy had so far put me in remission, killing off the last of the malignant lymphocytes with unrelenting force. But it had nearly wiped out my healthy blood cells, too. My counts of white blood cells, red blood cells, and platelets were almost mortally low; I had a fever that waxed and waned. Multiple antibiotics were flushed daily into my veins through an IV drip, as one white-coat after another came into the hospital room for a look. No one knew quite what to do—except keep me there.

I was not like my father then. I was not like young Brian Quinlan. I was not bighearted. I was not brave. I was bratty, insular, confrontational, and moody. Much about that stay in the hospital room I did not remember for years.

What I could not forget, however, was that I had been in the same room for two weeks, and that on this night I was angry about something my father had done. It wasn't anything, of course. He had been sitting down, reading a magazine, passing the long hours with his son, and he had fallen asleep. I am ashamed to say, I told him to get up and stand in the corner. And to stay there.

My father looked at me, nodded gently, and stood up in the corner. He did not move. When I awoke the next morning, he was still there. The biggest man I had ever known had stood in the corner all night because the son he thought was dying had asked him.

I wish I could say that it was the fever that made me do it. Remembering the incident now, some three decades later, makes my body shrivel in shame.

And at the same time, I cannot help but marvel at the man who would do anything to help his son feel powerful, feel unchallengeable, in a time of utter fear and weakness. I cannot help but be awed by his overwhelming bigness.

Part Two

The Myth of the Magic Bullet

Chapter 5

The Little Orange Pill

A
s immense as the human cost of cancer has grown over the past
century, there is a solution, say many in the research community.
And it takes the form of a little orange pill.

In the universe of cancer science, there is no brighter star than the
drug called Gleevec in the United States, Glivec in Europe—or as it is
known in the medical literature: imatinib mesylate. By whichever name,
it is one of the few actual breakthrough cancer medicines to emerge over
the past two decades.

The drug does something wonderful: it dramatically improves the outlook for patients with a rare form of blood cancer called chronic myeloid
leukemia, or CML. (Unlike acute lymphocytic leukemia—the disease
Brian Quinlan was diagnosed with in 2004—CML affects a type of white
blood cell known as a granulocyte. More often than not, it strikes in
middle age as opposed to childhood. As the word *chronic* implies, its progression is slow and deliberate, at least in the early going.) In 2000, a year
before the drug's US approval, some 2,300 Americans died of CML, or
roughly half of those who got the disease. By 2006, the death count had

dropped to 600. By 2009, despite a slightly greater number of new cases, the total had dropped even further, to an estimated 470. The change, essentially, was due to this one drug.

Beyond even that remarkable achievement, Gleevec is effective against a second, still rarer disease: gastrointestinal stromal tumor (or GIST).

These effects alone would have been enough to call any drug a success story. For cancer scientists, however, Gleevec's dazzle goes well beyond the remissions it brings to patients. The real power of the drug, they say, is in the *way* it works—or more to the point, in the extraordinary science that made it. Gleevec, according to one researcher, is "proof of principle that rationally designed, molecularly targeted therapy works."

This crisp summary is from Brian Druker, the doctor most instrumental in bringing the medicine to clinical trials, writing with two colleagues in a leading medical journal. The drug represents "a paradigm shift in cancer drug development," the researchers said, one they hoped would "pave the way for a new generation of specific, targeted therapies for the many malignant conditions for which no efficient drug therapy is currently available."

Such enthusiasm is muted compared with the assessments of many of Druker's colleagues. Nobel laureate Harold Varmus, who is now director of the National Cancer Institute, penned a buoyant essay in 2006 titled "The New Era in Cancer Research," a period of optimism in cancer treatment heralded by "the dramatic arrival of a near-miraculous drug, imatinib (Gleevec)." Another veteran scientist called the molecule, developed by the Swiss pharmaceutical giant Novartis, "prototypic of a hoped-for revolution in oncology therapeutics." A third told the *New York Times* that it was "the beginning of a sea change—and I am speaking conservatively—in the way we practice cancer medicine." A fourth put it this way: Gleevec "represents a monumental leap forward in cancer chemotherapy. It proves a principle. It justifies an approach. It demonstrates that highly specific, nontoxic therapy is possible."

So went the accolades up to the top of the cancer food chain. Andrew von Eschenbach, who served as the director of the National Cancer Institute in the heady days of Gleevec's approval and who later headed the FDA, summed it up in 2002: "Things like Gleevec are not success stories in the context of magic bullets, they are success stories in proof of principle. If you can do it for that tumor, then why not for others?"

Paradigm shift. Sea change. Leap forward. Near-miraculous. Revolution. Proof of principle.

Such reactions to a single drug, even a great drug, may now seem a bit breathless. But one would have been hard-pressed to find any prominent cancer researcher disavowing them in the first years of the new millennium. Top scientists, drug developers, and patient advocates alike repeated the refrain. When senior researchers spoke of their work in the lab, they often talked of scrambling after the "next Gleevec." Aspiring young postdocs routinely inserted references to the molecule into their presentations at meetings, as if to validate their own findings by inference.

The excitement was so contagious that, in May of 2001, it spread to the cover of *Time* magazine. To convey the message, editors needed but a handful of bright orange pills and a cover line that every patient in the world was grateful to hear: "There Is New Ammunition in the War Against Cancer. These Are the Bullets."

The drug had been approved on an "accelerated" basis by the FDA a mere two weeks earlier. (Tested on fewer than twelve hundred patients in a handful of early-stage clinical trials, it had not yet proven that it could keep patients alive longer, though it would do so in subsequent trials.) But even in the spring of 2001, the writers of *Time*'s cover story understood what the revelry at cancer meetings was about: Gleevec was a breakthrough "not only for what it does but, more important, for the revolutionary strategy it represents."

The molecule, in other words, was (and is) the natural extension of cancer research itself. For rather than poison any dividing cell, healthy or malignant, as most conventional chemotherapy does, this man–made agent homes in on a precise molecular target. As if by magic, the drug wipes out the fast-growing cancer cells without causing the grave side effects (nausea, hair loss, destruction of normal blood cells, organ damage) so common to old-fashioned chemo.

But it *isn't* magic. Gleevec's wondrous effect is not a product of incidental discovery, the story goes; it is a function of logical design, a specificity informed by decades of basic research into the inner workings of human cells. Here, after all, is not just a single, death-defying medicine, but rather a template for drug development that can be copied again and again in one form of cancer after another.

The story mesmerizes not only cancer scientists, but also patients and advocates, drugmakers and government regulators, politicians and reporters. Of all these groups, in fact, probably the last have been most taken by the narrative. One writer at the normally sober *Fortune* magazine went so far as to call Gleevec a "marvel of medical alchemy" and "the first smart bomb in the war on cancer," describing its journey to the clinic as "a heroic saga indeed."

That journalist was me. (In 2003.) I had managed to squeeze such hyperbole into a blurb of just 135 words. (I had reviewed a book on Gleevec's discovery written by Daniel Vasella, who at the time was CEO of Novartis, the drug's manufacturer.)

But then, it is no secret why so many of us succumbed to its allure: *The Gleevec Story* is a tale of unassuming geniuses, bold discovery, and true grit. The heroes are genuine and modest. And most important, it tells us what we want to hear: that there will soon be simple, easy cures for every type of cancer; that we will be able to pop a pill and reverse any fast-growing tumor, just as millions now control their blood pressure and cholesterol.

Once again there is a catch. This one, though, has less to do with the Gleevec drug than with the narrative surrounding it. For as lifesaving as this molecule is, *The Gleevec Story* is deadly in its seduction: sirenlike, it has taken the global cancer-fighting enterprise down a perilous path—a path that can never lead us to victory in the war on cancer.

To understand why, however, it helps to hear the tale from the beginning. For hidden within this saga are clues to the true wiliness of our cancer foe, and to the real-world flaws of this long-promised paradigm.

In the spring of 1950, a second-year medical student at the University of Pennsylvania burst into his professor's office and told him, "If you give me a job for the summer, I can solve your cancer problem." Peter Nowell, then all of twenty-one, bigheaded and jocular, got the job.

Unfortunately, the promise was harder to keep. "That was the year the

Phillies won the pennant," Nowell explained in an interview, not long before his eightieth birthday. "And I got married that summer. So I got distracted."

Then came the "Doctor Draft," which conscripted thousands of new medical corpsmen into service during the Korean War and brought Nowell to a naval defense laboratory in San Francisco, studying the effect of radiation on mice. "I served my country by doing five thousand mouse autopsies," he quipped. Then came five children in a five-year span. And then came a chance to make history.

It was 1959. Nowell had returned to Philadelphia a couple of years earlier, securing a small lab space in the department of pathology. His aim, generally, was to learn something about leukemia at the cellular level. Despite the introduction of powerful DNA-destroying poisons such as methotrexate that had shown some promise against the disease, leukemia remained invariably fatal.

Nowell had no specific hypothesis to chase down. The plan was simply to do morphological studies—that is, to observe the way leukemic white blood cells appeared under the microscope. That meant getting samples of patient blood (often drawn hours earlier at a hospital across town), separating the leukocytes from the masses of red blood cells, carefully drying the cells of interest onto glass slides, and staining them with dyes that highlighted various cell structures. The next steps were to watch and wait and watch some more to see if anything interesting popped up.

One day something did.

After staining his cultured cells, he rinsed off the slides in tap water. Later, when he looked at the strip of glass under the microscope, he found dividing cells with visible chromosomes—strands so clear he could count them. The tap water had the effect of diluting the salt content in the culture solution, causing the DNA innards of the cell nuclei to swell. The chromosomes were still a jumble of tiny, bent hash marks and even tinier blotches, but they weren't clumped together. The individual strands were distinct. Nowell had never seen anything like it.

Without knowing it, he was reliving the accidental discovery made seven years earlier in the lab of the cell biologist T. C. Hsu. One morning,

Hsu had likewise found himself staring at human chromosomes that were "suddenly beautiful," as he put it. Doggedly, he had retraced the steps leading up to the miracle: Someone, presumably a lab technician, had diluted a rinsing solution used to pretreat slides with distilled water, lowering the concentration of salt. With less salt in the rinse, the cells on the slide sucked up more water, causing the chromatin fibers in the nucleus to bloat. The unknown assistant never owned up to the mistake. Hsu went on to publish the new "hypotonic" technique in the *Journal of Heredity*, ushering in a new golden era in human cytogenetics, as the study of chromosomes began to be called.

If Nowell had known the lesson of Hsu, however, he had forgotten it. While his reaction to the clarity of the chromosomes was the same as his predecessor's—"Beautiful!"—there was one problem: Nowell wasn't a cytogeneticist.

The study of human chromosomes was still a young science. The stunning work by Tjio and Levan, announcing the correct number of chromosomes, had been published just three years earlier, in 1956. Only three years before that, the twisting, helical structure of DNA itself, the precious molecule sheltered within these twenty-three pairs of chromosomes, had been revealed by James D. Watson and Francis Crick. And while, by now, both discoveries had attained the status of settled knowledge, there was little else in the realm of cytogenetics upon which scientists could agree.

This wide-open steppe of uncertainty included not just the question of how chromosomes worked, but also how to study them in the first place. Tjio's proficiency in freezing the fragile strands in metaphase had been lauded by colleagues. Technique, though, was easier to read about than to master. Nowell needed help. He found it in graduate student David Hungerford, whom he borrowed from a colleague's lab at the Institute for Cancer Research (now Fox Chase). It seemed a fortuitous pairing: Hungerford, who was actually a year older than Nowell, was looking for a good thesis project with which to earn his PhD; Nowell needed a good set of eyes.

———

Hungerford was sure he'd seen something strange under the microscope and called over to his colleague. Nowell peered into the ocular. Now, both of them saw it: One of the forty-six chromosomes in one particular cell appeared smaller than it should be.

At first, Hungerford thought it might be a Y chromosome. Males have an unmatched pair of sex chromosomes—one X and one smaller Y. (Females have two Xs.) And these cells, after all, had come from a male leukemia patient.

But after further examination, both researchers could spot the normal Y in the samples, along with the corresponding X. One by one, they matched the nonsex chromosomes to their mates.

Human development is an orchestral fantasia, replete with jaw-dropping wonders and long-standing mysteries. The process begins, though, with a single fertilized egg cell called the zygote—its nucleus, unlike that of every other egg cell, now suddenly packed with *two* sets of twenty-three chromosomes. In perfect equanimity, one set hails from the ovum itself—a genetic legacy from the mother; the other, from the father by way of his sperm. With the exception of the sex chromosomes, each chromosome in the zygote is matched with its counterpart. The sibling strands are not identical, but rather *homologous,* to use the biological term—they are similar in size, shape, and function the way a left hand is to a right. Generally, in other words, one can tell which strand corresponds with which.

Nowell and Hungerford took turns at the microscope, each succeeding time counting ever more carefully. Twenty-one of the pairs synced up in shape and size. Plus the X and Y. That left one pair that didn't seem to match. The remaining chromosomes were runts. But even so, one homologue was seemingly shorter than what had to be its mate.

Neither man could be sure at first. Though the strands were now relatively engorged, they remained blurry ink stains under the bright lamp glow of the microscope. And the smaller ones were mere jots of black, like the smudge of a felt-tip pen. The cells had come from a man diagnosed with chronic myeloid leukemia. What the researchers needed were cells from another patient with the same disease. Nowell cultured a second batch in the same way and gave them to his eagle-eyed partner to view under the lens. Both men saw the same thing: in one of the tiniest pairs of homologues (later to be known as chromosome no. 22), one strand was shorter than its partner.

Excitedly, they scoured the cell nuclei of an additional five patients with CML, and behold: the pattern held. Of the seven, five were men and two were women. Some were asymptomatic; others were in full-blown blast crisis, the final and most accelerated stage of the disease. In none of the samples could the researchers find any additional consistent chromosomal irregularities—at least not in the straightforward dimensions of size and shape. What was more, in the same blood samples, some cells did not have the tiny chromosome no. 22. Their genetic complements, as far as Nowell and Hungerford could tell, were normal. This suggested that the oddity was somehow acquired in a subset of cells.

Finally, the change appeared specific to cases of CML. As with other acute forms of the disease, chronic myeloid leukemia was marked by a frightening proliferation of white blood cells—though, in this case, the transformed cells were able to differentiate into maturity and function to some extent. (Not until the terminal "blast" phase, typically several years into the disease's progression, did immature cells swarm the peripheral blood.) When the researchers checked samples from patients with other forms of leukemia, however, the abbreviated strand was nowhere to be seen.

The findings, as the pair wrote in 1960, suggested "a causal relationship between the chromosome abnormality observed" and CML. That simple observation would change cancer science forever.

It took a dozen years and another change of eyes to make sense of Nowell and Hungerford's discovery. By 1972, the story had moved from Philadelphia to the south side of Chicago, where Janet Davison Rowley worked in a university hospital. Rowley was a cytogeneticist. A decade earlier, she had received a training fellowship from the NIH to study DNA replication in Oxford, England. The experience had transformed her, and she had returned to the University of Chicago with a new passion—eyeballing human chromosomes under a microscope—and she had been pursuing that obsession ever since.

After the initial excitement of Nowell and Hungerford's finding, most cytogeneticists had moved on. The so-called Philadelphia chromosome seemed to be a rare, and likely meaningless, anomaly. But now, Rowley had found another piece of the CML puzzle.

Like Peter Nowell, Rowley was a medical doctor who had chosen a career of scientific research over clinical practice. Also like her Philadelphian colleague, she had raised a big family after earning her medical degree. But in contrast to Nowell, Rowley—who had begun college at age fifteen, received her medical degree at age twenty-three, and married the very next day—chose to put her research career on the slow burner, working only part-time until the youngest of her four sons was nearly a teenager.

The late start made academic status harder to come by. Rowley was fifty-two years old, had been "first author" on dozens of papers, and had several major discoveries to her name by the time she was named a full professor. The biggest of these discoveries, certainly, related to Nowell and Hungerford's minute chromosome. Using a new staining technique that "banded" each strand into alternating strips of light and dark segments, she determined where the missing piece from Philadelphia chromosome had gone.

Each chromosome had two arms: a short arm called p and a long arm called q. In these cancer cells, the bottom half of the long arm of chromosome no. 22 had been pinched off and glued to the long arm of chromosome no. 9. That made no. 22 much shorter than normal, and no. 9 a bit longer. In the fleeting instants of cell division, a portion of no. 9 had *also* migrated onto no. 22. The swap, which Rowley christened a "reciprocal translocation," wasn't equal: The former got a greater share of nucleotides in the exchange.

What the Philadelphia chromosome got, however, was the blueprint for a microscopic monster. This snippet of DNA, now fused to the butt of a broken chromosome, was capable of upending the carefully regulated cycle of cell development. This bizarre, nearly unnoticeable, swap of genetic material could kill a person, though it would take another dozen years and dozens of researchers to solve the mystery of how.

The parcel of genetic material jettisoned from its home on chromosome no. 9 was part of gene called Abelson, or *abl* for short. Genes themselves do not "do" anything, it is worth pointing out—except carry the sacred plans for assembling proteins: the molecules that perform most of the work in the body and build its cellular structures. Nor, surprisingly, does every stretch of DNA bear the blueprints to make even a protein. (The overwhelming share of twisting nucleotides, tucked away in the chromosomes, do not encode for these workhorse molecules; their precise purpose, in fact, remains one of the enduring mysteries of biology.) But *abl* did. It held the plans for a protein involved in a host of key processes, from how the cell divided to how it differentiated (took on a specialized role in the body).

Researchers gave the spot where *abl* ended up on chromosome no. 22 the unwieldy name of Breakpoint Cluster Region, or *bcr*. No one was yet sure whether it was part of a gene or not. A group of Dutch researchers, though, had shown that in the Philadelphia chromosome, the head of *bcr* was connected to the tail of *abl*.

That is how science works . . . when it works well. One researcher (or a team of them) alights upon something interesting and often generates a hypothesis; another builds upon the newly discovered model (or disproves it) with an additional finding; which, in turn, launches an investigation by a third group. The bricklaying is as much competitive as it is collegial, but the knowledge that emerges tends to be sturdier, as a result.

So it was with the Philadelphia chromosome. In 1986, David Baltimore, in Cambridge, Massachusetts, led one of the key laboratories in the race to decipher the *bcr-abl* translocation. Baltimore had already shared a Nobel Prize in 1975 for his codiscovery of a remarkable, dogma-defying protein called reverse transcriptase. He was unquestioned royalty in the realm of biological science, and his crack team of postdocs were now leading the charge on *bcr-abl*. They had even converged on a strange protein that the fusion of genes appeared to encode. One and a half times larger than the normal protein associated with the Abelson gene—the eponymously named BCR/ABL*—was a hybrid, just like the gene. What was

*Yet another confusing aspect of biology is that genes and proteins often share the same name. To distinguish between them, I have rendered all genes in italicized lower-case letters and all proteins in roman capital letters.

still wholly unclear, however, was *how* this protein could turn normal white blood cells into leukemic ones.

It had taken more than a quarter century from Nowell and Hungerford's discovery to come this far—and the disease called chronic myeloid leukemia was only just beginning to reveal its secret.

The monster BCR/ABL shared one trait with the normal Abelson protein. As Owen Witte, a researcher working in David Baltimore's lab, had shown, each was a special kind of protein called a kinase. The revelation wasn't minor. For biologists, identifying the mutant BCR/ABL as a kinase was equivalent to a police detective discovering that a murder suspect was holding the keys to the victim's house and a bloody knife in his pants pocket. When it came to the crime of cancer, kinases had both the means and the opportunity.

That was due to the critical role such enzymes play in the life of a cell. Kinases serve as mobile transfer stations in a sprawling network of intracellular communications. Many of the messages they transmit tell the cell when to grow and divide. Some kinases initiate the signals; others act as receptors, receiving the messages and forwarding them. What transpires between the enzymes is an elaborate relay race, with each protein passing a baton of information to the next molecule in the chain.

The communication comes through a process called phosphorylation: one kinase transfers a phosphate group—a compact ring of oxygen surrounding an atom of phosphorus—to a second molecule, giving the latter a jolt of chemical energy, and setting it into motion. The second kinase transfers the phosphate to a third, and so on, prompting a frenetic relay that ultimately carries the signal into the cell nucleus. In the end comes a change in behavior: the cell begins the careful process of copying its chromosomes, for instance. Or it releases a needed hormone. Or it performs yet another function critical to the life of the organism. Or it commits suicide.

With such high-stakes consequences, limitations were built into the signaling. The baton pass has to occur in a certain way: the receiving protein can accept the phosphate group in just one type of locale—at a specific amino acid jutting out from the molecule. Some kinases are phosphorylated only at the amino acid serine; others, at the amino acid threonine. Finally, a select group did the handoff at tyrosine. This seemingly arbitrary protocol matters a great deal, although during the late 1980s scientists were only just beginning to figure out its rules.

If nothing else, there was an accumulation of anecdotal evidence to suggest that the last-discovered and smallest subset of these kinase enzymes—the tyrosine kinases—played a formative role in cancer. They were popping up like crazy in the scientific literature.

In the case of chronic myeloid leukemia, a model for disease progression was at last coming into focus. The process began with a single cell—the one where the reciprocal genetic swap had first occurred. The hybrid gene continually instructed its cell to make lots of the BCR/ABL protein. This protein, a tyrosine kinase, set in motion a chain of signaling that started, and restarted, the cell division engines. Copies and more copies of the cell were made. And since each new generation of cells inherited the accidental gene along with the rest of its parent's genetic blueprint, the process fed upon itself. In time, the clones would become so plentiful that they would crowd out the remaining, functioning cells in the bone marrow and blood.

That was the terror of leukemia. It all started with a lone accident in a single cell. The challenge now was to find some way to stop it. The ideal way, it seemed to several groups of scientists, was to somehow interrupt the chain of signals begun by this mashed-up protein called BCR/ABL.

Medicinal chemists design drugs with one eye ever fixed on navigation. The compounds they build have to pass through a realm that is ever changing, held together by weak chemical bonds and charged atoms racing from one element to the next. To have any hope of reaching their targets, the agents first have to negotiate though a wonderland of contortionist proteins and barely penetrable membranes, of impossibly shaped crystals and floating radicals that are poised to attack anything in their path. The mission, often, is impossible.

To improve the odds of success, such chemists study charts and maps—learning how certain drug types bond with their targets, which shapes of molecules tend to be absorbed into the bloodstream, and which do not. They rely on known molecular templates—those chemical entities that have often fared well as pharmaceuticals. But as with any great navigator, the best drug designers depend on something that can be neither studied nor taught: they are guided by *feel*.

Jürg Zimmermann, a thirty-three-year-old chemist working at the Swiss drug company Ciba-Geigy, had that feel. Almost from the start of his days at the company, Zimmermann began tinkering with a class of molecules called phenylamino-pyrimidines (PAPs), which had been shown to fight inflammation in laboratory animals. The idea to test the molecules against kinases, though, had come from a professor at the nearby University of Basel. Ciba-Geigy had a few PAPs lying on the shelf, so the young chemist began to see if any inhibited these crucial signaling proteins. Serendipitously, one of the compounds worked against BCR/ABL.

When he told the news to the leader of his development team, Nick Lydon, the response was enthusiastic. Lydon, a biologist from the UK, instantly understood the significance of Zimmermann's find. BCR/ABL was the driving protein behind CML; a molecule that inhibited this kinase should curtail the growth of the cancer, if not stop it in its tracks. But the trick would be in "optimizing" the compound so that it shut down the mutant protein and no others. And this process, thought virtually everyone in the scientific community, was impossible.

One kinase signals another through the transfer of a phosphate group. But phosphorylation isn't merely a process by which proteins communicate. It is the economic soul of all living creatures. It is the means to a bristlingly efficient marketplace that makes possible nearly every muscle movement, nerve impulse, and biochemical reaction in a cell—almost everything, in other words, that requires the exchange of energy.

What makes this global market possible, in turn, is that the parties to these myriad transactions use a single, universal currency, the way banks and treasuries across the world exchange US dollars. In all creatures large and small, this currency is a molecule known as adenosine triphosphate, or simply ATP.

When food is broken down, its energy is extracted and preserved in molecules of ATP. But the storage is only temporary. This biological fuel is immediately used in the body's trillions of cellular engines—and in enormous quantity as well. In an average day, a 150-pound human being burns through nearly his or her body weight in ATP. Yet, at any given moment, he or she has less than two ounces (around fifty grams) of the molecule on hand. This incomprehensible gap is filled by an extraordinary recycling system.

It works this way: Adenosine triphosphate has a tail of three consecutive phosphate groups, held together by high-energy atomic bonds. When the bonds are broken through a chemical reaction, one phosphate group is freed to hitch up with another molecule, and energy is released. Losing one of its phosphates, ATP becomes ADP (adenosine *di*phosphate). But soon, in a separate chemical reaction, ADP acquires another phosphate from a different donor and starts the process all over—a cycle that is repeated, for each ATP molecule, some thirteen hundred times a day. This signaling cascade is what the Swiss chemist and the British-born biologist were thinking about messing with.

Shutting down the kinase connection in chronic myeloid leukemia meant finding a molecule that could wedge itself into the same "pocket" designed to embrace ATP. In the case of the BCR/ABL protein, that receptor was shaped by the welcoming arms of the amino acid tyrosine, which narrowed down the list a bit. But even so, that left scores of healthy kinases—those critical for life itself—which might accidentally be gummed up as well.

How could any drug fit neatly into a phosphate docking station that was part of a biological process so elemental and constant, and yet still be unique enough *not* to fit into any other? That was the question that kept every drug company from attempting to target kinases, even though, by all appearances, these phosphoproteins were at the heart of so many cancers—and perhaps all of them. That was the question that made Lydon's development team outliers at Ciba-Geigy in the first two years of the 1990s. "We almost cannot admit that today," Zimmermann told an interviewer in 2003. "[But] there was never a major project on inhibitors of BCR/ABL. All the experiments were done on the side and were received with a certain indifference."

————

Nick Lydon would never have been so primed to develop a drug targeting BCR/ABL if he had not met Brian Druker. Druker was a young medical oncologist—a physician who actually took care of patients—doing a research fellowship at Dana-Farber in Boston. The head of Druker's laboratory, Tom Roberts, was studying tyrosine kinases, so that was what Druker studied, too. Upon starting his fellowship, he had been given a daunting task: to develop an antibody that would allow researchers to detect the activity of tyrosine kinase in a cell. The project took two years, but when he'd at last produced the antibody assay in 1989, Druker— then just thirty-three years old—was in the middle of a global research scrum. He had something everybody in the field of kinase research wanted.

"Because of that," Druker recalled in an interview, "hundreds of collaborations opened up. I was working with immunologists, platelet biologists, B-cell* signalers, T-cell signalers. People from around the Harvard campuses would come to me for some antibody, or to get some advice, and it really opened up a lot of avenues for me." The most important of these relationships began when Nick Lydon from Ciba-Geigy came to work with Tom Roberts. Lydon had a molecule that shut down tyrosine kinase phosphorylation, at least in a petri dish. He was eager to take the testing to the next level, to see how well it worked against a sophisticated model of cancer. So Lydon and Roberts set up a collaboration. "And since I was the only doctor working in the lab," says Druker, "Nick asked what disease I thought would be approachable." Druker had been thinking about the answer long before he was asked. "Chronic myeloid leukemia," he said. CML.

At the start of the 1990s, no more than a third of those diagnosed with CML lived five years, a survival rate that had not improved in twenty years. Something had to be done to change these terrible odds. If a targeted kinase inhibitor was possible in any cancer, thought Druker, it was here.

In the summer of 1993, Druker traveled to Basel to meet with Nick Lydon's team at Ciba-Geigy. Straightaway, Lydon handed Druker four

---

*B cells and T cells are types of white blood cells central to immune response.

compounds to test against cell models of CML, using his sensitive antibody assay. By the following February, Druker issued a report. Of the four compounds, the best was the one called CGP57148B.* As is nearly always the case in drug development, an overwhelming number of compounds fail early in testing: they prove too toxic or don't last long enough to do the job. (Many drug candidates fail because they are eaten up by gastric juices or rapidly destroyed by metabolism in the liver.) An agent can bind to the wrong proteins or it can turn out to be metabolically unstable. So much can go awry that drug developers rarely let themselves get excited. But CGP57148B was unusually promising. Not only did it stop the growth of more than 90 percent of the leukemia cells studied in glass dishes under the microscope, it did so while sparing normal cells.

The sheer marvel of the molecule, though, was that it appeared to follow the exact "flight plan" that the scientists had charted: the drug bound to precisely the right cellular pocket, wedging itself smack in the middle of the terrible signaling cascade. Without these continuous instructions to grow and proliferate, the cancer cell died.

The impossible mission now seemed the faintest bit possible. The Ciba-Geigy team was optimistic enough about the drug to give it a slightly more manageable name, STI571. (STI stood for "signal transduction inhibitor.") Animal tests followed in the following year. Again, the researcher verified that the compound was shutting down the disease—leukemic cells were vanishing from the blood and, eventually, from the bone marrow as well.

Druker was ready to begin the first stage of human testing—Phase I trials—when there came a series of snags. The first obstacle had little to do with the drug itself. In March 1996, Ciba-Geigy announced a merger with another Swiss drug firm, longtime rival Sandoz, forming a behemoth called Novartis, with a market value of some $80 billion. Dozens of exploratory programs were downsized or phased out in the integration. Nick Lydon's kinase program had barely been on the radar as it was. Now,

---

*Every molecule in the testing stage had a jumble of letters and digits for a name; it was one more reminder for developers not to get too close to their study subject. CGP stood for "Ciba-Geigy protein."

due to internal competition, the effort sunk even lower on the priority list.

That concern, however, was nothing compared with what happened with the dogs. Eight months after the merger announcement came the first reports of serious side effects with STI571. When given low dosages of the compound, dogs (as with the prior animals that had been tested) appeared to have no worrisome reactions at all. That changed as the researchers gave higher concentrations of the drug. The animals' livers began to show damage that worsened with each climbing dose. Liver toxicity was enough to derail any investigative compound.

In Druker's view, the liver issue was manageable. In a clinical trial, after all, doctors could get an early warning of any problems by checking the patients' liver enzymes daily; at the first sign of concern, treatment could be halted. Besides, thought Druker, this case warranted some risk. "I'm an oncologist," Druker fumed. "I've given way more toxic drugs than this thing. I have patients in my clinic who are going to die, so what are we waiting for?"

Nonetheless, executives at the newly formed company began to get cold feet. As it was, many of the higher-ups at Ciba-Geigy had never quite believed in the vision of a *target-specific* kinase inhibitor. And yet one more obstacle loomed—one bigger than even liver toxicity: money. Even if the drug worked, thought many in the new company's executive ranks, the projected market for the drug was far too small for the R&D investment ever to pay off. This was no idle concern. Novartis is a public company, whose shareholders demand a sufficient return on investment. The United States had fewer than forty-five hundred annual cases of chronic myeloid leukemia during the mid-1990s. Human trials could cost the company tens, if not hundreds, of millions of dollars. Given the novelty of the drug's biological mechanism, moreover, anything could happen in the way of adverse effects. This terrain was uncharted. The FDA would surely insist that the trial investigators be extra cautious in evaluating every patient. That meant more costly medical tests (including possible hospital stays for the first trial participants), more oversight, slower enrollment of the patient trials. All of these things meant more money in the hole for Novartis.

Druker argued that the small size of the patient population was misleading. If STI571 worked, it would be hailed as a glorious proof of principle: it would revolutionize therapy across the full range of cancers. And CML was the perfect disease on which to test the theory: in its chronic (or early) phase, the disease was relatively homogenous as cancers went. With few exceptions, a single destructive protein drove the destruction of cells.

If ever there was a test case for "targeted" cancer therapy, this was it. Blocking a single kinase, Druker asserted, should be enough to flip the disease switch to the off position. And if it wasn't enough—if for some reason the target was wrong or incomplete, or if the drug missed its target—the investigators would know immediately.

As the company's then–CEO, Daniel Vasella, recounted, Druker was passionate. Novartis bought the argument. Two years later, in June 1998, the first human trial began.

The aim of a Phase I study is not to see if a drug works, but rather to determine if it's safe and what the optimal dosage might be. The compound is, at first, given in tiny concentrations, then the amount is scaled up until patients begin showing significant side effects, what researchers call the maximum tolerated dose.

By now, Druker had left Dana-Farber for the little-known Oregon Health & Science University in Portland, where he was named the study's lead investigator. Partnering with him were two physicians at much larger centers: MD Anderson in Houston, and UCLA.

The first three patients in the Phase I were given a minuscule dose of 25 milligrams a day. Nothing happened. The next month a few more patients were given 50 milligrams. But by the sixth month, with the dose now at 250 milligrams a day, everyone in the trial was responding. White cell counts that had been as high as 200,000—some twenty times the normal level—plunged to healthy ranges. And so far, there were few major side effects to report.

Of the fifty-four patients given at least 300 milligrams a day, blood counts in fifty-three reverted to normal. All but two of these patients continued to be healthy nine months later. More amazing was that seven patients experienced what was termed a "complete cytogenic remission"—that is to say, their white blood cells no longer showed evidence of the Philadelphia chromosome. Their genes, in effect, were normal. No one in the cancer world had ever heard of a brand-new drug yielding such uniformly and overwhelmingly strong responses in a clinical trial. That this was a Phase I study made the outcomes all the more unbelievable.

The second phase of clinical trials, conducted in three separate studies at more than two dozen cancer centers in six countries, proved equally remarkable. Those with early-stage disease (for whom the traditional therapy no longer worked) had the best results: 95 percent of patients had their blood purged of leukemic cells, an outcome that was known in the jargon as a complete hematologic response. Six in ten had a major cytogenetic response as well—that was, a substantial reduction in cells containing the Philadelphia chromosome. After more than two years of observation, a small number of patients relapsed, but the proportion was low in comparison to the then–standard treatment of interferon alpha.

A natural human protein discovered in 1957, interferon had been used in various cancer-treatment regimens since the 1970s. While its effects were not fully understood, the protein elicited an immune response that both interfered with certain cancer cells' ability to grow and summoned "killer" immune cells to attack. As with Gleevec, interferon had been the "it" drug of its generation: *Time* magazine had put it on its cover in March 1980. And interferon did cure some patients; in others, it caused brutal flulike symptoms but left the cancer raging.

None of the Phase II studies had been designed to compare survival outcomes between interferon and STI571. Nonetheless, one had only to look at the data to see that patients on the Novartis drug would fare better. The side effects of this targeted agent, moreover, were negligible. On top of that, the new kinase inhibitor was an oral drug. A *pill.* (Interferon had to be delivered by injection.)

A Phase III trial was already in the works, but there was little question that STI571 would be approved for marketing without waiting for the results. The speed of the FDA announcement, however, took even Novartis by surprise. The company got its answer just seventy-two days after filing a drug application—a record. It was barely enough time for Novartis executives to settle on a trade name for the medicine.

The US government went so far as to call a press conference. Rick Klausner, then director of the National Cancer Institute, told the assembled crowd that the drug was "a picture of the future of cancer treatment." The secretary of health and human services, Tommy Thompson, celebrated Novartis's targeted kinase inhibitor as "the wave of the future." It was the first time that anyone could recall a cabinet secretary attending the announcement of a drug approval. But then, everything about Gleevec, it seemed, was different.

The wonderful story of Gleevec—and it *is* wonderful—has since become the central tenet in a new theology of cancer science. Beyond a medicine, it is now an allegory. If we follow this model, the moral goes, we will defeat terrible malignancies, one by one—and we will do it not through blunt and brutal force (as with traditional chemotherapy), but by mastering the same molecular tricks that the cancers themselves use. *The Gleevec Story* says: damn the soaring cancer burden; we are on track to winning the war!

But the message, while convincing to many in the cancer research community and reassuring to patients, is wrong. The Gleevec paradigm is not likely to get us to victory in the war on cancer. It may even be drawing us further from that goal.

The reason rests, in part, with why chronic myeloid leukemia was such a good test case for a targeted kinase inhibitor in the first place: CML is a rarity among cancers. Its mechanism of transformation is not only well understood, but also simple compared with that of most cancers. In CML, a *single* hybrid kinase protein causes the leukemia, and the telltale gene aberration that produces the wayward signaling protein has been known for many decades. Cases of this leukemia that are still in the early, chronic phase are, moreover, believed to be among the most homogeneous of any cancer: Relatively few of these Philadelphia-chromosome-positive (Ph+) cells are beset with additional mutations.

And herein lies the problem: the quality that made early-stage CML an ideal test case for a targeted kinase inhibitor—its *uniqueness*—also makes the strategy harder to replicate in nearly every other cancer. Gleevec is the exception that reinforces the sobering rule.

Some top cancer biologists argue that solid tumors—cancers that grow out of the cellular linings of the lungs, breasts, colon, pancreas, and other major organs—are also, in many cases, driven by a single cancer gene. The theory is known as oncogene addiction. By that popular notion, if such a driving gene (or its protein product) can be shut down with a targeted inhibitor like Gleevec, even the major fatal cancers can be stopped. That is the hopeful scenario that the Gleevec paradigm carries with it.

But a raft of evidence supports the opposite conclusion. Most cancers are shaped by forces that go well beyond any lone gene or protein. These still-mysterious factors—the increasing instability of a cancer cell's DNA, the hyperspeed evolution of drug resistance, the uncanny endurance of cancer "stem" cells—make it unlikely that most of the common malignancies will ever be halted by a single molecularly targeted drug, or two, or three.

This assertion is not the expression of cynicism, but rather of history—the same history that gave us Gleevec.

For a glimpse of this evidence, one has only to revisit those heady days of the mid-1970s, when scientists such as Janet Rowley in Chicago were filling the medical literature with reports of chromosomal anomalies and their apparent links to specific cancers. Rowley, of course, had been the first to detail the DNA swap that gives the Philadelphia chromosome its monstrous appetite. In 1973, even before her famous *Nature* paper on chronic myeloid leukemia, she published a study on CML's more aggressive cousin, acute myeloid leukemia. Rowley had found a translocation that appeared so frequently in AML cells that it could not have been pure accident. The swap was between sections of chromosomes no. 8 and no. 21.

This aberration, however, did not earn a nickname like the Philadelphia chromosome. For soon it became clear that it was but one of many karyotypic changes seen in AML. The malignant blood cells of a number of patients had gained an extra strand of chromosome no. 8; several others had lost all or part of no. 7; a few more had swaps between chromosomes no. 6 and no. 9; and there were other kinds of changes. It was as though each aberration (or many of them, at least) gave rise to a slightly different disease. They all *looked* like AML and behaved like AML, but each had characteristics that distinguished it from its cousins—making one more resistant to treatment than another.

In those cancers that evolve from a different class of white blood cell, lymphocytes, the number of distinct chromosomal patterns recorded was far greater. And this is a mere taste of cancer's full palette of diversity. When it comes to solid tumors, the malignancies that make up the bulk of cancer incidence, the sum of distinct genetic subsets for any lone disease site can be staggering. In fact, even to use the word *subset* is a little bit misleading. Many cancers, by the time they are diagnosed, are mélanges of genetic destruction. Each case is unique, a class of one. (The term preferred in the academic literature is *heterogeneous*.) An individual cancer might well begin with a single genetic mutation, but the damage keeps piling on with time.

Details of this heterogeneity can be seen in a well-cited 2006 study led by cancer geneticist Bert Vogelstein of Johns Hopkins. Vogelstein and more than two dozen colleagues examined some thirteen thousand protein–coding genes in tumor specimens from eleven women with breast cancer and eleven others with colon cancer. What they found was that all twenty-two of the samples might well have been different diseases—at least genetically. That was especially the case when it came to breast cancer.

On average, each of the breast cancer specimens examined by the team had mutations in twelve different "candidate" cancer genes—those which, based on previous studies, were considered most likely to be involved in tumor generation and survival. No single specimen, however, had more than a handful of candidate genes in common with any other. Each, as Vogelstein's team wrote in the pages of *Science,* carried its own distinct "mutational signature"—a fingerprint left at the scene of the crime.

Even that, however, was actually a conservative reading of breast cancer diversity. For in addition to the 122 "validated" cancer genes that were mutated in this small sampling of tumors, the researchers dismissed another 550 or so miscoded genes as probable bystanders. (Counting these so-called passenger mutations along with the putative "drivers," as the two classes were known, individual tumors had roughly ninety genetic glitches apiece.)

That any two breast cancer patients are liable to have different mutational signatures is complicated enough. But more challenging, from a treatment point of view, is that individual patients often have widely variant mutations in different cells within the same tumor—or in multiple tumors in their bodies. For patients with cancers of the pancreas or ovary, heterogeneity within a person's tumors is often so pronounced that it is possible to count unique mutation signatures in thousands of cells. In the "same" tumor, one cell hardly resembles the next.

"The heterogeneous nature of cancer is what is the major, major, major obstacle to easy therapy," says Isaiah "Josh" Fidler, a legendary researcher at MD Anderson. "The fact that cancer cells give rise to variants so easily, so repeatedly, so fast. And so predictably, mind you."

The danger of the targeted drug revolution—of *The Gleevec Story*—is that it oversimplified cancer, treating the disease as an orderly march to disorder, the result of a lone, driving genetic aberration. That is not the case with the vast majority of cancers. The malignant cells that resist one treatment after another are in the throes of civil war. Their cellular genomes are often in full-blown anarchy.

The same holds true, it turns out, even for the later stages of CML. When, in early testing, clinical investigators gave the miraculous kinase inhibitor to patients with advanced disease—those who were either in the "accelerated" phase or in the terminal stage called blast crisis—the drug worked only for a short time or not at all. In some cases, the genetic damage (in even a fraction of cells) is such that Gleevec has trouble docking into its molecular berth from the start. Clinical scientists call this dilemma refractoriness or primary resistance, and an almost imperceptible change to a single amino acid in the drug's binding pocket can cause it. Alternatively, another mutation might result in multiple copies of the *bcr-abl* gene, which then spins out so many copies of the protein that it is impossible to block them all. In later stages of CML's progression, such primary resistance (from either cause) is, again, the rule—not the exception. For some 80 percent of patients in the accelerated phase of the disease, even Gleevec cannot purge the bloodstream of BCR/ABL.

A second barrier is clinical or secondary resistance: New mutations arise as a result of the treatment, causing patients to relapse. The problem is as ancient as chemotherapy itself and as predictable as resistance to antibiotics is predictable: single drugs "select" for resistant cells. Gleevec kills off most of the leukemic cells, but the ones it cannot kill quickly proliferate, becoming the new dominant "clones" in the bloodstream. It is yet unknown what percentage of patients on Gleevec will develop drug-resistant clones, but many clearly will. This group, sadly, includes patients who are responding well and in the early stages of the disease.

Second- and third-generation CML drugs, operating on the same principle as Gleevec, can sometimes reverse the reversal, blocking the BCR/ABL protein in other ways. But once a patient is on his or her third inhibitor, the responses are "usually not durable except in occasional patients" in chronic phase, as one group of leukemia researchers at MD Anderson Cancer Center recently found.

What the laboratory of the clinic has seemed to prove, perhaps more than anything else, is that cancer is an evolutionary process, albeit one played out in the universe of a single organism. In the evolution of species, new traits, selected over tens of thousands of years, give one lineage a survival advantage over another; in cancer, selection is sped up to the frantic pace of cell division.

Cancer's great challenge, at its core, is not *specificity*, but rather *complexity*. The fundamental barrier to success is not the unique shape of each signal receptor in every resistant cancer cell; it is coming to terms with the fact that cancer is a disease of progressive, unyielding, mind-boggling heterogeneity.

There is no magic bullet for that.

Chapter 6

Missing the Target

The development of chemical means for restraint of neoplastic disease has passed through two well-defined phases. It is now entering a third . . . with the study of substances which injure selectively by virtue of biochemical specificities of the target cells. . . . This selective effect may well be truly specific cancer chemotherapy, now just in its earliest inception, but bright with promise for the future.

—C. P. Rhoads, director,
Sloan–Kettering Institute for Cancer Research,
"Rational Cancer Chemotherapy," *Science*, January 15, 1954

Nowhere is the hope of the Gleevec model more intoxicating than in the case of breast cancer; and nowhere is the failure of the Gleevec paradigm so plain to see. Among the major solid tumors, breast cancers offer the most tantalizing array of molecular targets; and over the past two decades, more targeted drugs have been developed for, and tested in, women with breast cancer than patients with any other disease. Not everyone labels the drugs as "targeted" per se. But that is what they are: virtually all of the medicines used in breast cancer treatment today were developed, like Gleevec, to interrupt a particular signaling pathway—and in many cases, to seek out a specific molecule—critical to the survival and proliferation of malignant cells. Each was designed to hit a biological bull's-eye. This holds true even for some of the oldest of breast cancer agents, those that block the hormone estrogen.

Estrogen, of course, is the female sex hormone. It regulates the growth and development of cells in a woman's reproductive organs. But it is also a kind of universal remote control, affecting tissues throughout the body—mostly in women, but to a surprising degree in men as well. Estrogen protects the heart, for instance, in a slew of ways: by raising "good" cholesterol and lowering the "bad," by widening blood vessels, and by slowing the inflammatory response that ultimately leads to atherosclerosis. It helps maintain bone strength and triggers a range of responses in the pituitary, hypothalamus, and brain, switching on or off more than four hundred genes in all.

That one hormone can do such myriad things in so many parts of the body is a tribute to the silent partners in this undertaking: the estrogen receptors, which take on different roles depending on their location in the body. The receptors are the way stations that receive and transmit the hormone's signals to elements in the cell nucleus, which then either promote or prevent the transcription of certain genes. (Genes, in turn, are copied into nucleic acids called messenger RNA, which are then "translated" into proteins—which often serve as message-passers in their own right, or as enzymes that help bring about additional chemical transformations.)

Estrogen is thus at the head of what seems a never-ending chain of command. Or rather, dozens of them. And a few of those chains, it turns out, boost a woman's risk of getting cancer.

The hormone does not transform cells quite the way that the mutant BCR/ABL does in the case of chronic myeloid leukemia: it is not an unnatural protein that causes cells to enter into unbroken replicative loops. Its effect is more indirect. Estrogen, in some human tissues, causes cells to grow and divide. When estrogen peaks monthly in women of childbearing age, its molecules bind to the appropriate receptors in the breast—in cells of the milk duct, for instance—transmitting instructions for those cells to proliferate. (If the woman later becomes pregnant, her breasts will be prepared to produce milk for the infant.)

The problem is that this normal, even healthy, cell cycle can be treacherous, too. The choreography of cell division is a high-precision acrobatics—one nearly perfected over tens of millions of years of practice. But once in a rare while a tiny error occurs in execution. Somebody misses a grab and falls off the trapeze. In cell division, when the genome of one cell has to be doubled in a flash and delicately pried into two, such an error generally results in a mutation, an alteration to a cell's genetic code.

This is how cancer's subversion begins: a part of the DNA in the nucleus of a single cell is damaged or removed or rearranged or overproduced in just the wrong way. A mutation might be as infinitesimal as the snipping of a lone nucleotide (one of the so-called letters in the genetic alphabet) in a rambling stretch of DNA. Or an entire gene might be lost during mitosis—or perhaps copied too many times. The same can happen to an entire chromosome, deleting (or multiplying) the effects of thousands of genes in one fell swoop. Or sections of DNA from genes on far-flung chromosomes can meld together, as is the case in CML.

Any single one of these changes is certain to be imperceptible in the enormous scale of the human body. Most, in the end, have little or no effect. The cell with the mutation dies as the result of its damage, or the alteration is repaired as quickly as it arises. If neither of those scenarios occurs, another fail-safe will likely be triggered: urgent signals will be sent, and within moments the hobbled cell will initiate its own death. That is what happens almost all the time.

Infrequently, though, a series of unfortunate events ensues. A mutation arises in precisely the wrong spot—one that alters, for example, a key protein involved in the regulation of the cell cycle—and thereafter, in a surfeit of bad luck, every one of the fail-safes fails. The damaged cell survives and keeps dividing, making copies of its imperfect self.

Even that is not cancer, however. Not yet. For a cancer to develop, another rare mishap has to occur . . . followed (in nearly every case) by another . . . and another . . . and another. It typically takes several billion–to-one-shot mutations to turn a normal cell malignant and give it the capacity to flourish and spread in the well-defended domain of the human body. One mutation, for example, has to disable the mechanisms that tell the cell to stop dividing. Another has to stop the renegade cell from killing itself. One more lets it adapt to an environment with little oxygen and few nutrients—a requirement for most growing solid tumors. Still others are needed for the already dysfunctional cell to break away from its initial site and colonize another organ or tissue in the body, a complex endeavor called metastasis. And strange as it might seem, all of these mutations happen utterly *randomly*.

Cancer, in short, is a preposterous accident of biology, a flowerpot falling from a tenth-story windowsill.

That is not to suggest that there aren't things outside the body that contribute to, or even precipitate, such random errors. External factors (a virus, in some cases, a zap of radiation, chemicals in cigarette smoke, or some other potent carcinogen in the environment) invariably play a role in the breakdown as well, helping to cause the scattershot genetic damage either by throwing the process of mitosis off kilter or by damaging a cell's DNA directly. But there are also plenty of routine dangers as well, near-constant threats lurking within and around the cells themselves. Here, in the cellular milieu, assaults are not so much random as they are wanton. Roving molecules, known as reactive oxygen species or free radicals, bind to invading bacteria and destroy them—but also, quite frequently, clamp on to the wrong targets, which can include even a cell's DNA.

The onslaught is not the attack of disease. No, this is rather the bruising manner of life itself. And its implications are sobering: random or not, there is no avoiding genetic damage altogether. At any given point, in at least one of our living cells, the spiraling, twisting, folded up, carefully guarded blueprint of DNA is being assaulted in some way.

Which brings us back to estrogen. The hormone raises the risks of genetic injury even further in at least two fundamental ways. By thrusting cells headlong into their division cycle, estrogen increases the chances of a random genetic glitch. And alternatively, if the breast (or another estrogen–receptive organ) is already harboring a cell set on the course of malignancy—its DNA damaged in any part of the melee described above—exposure to the hormone makes it even more likely that the cell will proliferate.

For any one cell the risk of such an unfortunate combination of genetic mutations is minuscule. But many billions of breast cells are exposed to the risk anew every menstrual cycle, which itself repeats several hundred times over the course of a woman's reproductive years. The risk adds up over time, extending past menopause, even after the monthly estrogen cycles have ended, and peaking in the sixth or seventh decade of life. (A quarter of all breast cancer cases are diagnosed in women age fifty-five to sixty-four.) Each year, that risk catches up with more than a million women around the world in the form of an invasive breast cancer.

Some 70 to 80 percent of these cancers are responsive to estrogen's growth signaling at the time they are diagnosed. (These are called estrogen–receptor-positive, or ER+.)* And most of these seem to be driven by the hormone. In such cases, it is as though the tumors are cars whose gearshifts are jammed to the "drive" position and whose accelerators are likewise pinned to the floor. With a little bit of combustible gasoline to provide the energy, the cars go.

Estrogen is the gas.

It was the understanding of such mechanics, revealed over a hundred years of study, that led to the first targeted drug intended specifically for breast cancer: an agent that, quite miraculously, seems to sever the link between breast cancer cells and their ample supply of fuel. The drug is called tamoxifen.

Tamoxifen is known in the lab as a selective estrogen receptor modulator, or SERM. Its basic mechanism of action is mimicry: the molecule resembles the female sex hormone so closely that it can fit snugly into the receptor pocket sought out by the actual hormone. Tamoxifen is not so identical that it triggers the same reaction in the receptor (not in the breast, anyway). But with the impostor wedged into the hormone's docking site, estrogen itself cannot bind—and that, in turn, blocks the growth commands from getting through.

---

*A second female hormone, progesterone, is also implicated in many breast cancers. While estimates vary, about two-thirds of breast cancers appear to have functional protein receptors for both estrogen and progesterone and are called hormone-positive or hormone-sensitive. In some cases, women test positive for estrogen receptor (ER+) and negative for progesterone receptor (PR-); but the reverse is far less common. Roughly a quarter of newly diagnosed women test negative (ER–/PR–) for both hormones. In each case, however, the degree of receptor positivity, and variations within tumors, influence how hormone-sensitive the disease is—and, as a result, how it responds to hormone-blocking therapy.

Other drugs, known as aromatase inhibitors, try to shut down estrogen in a different way: interrupting the flow of gas by targeting one of its sources in the body. Estrogen is made primarily in the ovaries, a supply that turns off at the onset of menopause. But even then, the body produces the hormone in small amounts through a roundabout mechanism. Certain tissues in the body convert androgen to estrogen with the help of an enzyme called aromatase. It is only a tiny bit of gas, but even a little gas can be enough to drive some breast cancers. Aromatase inhibitors choke off that supply of estrogen by blocking the enzyme needed to make it.

Of course, powerful as it is, estrogen is not the only agent that can drive the growth of a tumor. Critical to the development of many breast cancers is a wholly different signaling network: an extended family of proteins that interact with four sibling receptors on the outer membranes of many cells. These are the epidermal growth factor receptors, known by the acronym EGFR. When functioning normally, this enormous complex of molecules regulates much in the life of a cell—from when and how the cell grows to how it moves and interacts with its neighbors. The genes that code for proteins in these signal cascades are thus vitally important. When nearly any of them is damaged, the result can be disastrous.

Mutations in some part of the EGFR network are found frequently in breast cancer (as well as in lung cancer and other malignancies). So it is not surprising that researchers and drug developers have made targeting these interconnected pathways a priority. EGFR inhibitors are the most studied and celebrated cancer drugs in use today, and the most storied of the lot is Herceptin.

Technically speaking, Herceptin is not a "drug." Unlike traditional forms of chemotherapy, this molecular weapon is a man–made antibody, a biologic agent as opposed to a chemical one. Antibodies are immune-system proteins that zero in on bacteria, viruses, and other foreign invaders by recognizing specific proteins on their cell surfaces. The match is like true love: each antibody is destined to bind with one specific protein, called an antigen. Once attached, the interlocked pair of antibody-and-antigen poke out like a signal flag from the cell membrane. And that's exactly what it is. Other immune system cells see the jutting marker, identify the trespasser as an imminent threat to the organism, and attack.

The antigen to which Herceptin attaches, however, is no invader, but rather the second of the four epidermal growth factor receptors mentioned above. It's called by a variety of names in the oncology community, from HER2 to ErbB2 to HER2/neu. (Cancer researchers have multiple names for everything.) What makes HER2 a seemingly ideal target is that somewhere between 20 percent and 30 percent of breast cancer patients have cells with a profusion of these receptors sticking out from their membranes. Ordinarily, a breast cell has fewer than a hundred thousand HER2 proteins, but a HER2+ (pronounced *HER-two-positive*) cancer cell can have upward of 2 million. While the mechanism differs from that of the jammed estrogen receptor, the result is similar: the growth-command signals from the activated HER2 sites keep coming and coming.

That is where Herceptin comes in. The man–made antibody zooms through the bloodstream looking for this one cellular protein. When it finds its mate, the antibody binds to it. Less understood is what happens next. Some HER2+ cells are no doubt recognized and killed by immune sentries. Other evidence suggests that the cells go immediately into arrest, an event that sometimes triggers their own death; still more evidence suggests that the antibody's clinging presence merely slows down the division cycle. The ultimate answer might well be a combination of these effects.

Clear, in any case, is that this biological "smart bomb," like Gleevec, works best in early-stage cancers, before the cells evolve and become harder to treat. But even in early-stage cancers, the drug's effect is generally modest: In women who test positive for the HER2 protein, Herceptin appears to shrink tumors in roughly a third—a response that typically does not last long.

In each of the examples above, the careful study of breast cancer biology yielded one molecular Achilles' heel after another: weak spots in the malignant cells that could be targeted by sophisticated drugs and antibodies. Long before Gleevec, this was the paradigm in cancer research. Even the more traditional chemotherapy agents, some of which were developed in the 1940s and 1950s and which continue to form the bulwark of breast cancer treatment, were likewise shaped by an understanding of cell biology. Their plans of attack had been equally well reasoned, even if the drugs' detailed mechanisms of action had yet to be mapped out at the time of discovery.

Decades-old compounds such as methotrexate and fluorouracil (5-FU), for instance, prevent the production of DNA in dividing cancer cells by binding to enzymes needed for the synthesis of its building blocks. Taxol and docetaxel—two major breast cancer medicines approved for use in the 1990s—kill cells by slamming the tiny spindle on which chromosome separation takes place. Now-ancient antibiotics called anthracyclines interfere with DNA replication by inducing structural changes in the strands themselves—a process called intercalation.

Each of these strategies remains as ingenious today as it was when first conceived. If the approaches of these drugs vary at all from modern ones, it is in degrees of specificity (cytotoxic drugs also kill a number of *normal* dividing cells), not in the logic of their battle plans. That is clear from the fact that drug developers are still avidly designing and testing new compounds that follow these same old lines of attack.

During the 1990s, the FDA gave its approval to no less than eleven new chemical or biological agents for the treatment of breast cancer, far more than it approved for any other disease. An additional six breast cancer medicines received the FDA's benediction in the decade that followed, including yet another drug that targets the estrogen receptor (Faslodex), plus a second-generation "Herceptin" (called Tykerb), and a well-hyped antibody (Avastin) that interrupts a cancer cell's ability to recruit new blood vessels to the tumor. The last of these has proved to be a mightier blockbuster than even Herceptin—with US sales surpassing $3 billion a year in both 2009 and 2010.

Given this prodigious output of targeted medicines, it may seem almost beside the point to ask whether they were actually boosting the life spans of breast cancer patients. If these breakthrough drugs had proven themselves in the laboratory, and in the rigors of clinical trials, and in the FDA approval process to boot, could there be any doubt that they were also saving lives?

Something, after all, was bringing down breast cancer mortality. After continuing to rise in the early days of the cancer war, the standardized breast cancer death rate had switched directions in 1990, swooning by nearly a quarter in the brief span of a decade. What else could have caused that turnabout except the new arsenal of drugs?

To its credit, the National Cancer Institute set out to answer that question, assembling a consortium called CISNET (for the Cancer Intervention and Surveillance Modeling Network) to examine the data. The enterprise took five years and included forty-three medical statisticians. When the team reported its conclusions in the pages of the *New England Journal of Medicine* in October 2005, no one could say that the analysis had been rushed.

Led by one of country's most prominent biostatisticians, Donald Berry of MD Anderson Cancer Center, the consortium comprised research groups from seven venerable institutions. Represented along with Berry's Houston center were the Dana-Farber Cancer Institute, Georgetown University, the University of Wisconsin at Madison, Erasmus University Medical Center in Rotterdam, the University of Rochester, and Stanford. Each of the seven research groups built is own statistical model, but in the end, with a few exceptions, arrived at a similar conclusion overall: drug treatment was responsible for a bit more than half of the drop in the risk of death during the period.

But the full story had one important nuance: of the portion of benefit attributable to drug therapy, more than half was apparently due to a *single* drug: the estrogen–blocking tamoxifen.

Tellingly, tamoxifen is not a new medicine at all. It was developed nearly a half century before the Gleevec era began, before even the modern breast cancer research-funding paradigm began. The billions of dollars raised by breast cancer marchers, racers, and pink-ribbon–wearing consumers did not give rise to this rare, life-prolonging cancer medicine. Developed in the mid-1960s by a British researcher who had been seeking a fertility drug, the compound was first approved as a treatment for advanced breast cancer in the United States in 1977 (four years after its approval in the United Kingdom). Nine years later, the FDA again approved tamoxifen's marketing, this time for delaying the recurrence of breast cancer in postmenopausal women who had undergone a total mastectomy. Then came five more US approvals (in 1989, 1990, 1993, 1998, and 2000) for various other indications in breast cancer—none of which, of course, made tamoxifen a new drug.

Yet what is perhaps most compelling about the CISNET study is not what it says about tamoxifen, but rather what it implies about *every other* agent in the fight against breast cancer—those myriad compounds that have set the research community abuzz, the ones that have already built up billions of dollars in sales: there is little evidence that they have had more than a modest effect on long-term patient outcomes. Taken together, this multitude of drugs has been responsible for about a quarter of the reduction seen in the standardized death rate.

So what accounts for the *other half* of the decline in the age-adjusted death rate—the half that cannot be traced to any change in therapy? The answer is earlier detection. Put simply, women who might once have had their cancer discovered only after the tumor had spread to nearby lymph nodes—or worse, to an organ beyond the breast—were now, more often than not, having their cancer caught in early stages of disease.

At the end of the 1970s, and even up through the start of the 1980s, only four of every ten breast cancers were diagnosed while still in a localized stage (Table 2). By the late 1990s, the share had risen to six in ten.

Table 2

Breast Cancer

Percent of Cases Diagnosed at Each Stage of Disease

	1977–82	1983–90	2002–8
Localized	40%	55%	60%
Regional	41	35	33
Distant	8	6	5
Unstaged*	11	4	2

*Disease in unstaged cancers is more likely to be advanced (metastasized).
SOURCES: ACS, *CA: A Cancer Journal for Clinicians*, "Cancer Statistics," 1986, 1995, 1996, 2009, and 2013.

Along with this trend has come a phase shift in the *size* distribution of breast tumors: The masses found on mammograms and ultrasound images have skewed smaller over the years—again because they are being caught earlier. "I saw breast cancers when I was an internist the size of a grapefruit," recalls John Mendelsohn, who served as president of MD Anderson Cancer Center in Houston from 1996 through 2011, and who did his residency at the Brigham hospital in Boston in the late 1960s. "Now, they're the size of a pea."

Tens of thousands of women who might once have missed (or dismissed) a two-centimeter lump in one of their breasts are now having tiny specks flagged by routine screening.

If the multibillion–dollar drug arsenal (post-tamoxifen) is responsible for a fraction of the decrease in breast cancer mortality over the past three-plus decades, something far more mundane, and far less brutal, is responsible for a much greater part: the mammogram. Extending regular breast cancer screening to more women has boosted overall five-year survival rates simply by moving more new patients into disease stages that have high survival rates to begin with—and by making it more likely that women within each stage have smaller (and perhaps less evolved) tumors.

Theoretically, at least, screening offers one more benefit: the earlier a tumor is diagnosed, the less likely it is that cells have broken away from the scrum and migrated to the lymph system, or the blood, or to some other secret redoubt in the body. Such adventurers, known as micrometastases, can make eradicating the disease agonizingly difficult.

Progress in the fight against breast cancer has come as much from dingy mammography centers in subbasements around the country as it has from research laboratories.

That is it. That is the whole story.

Well, not quite.

There is, indeed, one more twist in this sad saga, and here is where one of the critical failures in the cancer war can be found: mammograms are awful.

It appears likely that in some cases random screening "creates" tumors to treat—by flagging tiny groups of cells that are either not cancerous to begin with or are unlikely ever to expand or spread. The fear of cancer is so deeply rooted that rarely is a "spot" on an X-ray left untouched; not when the tissue in question can be biopsied and sent to the pathology lab.

Mammography screening has led not only to a surge of frightening false alarms, but is almost certainly tied (at least partly) to the sharp uptick of breast cancer cases since the early 1980s. Most of the lesions discovered are genuine cancers, and the patients have to be treated. Some are not—and unfortunately, those patients are treated anyway.

Such "overdiagnosis," as it is known, comes with tremendous costs, running the gamut from the physical and emotional to the financial. Surgery, the first response to a tumor, is an invasion—cuts made all the more personal by their location. (To many women, the removal of all or part of a breast feels as much a crime of intimacy as the disease itself.) Radiation therapy, which traditionally follows the more conservative breast surgeries known as lumpectomies, has its own serious dangers and lasting side effects. Cancer drug therapies, which course through the entire body, are inherently toxic, an adjective that applies to the newest targeted agents as well. Even mammograms themselves expose women to tiny doses of radiation, a risk that compounds with each new test.

Were these ample costs and risks mammography's only drawbacks, they might be enough to call the utility of across-the-board, random screening into question. (Such questioning lay at the heart of the debate that raged across the United States during the late fall and winter of 2009, when a government task force suggested that most low-risk younger women forgo getting their annual mammograms. Many patients and advocates were enraged by the recommendation, seeing it not as a protection, but as a veiled attempt to cut health care costs at the expense of saving lives.)

But the technology has another serious deficit as well: a failure that is manifest not only in mammography's role as random screener, but also in its use as a diagnostic aid. Even when authentic cancers are identified and removed, every imaging tool in use (mammography, ultrasound, MRI, and PET) is sometimes guilty of *under*estimating the disease's deadliness—of missing the most inchoate of killers lurking in the body.

These are the micrometastases noted above: cells of (presumably) the original mass that can migrate through the lymph system or blood, lie dormant for years, and later rekindle a tumor.

Many scientists believe that only rare lineages of these malignant survivors, known as cancer stem cells, can resist systemic treatment and seed new deadly colonies. But whatever the answer, some 30 percent of even early-stage breast cancers relapse—with the recurrence, in the majority of cases, happening in parts of the body far away from the initial site.

The implication is alarming, for it suggests that the metastatic process might already be under way, in some cases, early in the tumor's development, when the primary lesion is tiny. Most of these relapses occur within the first five years of diagnosis. And adjuvant (postsurgical) drug and hormone treatment *does* seem to lower the chances of such an event. But a significant amount of risk lingers on in the years that follow.

What neither mammography nor systemic treatment has been able to stop—and what the five-year survival rates, obviously, do not reveal—is that long after some women have entered into the ranks of "survivors," their breast cancers can still return. In one 2008 study, published in the *Journal of the National Cancer Institute,* researchers followed nearly three thousand early- and mid-stage breast cancer patients who had completed hormonal treatment or systemic chemotherapy at one of the top cancer research hospitals in the world, and who had apparently been free of disease at the five-year mark. Within the following ten years (or roughly fifteen years after diagnosis), 20 percent of the group had a recurrent lesion.

The message from all of the above is without a doubt strange and dispiriting: mammographic screening is responsible for roughly half of the gains that have been made in recent years in reducing the risk of breast cancer death. Yet this progress has come by using a technology so archaic and flawed that it cannot reliably identify which spots are malignant and which are benign, nor distinguish between tumors bent on aggression and those that ought to be left alone; it swings between "false positives" and errant reports of cancers swept clean; it can barely read the dense tissue that is prevalent in many younger women's breasts. Mammograms are hated by most; habitually avoided by many; uncomfortable, jarring, and sometimes painful. Every buzz of the machine's lead-cased armor signals a zap of one of the few factors that every expert (and layperson) in the world *knows* to be a carcinogen: ionizing radiation. And despite the recent advent of digital mammography (and a few tweaks here and there), the technology has not improved in decades.

Mammograms are awful.

The same can be said about the standard screening tool for prostate cancer. Prostate-specific antigen (PSA) tests—the blood assays that measure the presence of an antigen heavily expressed by many prostate cancer cells—are by no means as uncomfortable (or radioactive) as mammograms are. But they, too, are neither specific nor sensitive enough to be truly effective in screening for prostate cancer. The test is plagued almost equally by false positives and false negatives.

Given the complaints, it is understandable that some have lost faith in the salvation of "early detection" altogether in the fight against cancer. While the practice of screening has unquestionably reduced deaths in some cancers, it has been nowhere near effective enough to stem the tide of cancer mortality overall. Again, the test case has been breast cancer, which continues to claim the lives of more than forty thousand women in the United States each year. In the previous two decades, the annual death count has never once dipped below this threshold (Table 3). Among the dead each year are more than eight thousand American women between the ages of thirty-five and fifty-four. (That line has never been breached either during the past twenty years.) Breast cancer continues to take mothers away from children, steals sisters from sisters. It still butchers and disfigures and stabs at our collective soul. Early detection has not been able to prevent it.

Yet hope for the future lies, surprisingly, in this strategy—or at least in a version of it. The path to success, in fact, is clearly shown by two other decades-old screening practices: colonoscopy and the Pap smear.

The Pap test, in which cells are scraped off the uterine cervix and then examined under a microscope, was first adopted in the 1940s. Nearly by itself, it has cut the US death rate from cervical cancer by four-fifths. The colonoscopy—a test pioneered in September 1969 by New York surgeons Hiromi Shinya and William Wolff, in which the rectum and colon are examined with a lighted scope—has done more to reduce mortality from colorectal cancers than has any drug or other therapy ever devised.

Table 3

Breast Cancer
The Annual American Toll*

Year	Actual Number of Deaths	Crude Death Rate (per 100,000 women)
1970	29,652	28.4
1975	32,158	29.4
1980	35,641	30.6
1985	40,093	32.8
1990	43,391	34.0
1995	43,844	32.2
2000	41,872	29.2
2005	41,116	27.3
2010	40,996	26.1

Change in crude breast cancer death rate from start of cancer war (1970–2010): –8.1%.
*Female only. (Each year around four hundred men in the United States get breast cancer as well.)
SOURCES: Death counts and rates: National Center for Health Statistics (CDC); *Health, United States, 2008, 2010,* and *2011*; data for 1975 and 1985, National Vital Statistics System (see Notes).

Both tests catch early-stage cancers and so, in that sense, are tools for early detection, just as mammograms and PSA tests are. Both are physically uncomfortable and perennially avoided, and even expert practitioners in both procedures occasionally miss some deadly cells. In these respects, the tools are flawed, just as mammograms and PSAs are.

But there is a critical difference: Most of what the Pap smear and colonoscopy do is detect and remove groups of irregular cells that are not yet considered clinical cancer. Gastroenterologists, as a rule, remove any adenomatous polyp—a precancerous lesion on the lining of the colon—they find, ensuring that these buds of abnormal tissue cannot mutate further and become cancerous. The procedure does not guarantee that other polyps will not form later in the twists and turns of the colon, or even that every polyp has been found. But the practice reduces the odds that a cancer will develop in the near-term.

More than early detection, this practice is *preemption*. The aim is not to catch cancers early, but to stop them from forming in the first place—to interrupt this deadly process of evolution close enough to its beginning that it is possible, perhaps, even to reverse it.

As the lesson of breast cancer makes disturbingly clear, "early-stage" is often too late. By the time a tumor has reached a single centimeter in diameter—the size of a small grape—it is composed of roughly a *billion* cells. This population has, by then, gone through some thirty doublings from its original transformed ancestor: one cell replicating into two; two into four; and so on. By then, it is likely that this jumbled mass of generations has grown heterogeneous, that its constituent cells have become genetically variant in different ways.

By then, at the tumor's rough-hewn edges, a million cells per day are already pulling away from the mass, binding themselves to nearby blood vessel walls and shoving their way into the circulation. Out of this daily diaspora, perhaps no more than one is likely to survive the turbulence of the bloodstream, with its ever-present dangers. Only a fraction of survivors, furthermore, will have the necessary traits (and luck) to be able to seed a new colony somewhere else in the body. It is possible, though, that one has managed to do just that.

By the point at which a tumor is a mere gram in weight, treatment—with its potentially heavy costs and risks—is inevitable. And as the numbers in this chapter bear out, treatment does not guarantee a cure.

The answer, as many in the cancer research community knew in the early 1970s, at the start of the modern American cancer war, is preemption. This is the only way to tackle *both* ends of the growing cancer burden: the soaring number of new cases and the unending parade of deaths.

We *have* to pursue this strategy, even if current models make the prospect seem untenable.

And nobody knows this better, or speaks more convincingly of its promise, or speaks more harrowingly of our failure to implement it, than a scientist who made his career at the National Cancer Institute.

His name is Michael Sporn.

Chapter 7

Preemption

That the prevention of cancer will come there is no doubt, for man wishes to survive. But how long prevention will be avoided depends on how long the prophets of agnosticism will succeed in inhibiting the application of scientific knowledge in the cancer field.

—Otto Warburg,
"The Prime Cause and Prevention of Cancer,"
revised lecture, meeting of Nobel laureates,
Lindau, Germany, June 30, 1966

When I first met Michael Sporn, in January 2004, he was dressed in a dark green peacoat, green sweater, green check shirt, olive-green pants, and green knit hat with a green pom-pom dangling from a string. He looked like a leprechaun girded for winter.

I had driven up to Hanover, New Hampshire, to speak with him for an article for *Fortune* magazine. And when he saw me standing outside the local inn on the morning of our interview, he bounded through the snow from his Subaru Forester to greet me. The car was "his eighth straight Subaru," he volunteered just after saying hello, the corners of his mouth lifting into an unbroken grin.

Somehow, it was hard to picture this good-natured smirk of a fellow—a man who had owned eight straight Subarus—as being any kind of revolutionary. But that he was. Mike Sporn, graying, twinkling, was then a month shy of his seventy-first birthday. And if anything, he was more subversive than ever.

Like John Bailar III, the NCI statistician who had, in 1986, famously questioned the government's claims of progress in the war on cancer, Sporn had also challenged the gospel. He had sent his first broadside against what he calls "the cancer establishment" in 1996, when he was invited to write an essay for the venerable British journal *The Lancet* to mark the silver anniversary of the National Cancer Act. (The NCI director at the time had said the long campaign deserved a "birthday present" of a "pat on the back.") Sporn opened his own commentary with an epigraph from Charles Dickens's *Bleak House:*

> Dead, your majesty. Dead, my lords and gentlemen. Dead, Right Reverends, and Wrong Reverends of every order. Dead, men and women, born with Heavenly compassion in your hearts. And dying thus around us every day.

"This magnificent quotation," the scientist began, "provides a unique summary on the total success of the 'War on Cancer' during the past twenty-five years." The salvo was quintessential Sporn.

In his innumerable writings and lectures since then, he has found analogies to the failures of the US cancer program in Camus's *Plague,* the Lernaean Hydra, the guillotines of the Reign of Terror, and the intricate design of Byzantine mosaics. Where other scientists fill their PowerPoint presentations with charts and tables, Sporn prefers Renaissance paintings and classical sculpture. Elegant as the imagery is, though, the message behind it is often as blunt as the *Bleak House* passage. As Sporn told me several years after our first meeting, "The NCI clucks when the death rate goes down one or two points, but more people are dying than ever. Nothing is being done to stop this."

What makes the criticism sting, in particular, is that Sporn, who now holds an endowed professorship and runs a laboratory at Dartmouth

Medical School, has long been a prominent member of the cancer research club. After receiving his medical degree from the University of Rochester, he went to work at the National Institutes of Health, where he shone for thirty-five years before heading to Dartmouth. Along the way, he served as chief of the National Cancer Institute's Lung Cancer Branch and later ran one of the NCI's most storied labs. Like Bailar, he worked and thrived within the cancer establishment for decades.

But unlike Bailar, Sporn has largely gotten away with his truth-telling unscathed. That, for the most part, is due to the kind of researcher he is. Sporn is the sort of basic scientist other basic scientists look up to, one who has to date authored or coauthored more than five hundred research studies, perspectives, and reviews. But more telling than even the huge size of this output is its impact on the research efforts of colleagues: Sporn is among the most "cited" authors in the cancer field, a metric of peer approval that matters more than almost anything else in the culture of modern science. His writings, according to the official arbiter of such matters, Thomson Reuters's "Web of Knowledge," have been referenced in the published work of fellow scientists sixty-seven thousand times.

Sporn's impact, moreover, has been as broad as it is deep. While a dozen of his research papers have, individually, received over a thousand references from colleagues (a remarkable achievement), nearly 170 have been cited at least one hundred times each. Sporn's fellow scientists have cited his collective work no fewer than a thousand times per year, every year, since 1985.

Following the citation trail is itself a tour through cancer discovery, beginning with his seminal work on retinoids. Inspired by experimental work that had been done a half century earlier by Harvard's Burt Wolbach and Percy Howe, Sporn showed in the mid-1970s how cancer progression could be halted in some cases—and proper cell differentiation *restored*—by vitamin A and its chemical cousins. Such analogs of the vitamin, which Sporn termed retinoids (for their steroid-hormone-like signaling ability), could be synthesized in the lab to be thousands of times more active than the naturally occurring vitamin.

Since then, a number of leading investigators from all over the world had joined the quest and studied the effect of retinoids on cancer and other diseases, with varying degrees of success. Sporn, though, moved on.*

Just as famously, Sporn's NCI laboratory, along with another group at the Mayo Clinic, was the first to discover a protein "growth factor" called TGF-ß, which would prove from the start to be monumentally important in normal cell development, the healing of wounds, and cancer progression. Through the 1980s and '90s, he and his revered NCI collaborator Anita Roberts raced against a handful of rival labs to reveal the stunning complexities of this molecule, showing how it helped to suppress carcinogenesis in some contexts and foster it in others. In the end, the discoveries attributed to this duo of "TGF-ß pioneers" would be striking in number and significance.

With another accomplished scientist, George Todaro, Sporn formulated a hypothesis of "autocrine secretion" that laid out, as early as 1980, a clear framework for how cancer cells could produce the very protein growth factors, hormones, and other signaling molecules that inevitably allowed them to escape from normal growth controls.

The work would have been enough to distinguish any research scientist's career, earning Sporn the Medal of Honor from the American Cancer Society, the prestigious Bristol-Myers Squibb Award for Distinguished Achievement in Cancer Research, the Komen Brinker Award for Scientific Distinction, and prized lectureships at the AACR's annual gathering of cancer researchers. In 2004, even the NCI named its sometimes dissident alumnus its first-ever "Eminent Scholar."

For all his contributions to biology, biochemistry, and pharmacology, though, Sporn is still better known for something else. Rather than any one molecular discovery, it is an idea. The notion is so straightforward—so damned obvious, really—that it is easy to forget how revolutionary it was when he first proposed it in the mid-1970s: cancer, Sporn contended,

---

*In recent years, Sporn has developed new compounds in related chemical classes, called rexinoids and triterpenoids, which have been shown to be more powerful and selective as cancer-preventive agents.

could (and should) be chemically stopped, slowed, or reversed in its earliest *pre*invasive stages.

That was it. That was the whole radical idea.

Sporn was not the first to propose such an idea. Lee Wattenberg at the University of Minnesota had suggested the strategy in 1966 to little response. But Sporn refined it, pushed it, and branded it: To distinguish such intervention from the standard form of cancer treatment, chemotherapy—a therapy that sadly comes too late for roughly a third of patients to *be* therapeutic—he coined the term *chemoprevention* in 1976. The name stuck.

On first reading, the concept might seem no more than a truism. But to grasp the importance of chemoprevention, one has first to dislodge the mind-set that has long reigned over the field of oncology: that cancer is a disease state. "One has cancer or one doesn't." Such a view, indeed, is central to the current practice of cancer medicine: oncologists today discover the event of cancer in a patient and respond—typically, quite urgently. This thinking is shared by patients, the FDA, drug developers, and health insurers (who decide what to pay for). This is the default view of cancer.

And, to Sporn, it is dead wrong. Cancer is not an event or a "state" of any kind. The disease does not suddenly come into being with a discovered lump on the mammogram. It does not begin with the microscopic lesion found on the chest X-ray. Nor when the physician lowers his or her voice and tells the patient, "I'm sorry. The pathology report came back positive. . . . You have cancer."

Nor does the disease begin, says Sporn, when the medical textbooks say it does: when the first neoplastic cell breaks through the "basement membrane," the meshwork layers of collagen and other proteins that separate compartments of bodily tissue. In such traditional thinking, it matters little whether a cell, or population of cells, has become immortalized through mutation. Or how irregular or jumbled the group might look under the microscope. Or how otherwise disturbed their genomes are. As long as none of the clones have breached the basement membrane, the pathology is not (yet) considered "cancer."

For more than a century, this barrier has been the semantic line that separates the fearsome "invader" from the merely "abnormal." It is the

Rubicon of cancer diagnosis. From the standpoint of disease mechanics, the rationale is easy to understand, because just beyond this fibrous gateway are fast-moving channels (the blood and lymphatic vessels) that can conceivably transport a predatory cell, or cells, to any terrain in the body. Busting through the basement is therefore a seeming leap past the point of no return, a signal that a local disturbance is potentially emerging into a disseminating mob.*

But while invasion may define so-called clinical cancer for legions of first-year medical students, it is by no means the start of the pathology. Cancer is not any one act; it is a *process*. It begins with the first hints of subversion in the normal differentiation of a cell—with the first disruption of communication between that cell and its immediate environment. There is, perhaps, no precise moment of conception in this regard, no universally accepted beginning—which makes delineating the process that much harder. But most, if not all, types of "cancer" have their own somewhat recognizable stages of evolution along the route to *clinically* apparent disease.

"Saying it's not cancer until the cells are through the basement membrane," says Sporn, "is like saying the barn isn't on fire until there are bright red flames coming out of the roof. It's absolute nonsense!"

Long before a cancer cell becomes invasive it goes through a continuum of development, a process known as carcinogenesis. The precise molecular and physical changes vary from cell to cell, from one cell type to another, and from one tissue of origin to the next. But in the case of the major epithelial cancers (which account for the vast majority of all cancer deaths), the path to transformation seems to conform to one general rule: a group of normal cells gets stranger-looking as the progression wears on.

The first infinitesimal changes can be seen in a small number of cells in a particular organ, as they take on an irregular shape and orientation. In some cases, their nuclei bulge in comparison to the cytoplasm around

---

*Malignant cells that have not crossed this barrier are called in situ disease. The NCI's record-keepers, as noted in chapter 3, do not count such preinvasive (Stage 0) neoplasms in their annual tallies of cancer incidence.

them. Normal cells of the same lineage, in the same tissue, look generally uniform under the microscope. In the case of mild *dysplasia* (the word means "abnormal growth"), a smattering of cells do not.

Most often, mild dysplasia corrects on its own, replaced by a generation of well-proportioned cells. Occasionally, though, the progression continues, and a slight disturbance of order morphs into a moderate one. The boundary between such phases is a matter of judgment. (It is surprisingly common for two practiced pathologists to disagree on how atypical cells in any specimen are.) But dysplasia is often thought to be moderate when half the cells in a tissue look abnormal. The clumping appears stranger than in mild dysplasia. Nuclei, now packed with chromosomal material (chromatin), turn to dark blotches when stained on a glass slide.

Severe dysplasia is the next step in the continuum. Here, the entire layer of epithelial cells appears "disorganized," any semblance of order gone. Cells are frequently of different sizes and shapes and scrambled together every which way, their nuclear centers engorged with chromatin.

The border between this phase and the next—carcinoma in situ—is thin, if it exists at all. For under the microscope, the tissue has all the makings of a malignant lesion except that it has not yet invaded through the basement membrane. It is a "cancer in waiting," so to speak, though the wait might conceivably last forever. No one knows.

Given how blurry such dividing lines are, the entire spectrum of developmental phases is typically lumped together under a single rubric called intraepithelial neoplasia, or IEN.* But that's as far as the agreement goes. Pathologists argue over histology, the parameters of disorder, and the risks projected by each presumed degree of tissue irregularity. They speak in a babel of diagnostic tongues—with each organ site having its own unique argot. When it comes to IEN of the larynx, for example, no fewer than *twenty* classification systems have been put to the test over the years. Three are still in use today. Each breaks down the disease progression in a different way.

For all this fervent debate over the nature and inherent risk of IEN,

---

Intra, meaning "within," is the key. Such growths are still within the boundary of the epithelial layer.

though, all sides agree on one matter: the genesis of cancer is not merely a process (and a perpetually uncertain one at that), it is most often a slow-motion process, too.

The physical metamorphosis from one phase of dysplasia to the next is shaped and driven by an accumulation of changes at the molecular level, each of which is the result of an alteration in the coding or expression of a specific gene (or genes). Biologists and geneticists have spent the better part of four decades cataloging such molecular triggers. Many dozens of oncogenic pathways have now been plotted to a minute degree. But the factor implicated in carcinogenesis more than any other, it turns out, has little to do with genes or the proteins they encode. Cancer's great enabler is time. Time provides the opportunity for accidents, erosion, and random destruction. Time offers the chance for the orderly to break down. Time lets the damage from environmental carcinogens and mutagens accrue and compound.

A lethal cancer can manifest at any age—even in infancy, which is when many cases of neuroblastoma are seen.* But childhood cancers aside, the odds of developing an invasive malignancy increase with a person's age, as a rule, simply because there is more time for genetic accidents to happen, more time for entropy to run its inevitable course, more time for the continuous cycle of injury, repair, reinjury, and re-repair to go awry.

This is the long-enshrined "stochastic," or random, view of how most cancers form: the disease as a kind of Russian roulette of genetic injury. (When it comes to the relatively uncommon heritable cancer syndromes, mutations, typically in one copy of a critical gene, are carried from birth, sharply raising that person's risk of an early-onset malignancy.)

Over time, genomic damage and instability from all causes add up—to the point where four in ten Americans can be sure of a cancer diagnosis during their lifetime. While half of these cases will not be diagnosed until

---

*Neuroblastoma, a malignancy that develops in nerve tissue cells, is one of a dozen or so cancers that predominantly strike children. As noted in chapter 3, more than twelve thousand US children under the age of fifteen will be diagnosed with various forms of cancer in 2012—a number that has been rising dramatically, and inexplicably, for years.

patients are at least sixty-six years old (the median age of cancer "incidence" in the United States), it is folly to think that the process, in nearly every case, has not been under way for years, if not decades.

The parallels with coronary heart disease and hypertension, and virtually every other chronic ailment of advancing age, are hard to miss. A heart attack on the golf course is nearly always the culmination of a drawn–out process, a decades-long buildup of arterial plaque that may have begun, in some cases, in teenage years. Likewise, the diagnosis of an invasive cancer is the late recognition of a progressive disease long in development. If such is the case, Sporn reasons, it only follows that cancer ought to be interrupted or slowed or controlled early in that progression. That, after all, is precisely the strategy that has reduced the burden from heart disease and stroke so "miraculously" over the past half century.

"We do not generally wait until a person is in the midst of cardiac arrest to treat him or her," says Sporn. "We treat the patient at the first sign of early disease."

Statins are used to lower artery-clogging cholesterol in millions of people, even though not everyone with elevated levels of low-density lipoprotein ("bad cholesterol") is destined to die of a heart attack. Beta-blockers and other drugs are routinely, perhaps even too aggressively, used to counter high blood pressure. Blood thinners and anticoagulants are used to prevent clotting in those who are deemed "at risk." Irregular heart rhythms are stabilized, sometimes with risky surgery. Stents and other procedures are frequently employed in later stages of disease progression to prevent the heart muscle from being damaged. The approach is hardly passive; this prevention is interventionist in nature.

For nearly every major pathology other than cancer, a vigorous preemption strategy has governed. Doctors attack *pre*disease not only through chemoprevention, but also by having those with such risk markers as high LDL levels, blood sugar, or blood pressure make immediate, substantive changes in their diets and lifestyles.

One can only wonder what the result might have been had we tried a different tack fifty or sixty years ago.

That, indeed, is the what-if Sporn put to me as he drove me back to the hotel in his trusty Subaru, after the first of what would be nine years' worth of marathon conversations. "Imagine," said Sporn, "that instead of intervening early in the process of say, heart disease, we had poured tens of billions of public health dollars into developing better defibrillators . . . and faster ambulances to get heart attack victims to the hospital?" What if we had treated heart disease like an event to react to rather than a long process to stop at the beginning (or even in the middle)? What if we had approached this leading killer, in other words, the way we have approached cancer—how many millions of people would have died too soon?

Mike Sporn's heresy is that he began asking such questions in 1976. And that he cannot bring himself to stop.

Even in the early days of the cancer war, Sporn was not alone in his convictions. A cadre of preventionistas—including top-tier scientists such as Wattenberg, Waun Ki Hong at MD Anderson, Paul Talalay at Johns Hopkins, and the late I. Bernard Weinstein at Columbia University—helped make the case for realigning the nation's anticancer efforts to the goal of preemption. This was also the change that John Bailar was advocating when he wrote the first of his *New England Journal* articles questioning the US cancer strategy. In the generation that followed, the ranks of like-minded researchers grew to the point where the idea of detecting and treating precancerous lesions even began to take on an aura of fashionableness.

In 1976, Sporn and Emmanuel Farber, chairman of pathology at the University of Toronto, held a three-day "world conference" on the topic at the NCI—and one could have squeezed all the attendees into a school bus. A quarter century later, when the AACR held its own global meeting, scientists packed the halls. But perhaps the clearest sign that the revolution had arrived was in the rhetoric coming out of Building 1 of the National Institutes of Health. Shortly after he took the helm of the NIH in 2002, Elias Zerhouni told a reporter for the *New York Times:*

> For thousands of years medicine has relied on what? On the fact that you have a core of people to whom you come when a disease has declared itself. Well, by that time things are really way down the path of

destruction. So I believe strongly that in this century we're going to have to understand what I call the subclinical phase of diseases, where the disease is evolving in you but you feel nothing.

The message was a far cry from what Sporn had heard from cancer leaders a generation earlier. When he and Farber had asked Frank Rauscher, then head of the National Cancer Institute, to give some opening remarks at their 1976 conference, the director had brushed off the idea, calling precancerous lesions "unimportant." Zerhouni, however, could not have sounded more vigorous in his support for this decades-old notion, which he proudly adopted as his new "road map" for the NIH. When I later interviewed the former Johns Hopkins radiologist, who served as the NIH's director until 2008, he pulled out a Magic Marker and drew a long, accelerating curve on a whiteboard. The curve was carcinogenesis, he explained. He then scratched hash marks at several spots along the bend. These were the inflection points at which "cancer" would be preempted in the not-too-distant future, he said with swagger. All were below the curve's crest—which, in the diagram at least, represented invasion across the basement membrane.

On a whiteboard the strategy looks compelling, perhaps even obvious. Yet, as intuitive as the idea of cancer preemption is, as effective as the strategy has been in combating other major diseases, as frightening as the alternative (an ever-rising cancer burden) surely is, profound obstacles stand in its way, Sporn acknowledges. Three challenges must be overcome. The first is to identify people with precancerous lesions lurking somewhere in the body. The second is to discover how to stop or reverse their progression—and in a way, importantly, that does not in itself increase the cancer burden. And the third is to get over the fear of doing the second. Each of these barriers will take a herculean effort to surmount. The only reason to think that we can do it, says Sporn, is that we have no choice but to succeed.

Detecting invasive cancers in early stages of disease is agonizingly difficult, much harder than many, decades ago, thought that it would be. Few cancers in the lung, pancreas, liver, esophagus, stomach, or ovary are diagnosed before they have spread. Even with the aid of the Pap smear and colonoscopy—arguably the best "early detection" tools available—half of all cervical cancers in the United States, and a still-greater share of those in the colon or rectum, are not discovered today until they are relatively advanced.

Yet the preemption paradigm calls for an even more ambitious goal: catching *preinvasive* lesions, or IENs. The question is inescapable: If so many "actual" cancers are missed with current screening technology, how can the tiny populations of not-quite-malignant cells be found—and moreover, be found routinely, cheaply, and noninvasively?

Medical researchers have scoured human blood, urine, and saliva in a search for telltale molecules that might alert to a burgeoning cancer in the body. Cancers, after all, are directed by signals from within and without. Macromolecules—proteins, for the most part—convey each and every instruction. So it is here, in the uncharted seas of bodily fluids, that scientists have long expected to find the early-warning indicators of malignancy. Tens of thousands of investigators have spent decades seeking such microscopic red flags.* Candidates emerge on a near-weekly basis but, in the zeal of discovery, are just as quickly forgotten. Since 1990, more than 150,000 studies of would-be cancer "biomarkers" (including genes, proteins, and all else) have been cataloged by the National Library of Medicine's PubMed database.

The investment of time and public money, however, has brought us little closer to the goal. So little that the NCI was able to sum up its success in a 2008 "progress report" with a single sentence: "Yet, there are no validated molecular biomarker tests for the early detection of any cancer."

One hundred fifty thousand scientific papers, according to the government, have led not to a single FDA-approved, diagnostic molecular-based test for cancer, or at least any appropriate for widespread screening.

There are, to be sure, myriad tests to predict cancer risk. Researchers have zeroed in on a number of critical gene mutations and variations that make certain people particularly susceptible to developing one

---

*The name has evolved over the years, from *neoplastic antigens* in the 1970s, to *tumor markers* in the 1980s, to the more ethereal *biomarkers* of today.

malignancy or another. Women can learn, for example, whether they have inherited a rare mutation in a copy of any of two "tumor suppressor genes," BRCA1 and BRCA2, which would put them at far greater risk for getting both breast and ovarian cancer. (The US company that owns the patent on this gene test has set the price at more than $3,000, making this potentially lifesaving information far less accessible than it ought to be.) A separate crop of tests on the market offer predictions, based on the expression of dozens of genes in a tumor, of which patients' breast cancers are most likely to recur *after* remission. There is nothing, however, that can identify the disease early but for the much-disliked and fallible mammogram.

Other gene and protein tests provide valuable information—determining, for instance, who is likely to benefit from a given therapeutic agent (such as the HER2 receptor test for Herceptin), or who might suffer excessively from another. Biomarkers are now routinely used to fine-tune drug regimens for children with acute leukemia. Such tests are helping to forestall toxic side effects and predict nonresponders prior to treatment; some are clearly saving lives.

Best known of all, perhaps, are the tests to detect the recurrence of a cancer thought to be in remission. These protein assays, in some cases, can note the existence of a tumor sometimes months before it can be seen on a CT scan. But the grail of early cancer detection has still to be found. While a select few candidates have come tantalizingly close to fulfilling the promise, they have ultimately fallen short in either sensitivity or specificity: they miss too many cases or catch too many false ones. Or, as is typically the case, they do both.

Perhaps no marker illustrates the dramatic rise and fall of expectations better than Cancer Antigen 125. Isolated in 1981 by Robert C. Bast Jr. and colleagues at what was then the Sidney Farber Cancer Institute in Boston, CA-125 seemed to be the beacon that would illuminate hidden, symptomless ovarian cancers before they had the chance to spread.

Eighty percent of women with epithelial ovarian cancers (the most common form of the disease) have elevated concentrations of the antigen in their blood; an estimated 99 percent of apparently healthy women do not. CA-125 is, moreover, a huge molecule that, when shed from the surface of a tumor cell, circulates in the bloodstream for several days, making it easy to detect in a blood test. Such facts made the notion of a general screening program seem, at first, both feasible and affordable. But when it comes to biomarkers, even seemingly small gaps in predictive accuracy can expand into great holes of uncertainty. Such was the case with CA-125.

The initial issue concerned those women who tested positive. In roughly one of every seventeen women, high levels of the antigen were due not to ovarian cancer, but to a wholly different medical condition. Ailments that spiked the protein ran the gamut from common and benign conditions (endometriosis, pelvic inflammatory disease, ovarian cysts, adenomyosis, and uterine fibroids) to illnesses of the liver, pancreas, and kidney. The marker was also shown to be elevated in nearly a third of *non*ovarian malignancies.

Such false (and misdirected) alarms lead not only to further medical investigation and imaging but also to surgery, which is not only expensive, but carries its own risk as well. In a study of 5,500 Swedish women, random screening for CA-125 ultimately led doctors to perform 175 exploratory surgeries. During those operations, six cancers were found—just two of which were in a stage of disease that offered favorable odds for treatment.

Which brings up the other side of the standard biomarker dilemma: the prognosis for women who have low (or no) level of the antigen in their blood remains uncertain nevertheless. That is because this molecular dragnet often misses the cancers it is designed to catch: while roughly 90 percent of women with Stage II or higher ovarian cancers show elevated levels of CA-125 when tested in clinical trials, anywhere from half to three-quarters of Stage I patients do not.

The point of diagnostic screening is to alter the outlook for many individuals while keeping the cost of unnecessary intervention low. This biomarker, as with hundreds of other well-touted candidates, managed neither.*

---

*CA-125 is far more informative once ovarian cancer is diagnosed. It is used effectively to gauge response to treatment and to identify recurrent tumors two to three months before they are detectable by CT scan.

Much of the challenge of preemption, just as with early detection, has to do with biological scale. A single ovarian cancer cell has thousands of types of protein bumping and jostling in its cytoplasm or suspended across its membrane. Out of this swarm, a relative few are shed from the cell surface, or secreted, and eventually carried like jetsam into the rushing circulation. Among these are proteins that are common to all sorts of cells, including wholly normal ones. But perhaps a fraction of the lot are the smudged fingerprints of a thriving cancer.* As one might expect, bigger tumors slough off more of these telltale proteins than smaller ones do (and metastasizing cells lose more than their tissue-bound counterparts), which means that cancers in advanced stages have far more pronounced signatures than do tiny, localized masses. That is why early-stage ovarian cancers almost invariably slip past the molecular radar. And *pre*invasive lesions are even harder to spot.

Such daunting factors, however, do not mean that the idea of preemption is doomed from the start. Rather, the failed biomarker hunt demonstrates how poorly the search has been organized thus far. Indeed, there has been no actual search to begin with. Teams of volunteers have not walked arm-to-arm through the molecular woods, so to speak, as if looking for the body of a missing person. There has never been any real coordination of research teams or systematic follow-up on promising candidate markers. No one has been charged with the responsibility of *leading* the hunt—of saying, "Hey, you go this way, and I'll go over there."

As with so much else in the cancer research enterprise, the biomarker effort has been utterly decentralized, with the result equally predictable: as each investigator follows his or her own trail of bread crumbs through the dense forest, the ground simply fills with crumbs.

Many scientists engaged in the biomarker hunt are aware of the problem, as is the National Cancer Institute. In the fall of 2000, leaders of

---

*Proteins are not the only potential cache of biomarkers. Warning beacons might one day be found, for example, in the tiny complements of DNA in the mitochondria of cells or in patterns of gene methylation (i.e., which genes are "turned off").

the NCI's Division of Cancer Prevention offered an assessment of the biomarker campaign that was surprisingly scathing—at least by the docile standards of government officials:

> Researchers often compete rather than collaborate. This competition can create redundancy in research projects. . . . Information about biomarkers is not well organized, is often difficult to find, and is published in a large variety of journals and databases. . . . Among institutions, there are no uniform information storage schemes, complicating literature searches and data queries for biomarker information.

The critique appeared in a report announcing a new consortium of academic, private, and government scientists—christened the Early Detection Research Network—that was supposed to reverse all of these shortcomings. What was actually funded, though, were the same old studies in the same old ways. EDRN's proposal for liver cancer screening, for instance, turned out to be yet another clinical trial facing off two early-detection markers that had been parsed and tested and retested for decades. (One of them had been linked with liver cancer as early as 1963 and had already been put through at least twenty-two separate human clinical trials.)

Sporn and others, however, are convinced that biomarkers for early-stage—and, yes, preinvasive—disease can be found if the effort is managed well and focused relentlessly on the goal. Such were the guiding principles, after all, that led to the surmounting of an equally difficult challenge, the decoding of the human genome, a task completed in less than a decade and a half.*

Years ago, I asked Eric Lander, a professor of biology at MIT, founding

---

*The project was proposed in October 1986, but not funded by the NIH until 1990. The first draft sequence was published in *Nature* in February 2001; the public Human Genome Project, a community-orchestrated effort by some twenty laboratories and more than two thousand scientists around the world, was declared completed in 2003. Celera Corporation undertook a separate, privately funded, and self-managed effort to decode the human genome in 1998 and published its draft sequence in *Science* in February 2001, the same month as the public consortium's article.

director of the Whitehead Institute's Center for Genome Research in Cambridge, Massachusetts, and a leader of the Human Genome Project, how the genome feat was accomplished. Much of the credit, he said, was due to something that many people might find almost laughably prosaic, and even counter to the popular image of individual scientific pursuit: a weekly conference call. Every Friday morning without fail for seven years, a handful of project leaders got on the phone to discuss strategy, problems encountered, suggested fixes, and anything else that might move the project one or two steps forward each week.

> It was done because it got itself organized. You know, we got on the phone every goddamn week and we hated it. Because what a pain in the ass, but we managed this thing by close coordination. We argued, we fought it out, but at the end, there was a team. Yes, there were three or four big labs in the project, but those three or four big labs learned how to work as a team, and the funding agencies coordinated with the grantees and we got things done. We set ludicrous goals. They were audacious goals, so we could tell when we were a certain percentage away from a goal or a hundred percent toward a goal.

Likewise, on the cancer problem, said Lander, "We're not going to get there without that management. I'm still very much in favor of funding lots of bright young people and letting them do anything they want. But much of what's needed right now is to bite the bullet [and focus directly on] the problem." We can find the right biomarkers, but to do so will require a dramatic reorganization of the search enterprise. That, however, is just step one.

Assuming that such molecular beacons of precancer can and will be found, what then is to be done? As it is now, many early-stage and in situ lesions are overtreated, which has added tremendous cost, physical and emotional trauma, and risk to an already rising cancer burden. To take one example, women with ductal carcinoma in situ (DCIS), or Stage 0 breast cancer, opt for preventive double mastectomies twice as often as those women diagnosed with the same condition a decade earlier. The fear of the disease is so visceral that one in twenty women with preinvasive cancer in a single breast are willing to have both of their breasts removed.

Many, if not most, precancerous lesions either do not progress (carcinogenesis is suppressed by one mechanism or another), or they are restored to normalcy. The damaged tissue is repaired through largely the same systematic process initiated by any deep cut in the skin. It is healed. And therein lies one hope for chemoprevention, many scientists say.

To understand, one has to take another quick detour into the biology of wound repair. Healing entails several overlapping cascades of cellular and molecular actions, beginning with a series of rapid-fire events known as the inflammatory response. Capillaries nearby become permeable, as the walls of the tiny vessels open up just enough to let small molecules and infection–fighting white blood cells (neutrophils and macrophages) slip through and then migrate to the site of injury. Clotting factors go to work outside the vasculature, and certain adhesive glycoproteins are deposited, forming a temporary scaffold around the wound. Macrophages then release signaling molecules that bring yet another class of cells, called endothelial cells, to the scene. These cells proliferate to form new blood vessels, which in turn feed the injured tissue with essential oxygen and nutrients. (This process within a process is called angiogenesis; as will be clear in a minute, it plays a crucial role in cancer development as well.)

Also recruited to the site are connective tissue cells known as fibroblasts. The fibroblasts—together with inflammatory cells, fibrin, and other molecules derived from the protein–dense spaces surrounding the cells—create a "granulation tissue" that will become the foundation for the remodeled tissue at the site. A still more fibrous replacement, now dense with collagen, follows. Biologists call this event fibroplasia. Most people know it as scarring. The scar eventually contracts and fades, restoring the injured area to most (though not all) of its former functional ability.

This is the process of healing. But in the case of some early dysplastic lesions, healing goes deadly wrong. The notion, introduced in 1972 by the Scotsman Sir Alexander Haddow, and then resurrected years later by Harvard's Harold Dvorak, is that these same healthy and oft-repeated responses to injury are subverted in carcinogenesis. As Haddow formulated it, "The wound is a tumor that heals itself." (Dvorak's more well-known dictum, "tumors are wounds that do not heal," came in a *New England Journal of Medicine* paper in 1986.) The mistakes are mostly failures to end a mechanism that began appropriately: angiogenesis, for example, does not stop when it is supposed to (in no small part because tumors secrete chemical signals that keep the maze of spindly blood vessels coming). The vessels, for their part, continue to leak plasma proteins into the tumor. A frenetic three-way cross-talk between the abnormal cells of the lesion and the seemingly "normal" connective tissue nearby (the stroma) and the molecular soup that fills the space around these cells (the extracellular matrix) keeps the inflammatory and proliferative cycles going as it pulls the now-burgeoning tumor further and further away from its normal controls. An IEN thereby becomes a cancer.

In this light, it is clear to see that early carcinogenesis is not merely a continuum of disorder in a single cell (or in a zombielike population of cells); it is, rather, a conspiracy of sorts between the lesion and its immediate environs. It takes a village to raise a cancer. And if that is the case, many researchers contend, it ought to be possible to halt the cancer's development by fixing the neighborhood.

This idea is more than just theory. A hundred years of experimentation have demonstrated that cancers are as much a product of their "microenvironment" as they are of genetic mutations in the tumors themselves. One of the more famous of such experiments was done by Beatrice Mintz and Karl Illmensee at the Fox Chase Cancer Center in 1975. They showed that when tumors called teratocarcinomas were transplanted into healthy embryonal tissue, the abnormal clones reverted to a normal state.

But it was the work of Mina Bissell, a few years later, that most convincingly put tumor biology into its proper three-dimensional context. She immigrated to the United States from Iran in 1959, with the help of a high school scholarship, and enrolled at Bryn Mawr College. Then came Harvard Medical School (a PhD in microbiology and molecular genetics), two children, an appointment at Lawrence Berkeley National Laboratory (where she now holds the title "distinguished scientist"), and one of the more celebrated and revolutionary careers in cancer biology.

Along the way, she has become a one-name personage. To everyone in the cancer research community, Dr. Bissell is simply "Mina"—a name she pronounces with a profoundly long *Meee*, as if to stress there could be only one. Motherly, brash, and defiantly sure of herself, Mina began her trailblazing work with a set of questions that, at the time, sounded almost childlike in their innocence: If every cell in the body was born with the same endowment of genes, how did a nose cell know it was a nose cell? How did a breast cell remember whether it was a part of a milk duct, for example, or another functional unit of the breast?

Rather than search for an answer by examining gene mutations in cell lines, as so many of her colleagues were doing, Mina built a living model of the mammary gland in three dimensions—complete with a functional extracellular matrix (ECM)—and then examined the back-and-forth between the cells and their molecular scaffolding. (This 3-D "architecture," after all, is what makes a collection of different tissues an organ.) She studied communications as a whole, looking for broad patterns in the community of cells.

What she discovered ran counter to the established wisdom: cells receive continuous biochemical "cues" to their identity from components in the ECM. Each individual cell nucleus is directed, through a blitz of signaling, to maintain a gene expression signature that is specific to its role in the gland. It is not enough, then, to be the daughter of another breast cell; that identity has to be constantly relearned.

The implications of this revelation are profound: even a modest disruption in normal tissue organization can be enough to throw a cell's differentiation program—its sense of biological identity—out of whack and drive carcinogenesis. (Bissell and her colleagues demonstrated that as well.)

The research findings suggest there may well be an opportunity to interrupt the fledgling cancer process to prevent abnormal (dysplastic) cells from becoming aggressive invaders. Happily, this approach does not involve trying to kill the would-be tumor with toxic drugs or finding an ever-elusive combination of targeted agents to jam the cells' proliferation pathways (only to have the cells evolve around these blockades).

Such interventions do not have to be aggressive to be effective. It is conceivable, argue Bissell, Sporn, and many others, that a treatment directed against the "field" of the damaged tissue can be as gentle as slowing the inflammatory response associated with wound healing. (Aspirin and nonsteroidal painkillers, such as ibuprofen, do that to some extent.) An alternative plan—emerging, in part, from early investigations by Sporn and Anita Roberts—is to suppress a growth factor (TGF-ß) that is instrumental in both injury repair and tumor development. Indeed, some researchers, led by Paul Talalay of Johns Hopkins, believe that the best "chemoprotective" agents may ultimately not be drugs at all, but rather certain phytochemicals in foods and other natural products. Small, well-timed fixes to the neighborhood, in any case, may be enough to help the body do what it normally does on its own—that is to say, suppress carcinogenesis.

As with other therapeutic approaches, the strategy's success will ultimately hinge on timing. While there are rare reports in the medical literature of advanced cancers regressing on their own, the best chance of reversion, obviously, is before the area around the lesion has significantly deteriorated. The longer the destructive interaction goes on, the more likely it is the microenvironment will become irrevocably disordered, a phenomenon some have called "field cancerization." If precancer therapy is to be a viable strategy for reducing the cancer burden, treatment has to come very early.

And that brings up challenge number three.

No matter how "nontoxic" microenvironment-directed therapy may turn out to be, there will always be some risk associated with precancerous treatment. Risk is inherent in any intervention. An arsenal of biomarkers will, hopefully, help physicians determine which patients' lesions are most in danger of progressing over the near term and, therefore, suggest who would be a good candidate for chemoprevention and who would not.* But even when appropriate target populations can be identified

---

*As it is, without the benefit of such markers, certain individuals are known to be particularly susceptible to cancer—based on either hereditary factors or clinical ones: those infected with hepatitis B or C virus, or who have cirrhosis of the liver, for example, have sharply higher odds for developing liver cancer.

and the treatments are relatively benign, the strategy will still not be free of risk. Some people, inevitably, will not truly have aggressive lesions as supposed and will therefore have been treated needlessly. Some will have side effects. Out of that group, some will be seriously hurt or die from unexpected reactions to whatever therapy is administered.

Such is the reality for *any* drug treatment. Statin drugs, while lowering cholesterol counts, cause liver damage and serious muscle injury in some cases. Anticoagulants and blood pressure medications all come with profound risks. Vaccines (which, technically, are biological agents rather than drugs) can cause allergic reactions or other adverse effects. People get their shots and take their daily pills nonetheless, well aware that the alternative may be far worse.

Indeed, most of us are so comfortable with, or unwitting of, pharmaceutical risk that we expose ourselves to its uncertainty every day, even when the treated injury is minor. Aspirin use is linked to internal bleeding; sleeping pills can cause anaphylaxis or potentially bizarre behavioral problems such as "sleep-driving." And the leading cause of acute liver failure in the United States is not some exotic and terrifying virus, or alcohol abuse; it is acetaminophen, also known as Tylenol. Health care researchers now estimate that between 5 percent and 10 percent of all US hospital admissions are due to "drug therapy complications."

Risk is likewise inherent to any surgical procedure, even one as "routine" as a colonoscopy. The procedure saves lives, but once in a rare while a patient's large intestine is perforated. (There is a reason it is called invasive.)

Dangers both foreseen and unforeseen poke out of the dark corners of every conceivable medical intervention. When it comes to most cancer treatments, the dangers are well-known. But when it comes to *precancer* treatments, any threshold of risk is deemed too high. The disconnect in logic is strange, but real nonetheless. So whereas the idea of interrupting carcinogenesis by way of therapy is intuitively smart to many of the best minds in medicine and science, the thought of putting it into practice makes many of the same people thoroughly uncomfortable. "The issue here is you're talking about a well population taking a substance for their life, basically, or for prolonged periods of time," says Richard Pazdur, who presides over the approval process for cancer drugs at the FDA. "And obviously questions have to come in." Prime among them is, how can we treat "healthy" people when every potential intervention carries some risk? Many critics say we can't.

That widely held conviction is the single biggest impediment to a new and viable cancer-reduction strategy. That, right there, is the cancer war's Immovable Object. And even an irresistible force such as Michael Sporn has trouble pushing his way through it.

Over a period of nine years I have spent dozens of hours in conversation with Michael Sporn and exchanged hundreds of e-mails and letters with the man. His thoughts and memories unfold a history of cancer biology, one of improbable geniuses and the sometimes uncelebrated discoveries they made. Here is the story of optimism, of modesty, of hope, in the wisdom of the men and women of science. And at the end of the timeline is heartbreak.

Sporn has joked about the perennial lack of funding for prevention research ("We're still a minority viewpoint, but in terms of grant money, we're a superminority!"); he has cheerfully pressed his case for chemo-prevention in one scholarly article, speech, and government testimony after another. But he has been deflated by the mind-set, even among scientists and health policy officials, that people in the midst of active carcinogenesis are healthy.

"People do not wake up one day as 'healthy,'" he says, "and the next as 'having cancer!' Were the twenty thousand women told they had ovarian cancer this year *healthy* the year before, when they had no symptoms to speak of?

"There was a time when people were denying that adenomas [polyps] had anything to do with colon cancer because most adenomas do not go on to develop into colon cancer. Colon cancer only arises in a small percentage of polyps. This was a very, very big argument. And the modern corollary to this, to people who don't want any chemoprevention, is that you can't treat healthy people. 'Healthy people, healthy people. Dr. Sporn, how can you go treating healthy people?'

"Was Anita healthy in 2003?"

Anita Roberts had come to his NCI laboratory as a postdoctoral fellow in 1976. She had become his full partner in research, going on to earn fame for her pioneering work studying the protein TGF-ß, and had assumed command of Sporn's lab after he left. The pair published hundreds of papers together over a three-decade collaboration. On ScienceWatch's list of the fifty most cited researchers in the life sciences from 1983 to 2002, Roberts was one of only two women; Sporn was also on the list, naturally.

In March 2004, the sixty-two-year-old Roberts was told that she had an aggressive Stage IV gastric cancer. By May of 2006 she was dead.

The loss of his longtime friend and partner devastated Sporn. It was also a heartrending reminder of the cost of a mind-set. For even if doctors could have identified a precancerous lesion in Roberts's stomach five or ten years earlier, they would not have treated it. She would have been considered "healthy," after all—even colleagues at the NCI, who knew carcinogenesis was a process, would have sighed relief at the biopsy of a mere dysplastic lesion. "Thank God, it's not cancer," many would have said.

The view is so deeply etched into the cancer culture that it affects everything from the drug-approval process to clinical trial design, and reimbursement rules from insurance companies and Medicare. Current regulatory standards make it almost impossible to test chemopreventive drugs, let alone develop and market them. According to one pharmaceutical-industry database, only 1.5 percent of all drugs in active development as of 2004 had a prevention indication of any kind. The mind-set has frozen the science of chemoprevention in place, leaving even the growing ranks of believers in a kind of suspended animation. Theirs will continue to be a world of "task forces" and "working groups" and poorly funded "consortiums" until the risk equation is fundamentally rethought.

If we are ever to face the cancer burden head-on, the threshold for intervention can no longer be framed as one of risk versus benefit alone. The more important trade-off to consider here is risk versus risk: it is the uncertain risk of action versus the sure and devastating risk of inaction; it is the age-old contest between the sin of commission and the sin of omission. In this case, almost certainly, the sin of omission is the greater transgression.

Michael Sporn and others have shown what may be our most viable path forward, one that attempts to reduce the number of cancer deaths by reducing the number of people getting an invasive cancer in the first place. But even with a change of mind-set, it will not be easy to win the war on cancer. As will be argued in the chapters that follow, what is needed is nothing less than a cultural makeover throughout the national cancer enterprise. New ways of thinking, collaborating, and engineering solutions have to be absorbed by a profession that has long venerated individual pursuit. Infrastructure has to replace walls. And a renewed sense of urgency must challenge tens of thousands of scientists to reinvent academic traditions and funding methods that even many well-funded researchers concede no longer work.

The cancer burden has not gone away with the strategy we have pursued for forty years. It has grown larger, not smaller. It is time for a change.

Part Three

The Cancer Culture

Chapter 8

The Wrong Bill

Without Ann Landers, there would never have been a war on cancer. The ever-popular syndicated columnist had spent the month of April 1971 offering wise counsel to readers on their cross-dressing husbands, profanity-spewing bosses ("Wear earmuffs in the office" was her advice), rebellious children, and burgeoning ham-radio romances. The offering on Tuesday, April 20, therefore, had to have come as a surprise. That day, she began by warning readers who might be "looking for a laugh" to skip her column altogether. Instead, she wrote, she would offer them the chance to "be part of an effort that might save millions of lives," maybe even their own:

> How many of us have asked the question, "If this great country of ours can put a man on the moon, why can't we find a cure for cancer?" One reason is that we have never launched a national campaign, a united effort, against this killer disease.

The column, in Landers's earnest voice, was striking for its simple power. She offered a slew of frightening statistics, including the fact that "more Americans died of cancer in 1969 than were killed in the four years of World War II." Then, the pen pal of the lovelorn and the in–law-challenged morphed into something she had never before been: a political activist. Telling readers they had an "opportunity to be a part of the mightiest offensive against a single disease in the history of our country," Landers urged "each and every person who reads this column to write to his two senators at once—or better yet, send telegrams"—in support of a bill that was then being batted around a Senate subcommittee. "Your message need consist of only three words," she instructed: " 'Vote for S. 34.' "

The column, syndicated in hundreds of newspapers across the country, was reprinted as a full-page advertisement in dozens more. An avalanche of envelopes arrived on Capitol Hill. One senator from New Jersey received more than eleven thousand constituent letters in a single week. Three thousand five hundred arrived in the mailroom for Senator Robert Byrd of West Virginia. Senator Alan Cranston of California got sixty thousand urgent messages over a five-week stretch. Senator Charles Percy, who represented Landers's home state of Illinois, said he had "never had such a tremendous response from any other issue."

The cascade of correspondence into Senate offices prompted a few secretaries and clerks to post IMPEACH ANN LANDERS signs on their desks. But the senators themselves were no doubt more anxious than angry. They knew a hot-button issue when they saw one. Nobody was dumb enough to stand in the way of legislation aimed at eradicating the most dread of human diseases.

By the time the full Labor and Public Welfare Committee in the Senate took up Senate bill 34, the measure, introduced by the senior senator from Massachusetts, Edward Kennedy, had fifty additional senators listed as cosponsors. Members of the House, not to be outdone, submitted dozens of their own bills to compete with the Senate version. Within a few months' time, sixty-four different resolutions had made their way onto the committee docket, nearly all variations on a theme: the Conquest of Cancer Act, the Vincent Thomas Lombardi Conquest of Cancer Act, the Act to Conquer Cancer, the National Cancer Attack Amendments.

The idea of an all-out assault on the disease—a "war on cancer"—had stormed into the public consciousness, even as the country was mired in a bitter conflict overseas. The *real* war in Southeast Asia was sending body bags home every day; the actual horror of guns and grenades was being replayed each evening on the television news. Vietnam, in 1971, was an open sore on the national psyche. But rather than shy away from battlefield imagery, many in Congress embraced it, even drawing direct comparison between the dread disease and the conflict in Vietnam.

One was a staunchly conservative, thirty-six-year-old freshman named Jack Kemp. The former all-star quarterback of the Buffalo Bills had just been elected that region's representative. After just months in office, he was being hailed as the emergent star of his class. He was articulate and more than a little cocksure for a first-termer. Yet it must have surprised his House elders a bit when he appeared to lecture them in a subcommittee session: "Let me remind you that cancer killed eight times as many Americans last year alone than have been killed in Vietnam during the past six years."

Dick Shoup, a Republican colleague from Missoula, Montana, who had seen combat in both the Second World War and Korea, likewise bemoaned what seemed to be a broad undercounting of cancer's perennial toll. He demanded to know, why has the "public outcry against senseless death" been "so resolutely focused on the casualties of the Vietnam War?" Meanwhile, few had "marched down the streets of America demonstrating against a casualty list" that was so vastly larger.

As inflamed as the rhetoric might have seemed, the mortality data backed it up. According to death certificates filed and tallied by the federal government, 337,398 American men, women, and children would die from cancer during 1971—a total that was 143 times the number of US soldiers who would be killed in Vietnam during the same year. For those who questioned the fairness of comparing a casualty list of mostly older cancer victims to flush-cheeked men dying in war, the data showed another surprise. Over the previous decade—the bloodiest years of the Vietnam campaign—more Americans aged fifteen through thirty-four had died stateside, from cancer, than had perished with their boots on overseas.

The scale of cancer's death and destruction may have been beyond the yardstick of Vietnam or any other conflict in history. But Cornelius E. Gallagher, Democrat of New Jersey, had found a more appropriate parallel, he believed. The seven–term congressman, who had commanded a rifle company in General Patton's Third Army, warned his colleagues that the cancer threat was akin to the most ominous danger the country faced: nuclear war. Except, unlike nuclear war, cancer had "already realized its potential for destruction by taking the lives of millions of persons throughout the world each year."

Frustrated that he had tried "every possible parliamentary maneuver, every potential political squeeze, and every conceivable public outcry" to commit the nation to fighting the cancer menace, the congressman confided to his fellow members that he had done something radical to jump-start the effort. Gallagher, a ranking member on the Foreign Affairs Committee, had written Soviet premier Alexei Kosygin a long and impassioned letter, begging him to start a kind of arm's race for a cancer cure; Gallagher felt only an aggressive effort by the Soviet Union would spur America to action.

"Just as the United States could not afford a missile gap," wrote the congressman, "neither could we possibly afford a cure gap. If you announced the firm goal of cancer cure, we would obviously have to close the gap by working with equal speed and dedication towards that goal." The Soviet leader replied, curtly, that the American's suggestion did not seem "to be appropriate."

The overwhelming sense in Congress, and across America, was that something dramatic ought to come of the moment. Fear could be tethered to aspiration. The American nation could eradicate cancer through force of will, just as it had harnessed the awesome power of the atom, just as it had sent a man to the moon and back. That notion of a great cancer crusade was powerful enough to break, if only briefly, a three-year political stalemate between the Republican administration of Richard Nixon and a Democratic-controlled Congress. And on December 23, 1971, it even brought the thirty-nine-year-old Teddy Kennedy to cheer on President Nixon, as the latter signed the National Cancer Act into law in the State Dining Room of the White House.

That day, at high noon, the president addressed his invited guests and the television cameras in the back of the room:

> I hope that in the years ahead that we may look back on this day and this action as being the most significant action taken during this administration. As a result of what has been done, as a result of the action which will come into being as a result of signing this bill, the Congress is totally committed to provide the funds that are necessary, whatever is necessary, for the conquest of cancer.

Nixon then promised the American people that "all the agencies of government" were now "totally committed" to the nation's new anti-cancer crusade. Seconds later he offered "a presidential commitment" and another "congressional commitment" and on top of that "a government commitment" and then "a total national commitment" to the cause. Finally, in case the message had somehow been missed, he thumped the point again: "You will have, of course, the total commitment of government, and that is what the signing of this bill now does."

The war on cancer had begun.

Seated in the front row during the signing ceremony, however, was one man who knew the great crusade was a figment. There would be no cancer war. And he, more than anyone else perhaps, had been the one to bring the bill to the president's desk.

After his remarks, the president had beckoned Benno Schmidt to stand and receive one of the official signing pens. The special implements, with their tiny presidential seals, were considered such a prize that President Johnson used to conjure up as many as possible for each bill. (Johnson would often sign each letter of his name in a different pen—and, occasionally, *parts* of each letter in a different pen—creating a generous serving of memorabilia and endless photo ops for the archives.) Nixon had used just two this time, one for his first name and the other for his last.

"Benno," said the president, "you get the 'Richard.'"

Schmidt had chaired the grandly named National Panel of

Consultants on the Conquest of Cancer, commissioned by the Senate to study the cancer problem and to recommend a course of action. The stolid, six-foot-tall Texan had been an unlikely candidate for the job. He had neither scientific nor medical nor legislative expertise. He had never before crafted health policy, was known to neither the National Cancer Institute nor the research establishment outside of Bethesda. Nor had he ever held a management role in any federal agency. His highest position in government had been to serve, after the Second World War, as general counsel for an obscure outfit in the State Department called the Foreign Liquidation Commission.

Not only was Schmidt *not* a politician, but to the extent that his political leanings were known, he was a Republican. That alone would ordinarily have preempted him from the role of lead spokesman for the cancer legislation, because the most important listeners in the Ninety-Second Congress, the committee and subcommittee chairmen, were Democrats. What Schmidt lacked in insider knowledge and bona fides, though, he made up for in natural leadership skills. He had been a law professor at the University of Texas, then taught briefly at Harvard. With the arrival of the war, he had joined the army, rising to the rank of colonel.

A chance phone call in 1945 from financier J. H. "Jock" Whitney led him to Wall Street, where he once again shot up the ranks. He was now a managing partner at Whitney's investment firm in New York. In this capacity he had amassed a small fortune by offering seed financing to start-up companies, a practice that was just beginning to be called venture capitalism. (Schmidt, it was said, had coined the term.)

As for cancer, the little he knew about the disease he had learned serving as a trustee for New York's Memorial Sloan–Kettering Cancer Center, a role that had little to do with science or medicine and everything to do with money and management. Still, in the end, it was largely Schmidt who would guide the National Cancer Act through the congressional gauntlet; it was he who would bridge the gap between various constituencies on the Panel of Consultants, in the Senate, the House, the Nixon administration, and the parties outside of government, too.

The sad irony was that Schmidt knew, as he was collecting the president's pen and shaking Mr. Nixon's hand, that the legislation he was being credited for helping to bring to fruition had little chance of working. He had testified as much before Congress.

The problem was that Nixon had signed the wrong bill. The cancer legislation that the president had just approved was not the one recommended by the Panel of Consultants in its November 1970 report. *This* bill was not the one that had prompted hundreds of thousands of citizens to write and telegram their senators the following spring; it was not the proposal that had been debated by the Senate and eventually passed by a vote of seventy-nine to one.

While the bill had plenty of similarities to the Senate's original version—including roughly the same generous $1.6 billion appropriation—there was one crucial disagreement: the Kennedy bill would have taken the cancer effort out of the NIH, creating a NASA-like National Cancer Authority whose mandate would be to approach the problem like another moon shot, essentially applying a "systems" management approach to a systems problem. The bill Nixon signed left everything pretty much the way it was, only with far more money.

The citizens' committee led by Schmidt had done a careful study of the way cancer research was being marshaled by the National Cancer Institute, how inefficiently dollars were being doled out and how slowly new information was being factored into decision–making. The process was not only arduous, bureaucratic, and tradition–bound, it also seemed to float outside of any vision of what needed to be done to reduce the cancer burden. There seemed to be no accounting of the pieces of the puzzle that were still missing; no plan for how to solve the crisis; no sense of priority for which of the countless unanswered questions ought to be given immediate attention and funding. And since there had never been a genuine and comprehensive assessment of progress along the way, there was equally no mechanism for recognizing what needed to be fixed.

The committee had no confidence whatsoever that an intensified research campaign—even with ample new funding—could work if left within the management structure of the National Institutes of Health. On the contrary, the mission would have a much better chance of success, the group concluded, if it was directed by a newly created entity that was stripped from the NIH, and that operated in total independence from that agency's budget authority and oversight.

"We would have much preferred to reach the other conclusion and to have recommended the present setup," Schmidt testified:

> but after much study and consideration we concluded that if the Congress were genuinely committed to conquering cancer, this could best be done in a National Cancer Authority. If the salvation of this nation depended upon our success in dealing with the cancer problem, I doubt that anyone familiar with the situation would recommend continuation of the present organizational arrangements.

Schmidt was a compelling witness. But what made the assessment both credible and powerful were those who stood beside him. Among the more prominent members of the Panel of Consultants was Sidney Farber, perhaps the best-known cancer doctor in the world. Trained as a pathologist, Farber had developed a new type of chemotherapy, a drug that blocked the B vitamin folate, that had achieved the first true remissions in childhood leukemia. His discovery, and the boldness with which he had pursued it at Boston Children's Hospital, had made him a national hero.

Farber was joined on the committee by two fellow pioneers in chemotherapy, James Holland of Buffalo's venerable cancer center, Roswell Park, and Joe Burchenal, of Memorial Sloan–Kettering. The group included surgeons such as Lee Clark, who presided over the MD Anderson Cancer Center, in Houston, and Seattle's Bill Hutchinson, who had founded a research institute named for his brother Fred Hutchinson, the major league pitcher and manager who had succumbed to lung cancer at the age of forty-five.

Radiologist Henry Kaplan, at Stanford, had been recruited, as had Wendell Scott, of Washington University in St. Louis, then the editor of *Cancer*, the biggest medical journal in the field. Also in the mix were a number of basic scientists such as Harold Rusch, professor of cancer research at Wisconsin's McCardle Laboratory, Sloan–Kettering's Mathilde Krim—and the most celebrated name on the list, Nobel Prize–winning geneticist Joshua Lederberg of Stanford University.

Completing the impressive panel was an equal number of lay members, ranging from top business and labor leaders to major philanthropists. It would have been difficult for anyone to suggest that the group, particularly the scientists and physicians among them, were either naïve to the problems facing cancer research or ignorant of the enormous scope of the challenge. These were cancer warriors who had been in the trenches and seen the devastation of the disease firsthand.

All of them expected to receive at least a little criticism for their dramatic recommendation for a new NASA-like National Cancer Authority. This idea was big, after all, one that challenged the comfortable status quo. What followed, however, wasn't blowback. It was a hurricane.

On July 7, the Senate passed its bill, seventy-nine to one. On September 16, the bill was dead. Only one person knew it, however.

That morning, Congressman Paul Grant Rogers, Democrat of Florida, thumped his gavel on the great horseshoe desk in Room 2172 of the Rayburn House Office Building. It was 10:00 a.m. and the chairman of the Public Health and Environment subcommittee began his second day of hearings on the cancer legislation.

The day before had brought the president's emissary Elliot Richardson, the secretary of the Department of Health, Education, and Welfare, to offer his unqualified support for the Senate bill. Rogers had thanked the secretary and sent him on his way.

Now, it was time to take the measure apart. The subcommittee chairman was not opposed to legislation addressing "the cancer problem." But the idea of rubber-stamping a Kennedy bill gnawed at the conservative Rogers. The congressman, whose dark-rimmed eyeglasses and thick, gray sideburns made him look older than his fifty years, had never been a fan of the Kennedys, having been one of the few Democrats in national office to refuse to back the Kennedy-Johnson ticket in 1960. Now, the seven-and-a-half-term representative was determined to hold his own damn hearings and write his own legislation.

The first witness that Thursday morning would help in that regard. Senator Gaylord Nelson, Democrat of Wisconsin, had been the lone nay in the Senate's vote on the Kennedy bill. It was rare for a dissenting senator to attempt to scuttle a bill passed in his own chamber by offering a second round of testimony on the other end of the Capitol. And Nelson had not come to the House subcommittee without reservation. The Wisconsin senator, like most of his colleagues, had been deluged by mail on behalf of the cancer measure. (Nelson had received about six thousand letters.) But he had also gotten letters from key figures in science and medicine objecting to one of the Kennedy bill's central aims: to take the cancer research enterprise out of the NIH fold. The letters warned of disruption, wasteful duplication, and the dangers inherent in trying to produce scientific discovery by fiat. They warned that other disease groups would soon demand their own NASA-like missions. Some took it a step further, claiming that such an effort would destroy the NIH.

Other experts had contended, in testimony before the Senate, that there was no reason to do anything dramatic at all. The cancer problem was not yet ready to be managed. One professor at the University of California, a former federal health official, summed up the concern of many:

> Cancer is not simply an island waiting in isolation for a crash program to wipe it out. It is no way comparable to a moonshot, which requires mainly the mobilization of money, men, and facilities to put together in one imposing package the scientific know-how we already possess. Instead, the problem of cancer—or rather the problem of the various cancers—represents a complex, multifaceted challenge at least as perplexing as the problem of various infectious diseases. We do not know where the breakthroughs will come, and I think it would be a great mistake to begin to dismantle the NIH in favor of an untested approach.

Dr. Sol Spiegelman, the famous molecular biologist whose work would pave the way to recombinant DNA, told the committee, "An all-out effort to cure cancer at this time would be like trying to land a man on the moon without knowing Newton's laws of motion."

The Senate had heard these arguments, compelling as they were, and overruled them. As legitimate as the concerns might be, the present system clearly wasn't working. Cancer incidence and death had been rising furiously, and researchers seemed no closer either to understanding the disease, preventing it, or treating it effectively. Yes, there had been sporadic advances—including vastly improved treatments for childhood leukemia, Burkitt's lymphoma, Hodgkin's disease, and testicular cancer—but the overall battlefield had not changed for the better. Indeed, the available evidence indicated the disease burden was getting heavier. Cancer was now a greater problem of public health than ever before.

Nonetheless, the Nelson testimony provided Rogers with the rationale he needed to sink the Kennedy bill. And just as quickly as Ann Landers had changed the momentum in the Senate, another set of floodgates opened in the House. Rogers built on Nelson's concerns by inviting testimony from virtually every group in the country that represented academic scientists or physicians, all of whom singled out for attack the notion of an independent authority, which the Senate had proposed to call the Conquest of Cancer Agency (COCA). One by one, the groups sent strident letters, or witnesses, to testify against the Kennedy measure. Dr. John Hogness, president of the Institute of Medicine, an arm of the National Academy of Sciences, argued that the Senate bill promoted "fragmentation" of the scientific community and offered his support to an alternate bill introduced by Congressman Rogers. Thirteen scientists, including a number of Nobel laureates, signed a letter published in the *New York Times* saying that it was "hard to imagine a scheme with more potential for undermining the scientific integrity of the NIH."

The mighty Federation of American Societies for Experimental Biology (FASEB), representing six different guilds with some eleven thousand scientists, attacked the Kennedy bill, too, as did the Association of American Medical Colleges, speaking for its 103 schools, and the Association of Professors of Medicine, representing six dozen department heads. Leading physicians' groups, such as the American Medical Association and the American College of Physicians, weighed in with criticism. So did organizations representing pathologists, bacteriologists, and biochemists. Even groups of dentists and veterinarians contacted the Rogers subcommittee to slam the Kennedy bill and offer strong support for the House resolution. Dozens of cancer center directors, researchers, and professors sent separate letters—nearly all in similar language and format, as though following a template.

The barrage was so overwhelming that two of the members on Benno Schmidt's once-unanimous panel retracted their support for the Kennedy bill, claiming they had not understood the full ramifications of the autonomous cancer authority. Drs. Lederberg and Kaplan now preferred Rogers's bill, which left everything the way it was.

While many of the arguments were powerful, a subtext was easy to read. The scientists and clinical researchers who had fared well under the current collegially managed funding system—the tradition known as peer review—feared what a new, top-down authority would mean. There was even talk that the proposed COCA, like NASA, would use some sort of "contract" mechanism to pay researchers and others to complete specific projects. It was hard to imagine a concept more anathema to the scientific community.

"Much of the great progress we have witnessed derives from the now well-proved system of research grant awards through peer review," wrote the president of the National Academy of Sciences. "It is my earnest hope that this well-tried mechanism will be preserved."

The program specified in the Senate bill, wrote the director of the American Federation for Clinical Research, "proposes a deviation in the pattern of federal support of medical research which could be, in the long run, detrimental to the cancer program itself."

The director of the Fox Chase Center, in Philadelphia, got to the point: "The deficiency in cancer research rests in a lack of funds, rather than in agencies to dispense them."

The problem was *money*—not management. Medical science did not need to be pushed one way or another, they said; it did not need to be fixed. It needed to be left alone.

As with nearly every other major piece of legislation, the final language of the National Cancer Act was not determined in the open air of the House or the Senate, not in subcommittee hearings or in public debate, but in a nether realm of government called the conference committee. This committee was the proverbial smoke-filled room where the real power was concentrated, an institution that the Nebraska senator George Norris once christened the "third branch of Congress."

The Founding Fathers had never envisioned this intersection on the legislative path. The Constitution does not specify any formal process for hammering out the differences between the House and the Senate versions of a bill, instructing that each group must pass an "identical" measure before it can be offered to the president for his signature.

The cancer legislation that emerged from conference once again carried the name and number of the Senate bill. The language, however, was written by Rogers. The National Cancer Act had become a bundle of requisitions. There were orders to train an army of scientists, to build fifteen new centers for clinical studies, and to create an "international cancer research data bank" that would supposedly collect the untold bits of acquired knowledge, catalog them in useful ways, and disseminate the wisdom to physicians and scientists everywhere. The act established a prominent National Cancer Advisory Board, replete with citizens and scientists, to help guide the effort and, presumably, to prod the government bureaucrats into faster action. It also gave the director of the National Cancer Institute what seemed to some an extraordinary privilege: allowing him or her to bypass the normal governmental channels and submit an annual budget request directly to the president.

The stand-alone agency, the NASA-like mission that had so appealed to the Senate, was gone. There, in its stead, was a pile of cash. Cancer researchers in 1972 would have at their disposal close to double the money that had been granted just two years earlier. But that was a pittance in relation to what was to come. By 1976, Congress would double the NCI's kitty once again, to $762 million. Four years later, the cancer agency's budget would break the billion-dollar mark. It would have been hard for scientists in the winter of 1971 to imagine the scope of federal funding for cancer research four decades hence, when annual budgets would top $5 billion (and when grants from other funders both public and private would contribute twice that much to research efforts per year).

The cancer research community did not know what it had lost in the frenzied reconciliation of the two cancer bills. Nor, it seemed, did the members of Congress who stood behind the president after the bill signing, posing for photographers. But something substantial indeed had been swallowed up by the murky waters of the conference committee—something that went well beyond organization. What had been lost was the sense of mission.

The government had quietly dropped its commitment to an all-out, coordinated assault. Apart from the huge influx of money, the nation's new cancer effort was little different from the old one.

What had been lost was the *story.* The war on cancer was not a war at all. Nor was it the "moon shot" so many Americans had hoped for, and which the original Senate legislation, naïvely or not, had intended to launch. The new bill was the stuff of advisory boards and appropriations, of endless study and policy papers, of conferences and name tags. There were no deadlines, no accountability, no risk, no leaps into the unknown, no dark side of the moon.

The National Cancer Act offered no great crusade for the American people to share together. There was no story to tell. There was simply more money to spend.

Chapter 9

The "Door" Question

Mr. Sam Donaldson [news correspondent]: Dr. Klausner, if
these grant requests, that have gone through peer review,
that show some promise—and not someone saying let us flap
a bedsheet at the aurora borealis—were all funded, all ten
doors, how much money, sir?

Dr. Richard Klausner [NCI director]: We believe that to do that
would require a doubling of the NCI budget in three years.

Mr. Donaldson: Then let us do it. Then let us do it.

Hearings before a subcommittee of the Committee
on Appropriations, US Senate, May 7, 1997

The Senate hearing that morning in the Hart Office Building was
billed as a commemoration of the twenty-fifth anniversary of the
National Cancer Act. But each of the witnesses waiting to testify in Hart's
cavernous Room 216, as well as the assembled media, knew the point of
that morning's gathering was not to commemorate anything. The day was
about money.

This was the spring ritual known as markup, when Appropriations
subcommittee chairmen hold public hearings on Congress's twelve annual spending bills, reassign dollar figures to the president's thousands
of proffered budget items, dole out earmarks to the favored, squeeze the
disfavored, and openly revel in the power vested therein.

It was a heady time even for veteran Senate chieftains. But if Arlen Specter of Pennsylvania, chair of the health and labor subcommittee, now framed against an imperial marble backdrop, seemed especially jaunty this morning, it might have had something to do with the witness list. Rather than the usual humdrum assortment of agency officials and miscellaneous experts, the three-day roster of speakers for these "special hearings" boasted plenty of star power—enough that the second day of testimony, scheduled for three weeks later, would have to be held in Beverly Hills. (Sally Field, Diane Keaton, Olivia Newton–John, and Jack Klugman would headline that session.) As for today's lineup, the celebrities formed a more eclectic group, including golf legend Arnold Palmer, who had recently been diagnosed with prostate cancer and whose daughter had survived breast cancer. It was no secret why each of the speakers was there. Each had come to ask for more federal funding for cancer research.

Richard Klausner, the director of the National Cancer Institute, wanted more, too, of course. But Klausner, a well-respected cell biologist who had been thrust into the directorship of the National Cancer Institute less than two years earlier, was not allowed to ask—or not, at least, if proper protocol was to be observed. The National Cancer Act gives the NCI director the rare opportunity to present a budget request directly to the president, bypassing the ordinary chain of command—up through the director of the National Institutes of Health (the NCI is but one of twenty-seven research institutes and centers in the NIH), then through bosses at *its* parent agency, the Department of Health and Human Services, and so forth. But even then, there are rules. One cannot ask for the sky and the moon. The public's resources are limited. Every agency and cause has its own constituency, activist community, and lobby demanding a larger share.

Klausner had already submitted his "professional judgment budget" for 1998 to the White House, requesting a respectable 20 percent or so spike over the previous year's allotment of funds. The extra money, he testified, would "allow us to find what we believe are the immediately accessible and achievable opportunities." But that was not what either the senators or the crowd gathered in Hart 216 wanted to hear. Klausner's answer, it seemed, had been hemmed to the question of what the NCI could make do with—not to how much money was needed to satisfy every "blue sky" project and clinical trial on the agency's wish list.

Tom Harkin of Iowa, the senior Democrat on the subcommittee, explained the general disappointment in the crowd:

> You say, well, how much money do you need, and I say, I do not know, but I always look upon the research, Dr. Klausner, and we have talked about this before. It is like you have got ten doors, and those doors are all closed, and the answer may lie behind one of those doors. Well, if you are going to open one out of ten doors, your chances, your odds are what?—ten to one, nine to one that you are not going to find it. Those are overwhelming odds. Right now, we are funding two out of ten, two and a half out of ten, something like that, of—and those are the research proposals that have gone through the peer review process.

It was then that one of the stranger things to happen during a cancer appropriations hearing happened. An NCI director, probably much to his own surprise, revealed the magic number: the optimal funding level that would put cancer research where, at long last, it needed to be. The moment occurred when Harkin finished his remarks and noticed that one of the committee's prominent witnesses was twitching in his seat. The man was Sam Donaldson, the famously blunt ABC News correspondent, who was also a melanoma survivor.

> **Senator Harkin:** Did you have something, Sam, that you wanted to say?
>
> **Sam Donaldson:** This is a national emergency. And if you put it on that basis, Americans will respond. Because it is not something esoteric. Scientists tell us that if we do not get ahold of the hole in the ozone layer, it may kill us all. But it is not something people understand. Their mother did not die immediately, that they can see, from the hole in the ozone layer. But their mother died of cancer. Their best friend has it. They themselves may have it. Now, you gentlemen are on

the right track. Here is the question I would like you to put to Dr. Klausner. Not how much money can you *use*. He has got many considerations, as you well know far better than I, in how he has to frame his answer. Put the "door" question to him. Dr. Klausner, if we open all ten doors, how much money would that take?

He is freed now from having to worry about the other considerations and the other people that he has to worry about.

Senator Specter: Dr. Klausner, would you answer Senator Donaldson's question? [Laughter.]

Mr. Donaldson: Dr. Klausner, if these grant requests, that have gone through peer review, that show some promise—and not someone saying let us flap a bedsheet at the aurora borealis—were all funded, all ten doors, how much money, sir?

Dr. Klausner: We believe that to do that would require a doubling of the NCI budget in three years.

Mr. Donaldson: Then let us do it. Then let us do it.

Just one factor is holding back victory in the cancer war, say many generals and warriors alike, and that is a lack of money. The belief is so widespread, it has assumed the status of truism: we are ever so close to "a cure," the only thing that stands in our way is a paucity of funding for research.

That is what one invited speaker after another has, for years, been telling the President's Cancer Panel—whose role, per the National Cancer Act, is to gather testimony from experts on barriers to the cancer effort and report back to the president. Participants in the PCP's 2007 and 2008 meetings, for example, "were unanimous in their view that the US biomedical research enterprise as a whole was being starved of funding at a pivotal juncture." Years of "flat funding"—budgets that either had not been increasing or had been rising so modestly that they could not keep pace with the soaring cost of laboratory work—had resulted in "little or no growth in the number of grants awarded, curtailed and deferred research projects and clinical trials, closed or unrefurbished laboratories, and reduced staffing at many of the 3,000 institutions that conduct research with NIH grant funds."

That was the message when, in March 2007, a group of nine prominent "concerned universities and research institutions"* took the unusual step of publishing a twenty-four-page "statement" on research funding, entitled "Within Our Grasp—Or Slipping Away?" In one testimonial after another, star scientists spoke harrowingly of the funding crisis at the NIH and its flagship research center, the National Cancer Institute, and about what this would do to cures-on–the-brink. A year later, when a second collection of universities issued a follow-up statement, the appeal was more urgent still, as the title—"A Broken Pipeline? Flat Funding of the NIH Puts a Generation of Science at Risk"—made clear.

So, too, Congressman Brian Higgins of Buffalo, a junior member of the powerful House Ways & Means Committee, made the point in early 2010, telling congressional colleagues: "*The only failure* in cancer research is when we quit, or when we are forced to quit because of lack of funding." If US taxpayers were only to give the NCI enough funding to open "all ten doors," as Sam Donaldson put it a decade and a half ago, we would end the plague of cancer as we know it. That is the message: plain, simple, obvious. And yet it is also not true.

Unfortunately, a bounty of new funding for the NCI, welcome as it would be to thousands of cancer researchers, would do little to ease the national cancer burden. The truth—in 1971, as now—is that winning the war on cancer will not be achieved simply by a doubling or even quadrupling of dollars.

This statement is sacrilege. It goes against every talking point, every fund-raising letter, every urgent charitable appeal. Not a soul testifying before Congress in 1997, alongside Sam Donaldson, would have

---

*The University of California, Columbia University, Harvard University, Johns Hopkins University, Partners Healthcare (Brigham & Women's Hospital and Massachusetts General), the University of Texas at Austin, Washington University in St. Louis, the University of Wisconsin, Madison, and Yale University.

ventured such a thought, nor has anyone in any congressional hearings since. The dedicated academic scientists, whose work might well be sustained by such dollars, will scream and shout at the heresy. Advocates and volunteers in the cancer fight will rise up in arms. Many will see such a claim as an unwarranted attack on hope itself.

A lack of funding, however, is *not* the major barrier to progress against cancer. Nor by itself will "more research"—the corollary to "more money"—win the cancer war. At least, not *as long as the current systems remain in place.* This is not an attack on hope; it is a call for change.

To understand why, we have only to look at past funding for cancer research. From the founding of the National Cancer Institute, in 1937, through the end of the 1960s, Congress gave the agency less than $2 billion in total. In the decade of the 1970s alone, after passage of the National Cancer Act and the launching of the modern war on cancer, the NCI received more than $6 billion. Yet even this amount was modest in relation to what was to come. Total appropriations would double during the 1980s, to roughly $12 billion. By 1993, a single year's budget for the National Cancer Institute would begin to top $2 billion, more than what had been spent in the 1940s, 1950s, and 1960s combined.

Still, the rate of funding would accelerate. Between 1998 and 2003, the annual NCI allocation would leap from $2.5 billion to $4.6 billion, a five-year growth rate of 80 percent. It was not quite the budget doubling that Sam Donaldson had appealed for so eloquently at the 1997 Senate hearings (though Congress would indeed more than double its yearly allotment for NCI's parent, the NIH, during this time), but the implicit promise behind the dramatic boost was largely the same: the nation's cancer research enterprise would have enough money available, in theory anyway, for scientists to open most, if not quite all, of those "ten doors."

Of course, that would not be the case. There would always be more doors to open and more money needed to do it. So, as high as federal cancer funding got during the 1990s, Congress would, again, more than double that ten–year total during the first decade of the 2000s. After adjusting for inflation, the NCI's over $5 billion allocation in 2010 was more than five times the size of the one in 1970.* Funding for the National Cancer Institute has grown under Republican and Democratic administrations, under Congresses hewing to either end of the political spectrum, in times of war as well as peace, through boom periods and recessions. Cancer has always been a bipartisan disease.

The appropriation to the National Cancer Institute is the "official" cancer war chest. In reality, however, it is merely a portion of what is spent annually fighting the disease. While the NCI is the only center at the National Institutes of Health expressly devoted to the anticancer effort, it is not the only one that doles out money for the cause. A few of NCI's sister institutes award hundreds of millions of dollars in grants each year for cancer research. So do federal agencies outside of the NIH (such as the CDC, the Defense Department, and even the Postal Service). So do many state governments.

Matching this public investment is a private one that has gotten dramatically more ambitious since the cancer war began. The pharmaceutical industry now spends as much as $8 billion each year in the United States researching and developing cancer drugs—a sum that, among other things, pays for the lion's share of drug clinical trials for the disease. (After adjusting for inflation, that's roughly an eightfold increase over what the industry spent on cancer-related research and development in 1980.) The American Cancer Society raises an impressive $1 billion a year and spends almost three-quarters of it on anticancer programs. Several other nonprofit organizations contribute anywhere from tens to hundreds of millions of dollars each, while hundreds upon hundreds of other groups collect smaller amounts for the cause. As of the end of 2010, the Internal Revenue Service recognized 2,786 distinct cancer-focused charities.

All told, the money invested in cancer research in the United States exceeds $16 billion each year—more than three times the budget of the

---

*For comparison, the entire federal budget grew just over three times, adjusted for inflation, during the same period. Not included in the NCI budget figures for 2009 and 2010 are roughly $1.3 billion in additional cancer-related funding through the American Recovery and Reinvestment Act (ARRA), intended as a jobs stimulus program.

National Cancer Institute. The money has paid for some good science, created tens of thousands of jobs, and improved scientific understanding of cancer. Without question, some of those discoveries have saved lives. However, America's four-decade investment in cancer research—a total of more than $300 billion (inflation–adjusted) in taxpayer spending, private R&D, and donations—has not stopped, or even substantially slowed, the soaring cancer burden. "More money" has not solved the problem.

As argued in Part II of this book, the primary reason for this failure has been our nearly exclusive focus on trying to "cure" extraordinarily complex, advanced cancers through drugs that target one broken genetic mechanism or another rather than on trying to preempt those cancers from progressing in the first place. No amount of money can end the cancer problem if more people keep developing the disease. But setting that overarching issue aside for now, it is worth digging into another mystery: The billions of dollars spent so far have not, arguably, accomplished goals that might have seemed far more achievable, those where the connection between funding and outcomes would appear to be straightforward. The question is, why? Why, for instance, despite our substantial investment, have the professional lives of cancer scientists gotten *harder* over the past forty years rather than easier? (For we'll see in a moment that they have.) And more surprising, if the whole point of increased cancer funding is to open more of those Sam Donaldson "doors," why are so few new ones being opened from year to year?

In the answers to these two questions, I believe, are at least some of the reasons why just putting more money into the NCI's coffers will do little to speed progress—and perhaps even a few clues as to what we should do now.

On its face, the rationale seems uncontestable: increasing the pool of NCI grant money buys more unrestricted research time—more freedom, in short—for scientists to study the disease. Yet that is not the case. Cancer scientists today do not, in truth, have more freedom to study the disease than they did two generations ago. By nearly every measure policy experts use, "doing science" today is more difficult than it was then, starting with the most familiar challenge for any researcher: getting a grant. Though the overall NIH budget soared from $1.5 billion in 1972 to $30.9 billion in 2011, biomedical researchers now have less than half the chance they had in 1972 of securing significant NIH funding for their work. (That year, 41 percent of grant applications to the NIH were successful, compared with just 18 percent in 2011.) Current grant success rates at the National Cancer Institute are actually lower, hovering under 14 percent—or at half the level they were just nine years earlier, when the cancer agency had a billion dollars less at its disposal.

The dreary success rates have forced researchers to devote an ever greater share of their time to the grant application process rather than to doing science, says John P. A. Ioannidis, chair of disease prevention at Stanford University, and a professor of both medicine and health research policy at Stanford University School of Medicine. "It's a major problem," he says. "Probably scientists spend about half of their time writing grants, or thinking about grants, or reviewing grants, or managing grants, or administering grants, or dealing with nonscientific issues about grants. And all of that time is completely lost." The prospect of securing NIH funding has become so challenging, and the process so time-consuming, that many seasoned investigators with stellar résumés and long histories of grant success say they sense a hovering uncertainty when it comes to the future of their work, their laboratories, and their independence.

For younger scientists, though, it has reached a crisis stage. As the 2008 appeal from "concerned universities and research institutions" mentioned near the top of this chapter begins: "The most promising young investigators at premier academic research institutions are struggling under tremendous financial pressures. They are having a hard time getting their research done—research that could save lives. As a result, a generation of scientific discovery is at risk." In 1980, for example, new investigators got their first major NIH grant, essentially launching their so-called independent research pursuits, at an average age of thirty-six; today, it is forty-two. In 1980, more than four in ten NIH research project grants (RPGs) were awarded to a principal investigator under the age of forty. That share is now one in ten.

But scientists are not spending their thirties and early forties just applying for (and not getting) research grants; they are often looking for academic homes, too. Four decades ago, more than half of those earning a PhD in the life sciences secured a tenure-track faculty position within six years. That share has since fallen to about 15 percent. "Exceptionally bright science PhD holders from elite academic institutions are slogging through five or ten years of poorly paid postdoctoral studies, slowly becoming disillusioned by the ruthless and often fruitless fight for a permanent academic position," inveighed the editors of *Nature* in 2011, echoing the frustration of NIH director Francis Collins, who had published much the same lament in the same journal the year before. Collins, for his part, had merely echoed his own predecessor in office, Elias Zerhouni, and a fair number of blue-ribbon commissions. If the current trend continues, by one estimate, the number of investigators over age sixty-eight receiving NIH grants will exceed the number under thirty-eight by the year 2020.

Making it harder for young researchers, in particular, has been a flood of competition. The doubling of the NIH budget during the Clinton years, Zerhouni has pointed out, brought a parallel doubling in grant applications, the number rising from around twenty-four thousand in 1998 to nearly fifty thousand in 2007, with an increasing proportion of those coming from early-career scientists and newly minted PhDs. The surge in life scientists, however, has not just increased competition for grants all around, it has led to a second phenomenon: crowded laboratories. Senior investigators have absorbed most of these masses of unfunded postdocs, predocs, and fellows into their labs, finding modest research roles for brilliant, frustrated thirtysomethings. To accommodate these swelling labs and research teams, universities have grabbed a significant share of NIH dollars to expand existing research facilities and build new ones. The result of this crowding and expansion, seen in Figure 7, has been bigger, longer, and more expensive scientific projects—but not such a big increase in the actual number of them. That is how "more money" can end up opening relatively few additional research doors.

In 1975, the National Cancer Institute spent $131 million (or roughly $531 million in 2010 dollars) to fund 2,042 various scientific investigations, known in the jargon as research project grants (RPGs). Roughly a quarter of those awards (and 23 percent of all grant dollars) supported new investigative projects. In 2010, the institute devoted more than $2 billion to research projects in total, but it spent proportionately less (18 percent) on new investigations, funding 1,041 of such projects. The overwhelming share of the agency's grant money instead went to supporting continuing research efforts the NCI had approved in previous award cycles.

The size of individual grants has in the meantime grown substantially, rising some 70 percent for new awards on top of inflation. (In nominal dollars, the average new award has risen nearly sixfold since 1975.) This grant-size inflation, importantly, is not driven by the price tags for the state-of-the-art instruments of cancer genetics and molecular imaging— which might, were it the case, be alleviated by an infusion of money. The equipment of modern science accounts for just around 6 percent of the cost of running a lab. Today's cancer research teams spend most of their grant money (65 percent or more) on people—that is to say, on the salaries and benefits of the lead investigators, plus those for legions of postdoctoral students, research fellows, technicians, and administrative employees who work in support of the lab.

Figure 7

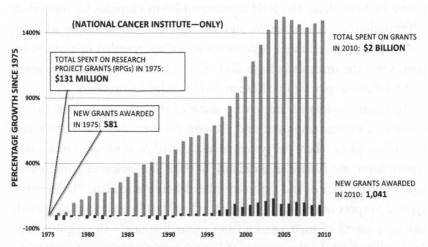

MORE FUNDING, YES — BUT FEW "NEW DOORS" ARE BEING OPENED

(NATIONAL CANCER INSTITUTE—ONLY)

TOTAL SPENT ON RESEARCH PROJECT GRANTS (RPGs) IN 1975: **$131 MILLION**

NEW GRANTS AWARDED IN 1975: **581**

TOTAL SPENT ON GRANTS IN 2010: **$2 BILLION**

NEW GRANTS AWARDED IN 2010: **1,041**

NOTES: Refers to new "competing" RPG awards, not grant renewals or supplementals; the NCI also funds continuing projects with "non-competing" awards. Counting all grants together, the NCI made 5,079 RPG awards, compared with 2,042 in 1975.
SOURCES: *NCI Fact Books* for 1977, 1983, 1987, 1993, 2002, and 2010.

Cancer investigators are not getting rich. Academic salaries are generally meager. Student debt, for postdocs and fellows, in particular, can be despairingly high. The problem is that, today, each NIH grant must feed more institutional mouths than ever—and that includes mouths that have only a tenuous connection to the research itself. Each research project grant from the NIH, for example, not only supports those in the lab (the "direct" costs of the study), but also an abundance of personnel at the institution where the research is being conducted (the "indirect" costs). Three of every ten dollars doled out by institutes of the NIH goes to reimburse universities and research centers for these indirect or "facilities and administrative" costs. The fees are used to keep the lights on in the lab, pay for common facilities, libraries, and journal subscriptions, and to cover the personnel costs of everyone from secretaries to deans.

Every university charges its own indirect rate, which it negotiates separately with individual government funding agencies (such as the NIH or Department of Energy) every few years. At Johns Hopkins, for example, the rate in effect in January 2010 was 64 percent, meaning that for every $100,000 awarded to a Hopkins grant applicant to pursue a specific project, an additional $64,000 (39 percent of the total award amount) is given to the university for common expenses. To put that in real-dollar terms: in 2010 alone, the NIH reimbursed Johns Hopkins for more than $200 million in administrative and overhead costs. The money adds up, as Congress's Government Accountability Office revealed in a recent report. Over the three years from 2003 through 2005, US taxpayers spent $12.5 billion to pay for overhead at NIH-funded institutions.

In theory, taxpayers are paying some of that money to keep young medical scientists employed and chasing the next big discoveries. But here is one place where the system breaks down. As made clear in a recent report from the American Academy of Arts and Sciences authored by four Nobel laureates and eighteen other leading scientists: "Universities typically expect or require . . . medical school faculty members to provide half or even all of their salaries from research funds." The requirements are hardly secret. In the nine years I spent talking with young scientists, few did not acknowledge, in some way, the pressure of having to "put up" (with an NIH research award) or "shove out," pressure that keeps the per-petual grant-writing cycle in motion.

The current system of research funding "is just a terrible economic model," says one of those young researchers, E. Ray Dorsey at Johns Hopkins—who, as it happens, knows something about economic mod-els. Five years after getting his undergraduate degree in biology at Stan-ford, he earned his medical degree from the University of Pennsylvania and an MBA in health care management from the Wharton School. Then he spent three years as a consultant with McKinsey & Company before doing his medical residency back at Penn. Imagine, says Dorsey, now forty, if we had the same system of funding and training in the air force as we do at the NIH:

> The air force might weed out some of its pilots. But it would be against the government's interest for most of the pilots it fully trains *not* to suc-ceed and *not* to fly planes. In academic research, you have people who do all this training—often ten years or more postcollege—and then end up not using it. And some of that training is sponsored by taxpayers, directly or indirectly. It's just not a good model. It strikes me odd that history professors get a large portion of their salary funded by university tuition. But medical school faculty have to fund one hundred percent of their salary, or a large portion of it [through grants and fellowships]. And that leaves medical researchers to spend a lot of their time raising funds, and less of their time doing the work they were trained to do.

One obvious cost is that many young investigators are growing so de-moralized that they are abandoning once-promising research careers. And some prominent cancer scientists say they cannot blame them. "For the first time in thirty-three years," Robert Weinberg, the legendary biologist and cofounder of MIT's Whitehead Institute, told thousands of attendees at the 2006 meeting of the American Association for Cancer Research, "I can no longer tell [young investigators] with a straight face to go into cancer research. Because for the first time in a third of a century, there doesn't seem to be much of a future for them."

The profound danger for all of us is that, as young investigators quit or are pushed to into "postdoc purgatory," as one scientist put it, the national cancer effort loses some of its best ideas and idea generators. "Younger scientists," says Dartmouth's Michael Sporn, are overwhelmingly more likely "to have the unorthodox, new ideas that we need in order to solve the cancer problem."

To illustrate the point, many within the research community point to a well-studied group of path-setters: those who have won the Nobel Prize. Between 1980 and 2010, ninety-six scientists received the Nobel Prize for work related to biomedicine, according to research by Kirstin Matthews and colleagues at the James A. Baker III Institute for Public Policy at Rice University in Houston. Six in ten of these laureates published their Nobel Prize-cited discoveries before the age of forty-two.* Yet, the more money that flows into the system each year, the less, proportionately, seems to go to those most likely to come up with revolutionary ideas.

The fix that most scientific leaders recommend, of course, is a circular one, and that is to increase research funding overall. But apart from that discussed above, there is yet one more reason even a giant boost in federal funding won't change the paradigm. And this also helps explain why much of the cancer research community feels starved for funds *and* why so few new scientific "doors" are opened each year. The reason concerns not how young or old the investigators are, but where they are: in short, we keep giving money to the same researchers, at the same small group of research institutions, with much the same research cultures and training. Is it any wonder that radically new approaches to solving cancer's biological mysteries—ones that, in effect, challenge the prevailing scientific views at these same research centers—do not often emerge? (And when

---

*More striking, perhaps, is when Nobel Prize winners actually came up with their ground-breaking insights. In a 2007 paper aptly titled "The Optimal Age to Start a Revolution," published in the *Journal of Creative Behavior,* cognitive neuroscientists Arne Dietrich and Narayanan Srinivasan recorded the age at which all 493 Nobel Prize laureates in physics, chemistry, and physiology/medicine between the years 1901 and 2003 first alit upon their paradigm-shifting ideas. The peak age was thirty-four. Only nineteen of the laureates (3.8 percent) were fifty or older at the moment of brainstorm, according to the scientists' own reporting (in Nobel Prize lectures, autobiographies, et cetera).

they do emerge, is it likely that grant reviewers from these same institutions will recognize their merit?)

NIH leaders and supporters routinely state that the health agency funds biomedical research at "more than 3,000" universities, medical schools, and other centers of science across the United States. (The actual number is closer to 2,600 today.) But this number has a big footnote. In 2011, the top 43 research centers got more funding ($12 billion) than did the bottom 2,574 institutions receiving any kind of NIH support, whether in the form of a grant, fellowship, or contract. Scientists at the 1,100 schools and centers on the bottom of the list split between them a mere 1 percent of the total research funding during 2011.

The same pattern can be seen in the prior year, when half of all NIH dollars went to just 37 institutions, and over 90 percent to the top 200. And so it has gone, at least as far back as 1987, when the General Accounting Office, investigating on behalf of the US Congress, reported a similar concentration.

The biggest institutional grant-getters almost never change from year to year. The six leading recipients of NIH money in 2011 are the same universities, if in slightly varied order, that led the list in 2010 and 2009; the ranking for 2008 differs by one name only. Likewise, in terms of National Cancer Institute funding alone, the same six research institutions* have led the list for years.

To those in the top tier, of course, there is nothing surprising about this record. The money goes where the best science and scientists are. As the CEO and faculty dean of Johns Hopkins Medicine told colleagues in 2005, "The NIH ranking is merely testimony to your hard work and commitment to excellence."

But there is, indeed, something remarkable about the NIH rankings that cannot be seen from a quick glance, and it sheds yet more light on why "more money" has not come close to solving the cancer crisis. Not only are the top dozen, or fifty, or one hundred ranks filled, year after

---

*The University of Texas/MD Anderson Cancer Center, Fred Hutchinson Cancer Center, Johns Hopkins University, Dana-Farber Cancer Institute, University of Michigan–Ann Arbor, and Sloan–Kettering Institute for Cancer Research.

year, by the same universities and research hospitals, so, too, have their relative positions on the list remained essentially unchanging.

Table 4

Top Recipients of NIH Funding

Institution	Rank*							
	2011	2010	2009	2008	2007	2006	2005	2004
Johns Hopkins University	1	1	1	1	1	1	1	1
Univ. of California–San Francisco	2	3	2	2	4	4	4	4
Univ. of Pennsylvania	3	2	3	3	2	2	2	3
Univ. of Michigan–Ann Arbor	4	5	4	4	6	6	7	6
Univ. of Washington	5	4	6	5	3	3	3	2
Univ. of Pittsburgh	6	6	5	7	7	9	9	8
Univ. of California–San Diego	7	7	10	12	12	12	14	12
Yale University	8	9	11	9	10	10	10	11
Washington University	9	8	8	6	8	8	5	5
Univ. of California–Los Angeles	10	10	7	10	9	7	8	7
Duke University	11	11	9	8	5	5	6	9
Univ. of North Carolina–Chapel Hill	12	12	13	11	11	14	16	16

*Out of the roughly 2,600 to 3,000 public and private research institutions that receive financial support each year. Does not include contract funding for Science Applications International Corp. (SAIC), a Fortune 500 company. Among its work for the federal government, SAIC operates a National Cancer Institute research center in Frederick, Maryland. Overall funding for some university research systems may be larger than it appears in this league table because funding is measured separately for each individual component. For example, if one counts together NIH awards to Harvard University Medical School, Harvard University School of Public Health, and Harvard University (each of which the NIH considers separate entities), "Harvard" would rank number 8 in 2011 funding, just above Yale. If one also includes in this total funding for Dana-Farber Cancer Institute and Massachusetts General Hospital, which many consider to be part of the "Harvard system," then Harvard would have garnered more than $866 million in NIH funding in 2011, placing it first on the list. SOURCES: NIH Reporter Tool (2004 and 2005); Blue Ridge Institute for Medical Research (2006 through 2011). The NIH stopped publishing such lists after 2005—a change it made in part because of "responses received from the grantee community suggesting that ranking tables were not necessary."

Most obvious in this regard is the reign of Johns Hopkins, which has received more research dollars than any other school each year since 1992, an unbroken streak of two decades. But equally notable, if less obvious, is that Vanderbilt University has, for four straight years (2008 through 2011), occupied the 15th spot on the rankings. The University of Louisville, likewise, was the 100th biggest NIH money-winner in 2011, just as it was in 2010; those same two years, Montana State University in Bozeman came in at position no. 195. And so the general patterns hold up and down the list from one year to the next.

The seemingly immutable nature of the grant-getting pecking order is not just a quirky phenomenon. It reveals something important about the medical-research-funding process itself: It suggests the system is neither as purely "science-driven" nor as merit-based as it has been held up to be. After all, if the peer-review process—the age-old method by which grant applications are evaluated—were truly blind to all but the quality of the proposals at hand, research awards would certainly be spread more randomly throughout the academic arena. Such randomness would at the least be seen within the top echelons of medical research, where institutions compete fiercely with one another for star faculty and prodigious grant-getters.

There would have to be one year when Johns Hopkins's NIH funding (hovering, since 2004, at $600 million a year) dipped below that of a rival—or one year when Stanford University fell lower than sixteenth place, or when Penn did not crack the top five. That such movement so seldom happens suggests that something besides the fickle hands of creativity and entrepreneurial spirit is driving the process: the system may not be rigged, in the familiar sense; but the status quo is nonetheless maintained by the traditions of an ancient academic culture—one that rewards a certain kind of science from a certain kind of investigator at a certain kind of institution and largely rejects the rest. (The extraordinary system through which this plays out will be revealed in the following chapter.)

Brian Druker, the scientist at the center of the development of the drug Gleevec, and now director of the Oregon Health & Science University's (OHSU) Knight Cancer Institute, says he has thought long and hard about the implications of the "haves and have-nots" issue in cancer funding. "You look at what comes out of the big research institutions and it's fabulous," says Druker, who left Harvard (and its affiliated Dana-Farber Cancer Institute network) for OHSU in 1993, and who would sixteen years later win a Lasker Award, what many consider to be America's Nobel Prize. "In part, I don't know that I could have done what I did had I not trained in the Harvard system, made the connections that I did, and gotten the background I did. On the other hand," he says, "I probably couldn't have done what I did if I didn't *leave* the Harvard system."

One of the problems that I have with the Harvards, the Stanfords, the Johns Hopkinses, is that it's almost the same as it is at the big drug companies, where there's this herd mentality: there's "a way" of approaching a problem and this is the way we approach it. And if you don't approach the problem this way, then what you're doing is of less value and will never work. It becomes a cookie-cutter approach to every problem, based on what a few of the top leaders are doing. A new technology comes on board and you see this enormous stampede where every lab at Harvard will have that technology and they'll be doing [the same types of experiments]. And for me, I needed to get off that treadmill and say, "You go do what you're doing. I have this idea I want to test out." And that worked out for me. . . . Sometimes [it's important] just getting out of that mix and being able to explore."

The funding system, however, makes it profoundly difficult for most scientists to do what Druker did, to go "explore." And it makes it hard for grant reviewers to see the explorers and paradigm-shifters at institutions well down the funding tier. There is surely a cost to this pattern, unknowable though it is. While one cannot prove what might have been, one cannot help but wonder how many worthy ideas and discoveries made by scientists at institutions lower on the funding tier have been overlooked over the past many years. Still, if history prior to 1970 is any guide, the number is bound to be significant.

In 1963, a thirty-six-year-old biophysicist named Barnett Rosenberg and two lab colleagues were studying the effects of electrical current on *E. coli* bacteria when they made a serendipitous discovery: the bacteria filaments became elongated, a sign that they were unable to divide. That phenomenon—which, it was later found, was caused by a salt produced by the platinum electrode, rather than by the electrical current itself— soon led Rosenberg and his coworkers to one of the most important cancer discoveries of all time: that a metal compound, called cisplatin, could stop cancer cells from dividing. In the decades since then, cisplatin and its analogs have saved tens of thousands of people from once-deadly testicular and cervical cancers and remain among the most potent cancer weapons available today. Rosenberg was at Michigan State University, then about as far from the cancer research epicenter as one could get.

Chapter 10

Publish and Perish

Leading the news section of the November 18, 1960, edition of the journal *Science* was an editorial lamenting the quality of television shows and warning of the dangerous tendency of TV commercials to employ "pseudoscience." Following that came a barbed commentary wondering if President-elect John F. Kennedy, who had squeaked into office by the thinnest of margins two weeks earlier, would live up to his science-friendly reputation. The fifty-one-page issue had sizable articles describing the genetics of an alga called *Chlamydomonas*, the radiation hazards that might await space travelers, the scent gland of the rice stink bug, and the effect of emotional stress on rats. Bringing up the rear of the magazine was a roundup of sixty-two abstracts that had been presented at the autumn meeting of the National Academy of Sciences. Among them was a report by two young Philadelphia researchers entitled "A Minute Chromosome in Human Chronic Granulocytic Leukemia." It ran only 238 words.

The two investigators, Peter Nowell and David Hungerford, reported seeing a chromosomal anomaly, a strand that was apparently shorter than it should be, in the white blood cells of a small number of leukemia pa-tients being treated at a Philadelphia hospital. Nowell and Hungerford could not be sure which of the twenty-three pairs of chromosomes these particular runts belonged to, though they suspected it was either no. 21 or no. 22. The study of human chromosomes was then in its infancy, with the true number of these gene-carrying strands in man established only four years earlier. And besides, the resolution of the microscope was such that the smaller chromosomes often looked more like blurry smudges on the glass slides than identifiable strands. They had no theory about why they might be seeing a shortened chromosome in patients with chronic granulocytic leukemia (now called chronic myeloid leukemia, or CML), no notion as to a specific, biological "mechanism of action" that might connect one with the other. And their sample size was too small to be sure they were truly seeing what they thought they were: the researchers had spied the diminutive strand in a mere seven specimens from patients with CML, after all. Their only "control" for the experiment was that they had not noticed the abnormality in the cells of patients with other forms of leukemia, of which they had examined but ten cases. Their discovery wasn't "hypothesis-driven"; it was happenstance. Their research goals, as Nowell himself would describe it years later, had been "fuzzy, at best."

What he and Hungerford had in 1960 was an unexplained coinci-dence. Yet it ended up published in the pages of *Science,* arguably the premier scientific journal of its day, with news of the finding spreading rapidly over the international grapevine of cytogenetics. Today, Nowell and Hungerford's 238-word "paper" revealing the existence of the "Phila-delphia chromosome" is among the most highly cited in cancer science.

When I asked Nowell about that initial study in a 2007 interview, he marveled at his good fortune. Had the same experimental report been sub-mitted today, he acknowledges, it would not likely have met the threshold for publication in any serious academic journal, let alone *Science.* Gracious and self-deprecating, the seventy-nine-year-old scientist was quick to at-tribute most of his success to the hands of his secret collaborators: "the Princes of Serendip," as he called them. "I have a lot to be humble about. I stumbled into the discovery of the Philadelphia chromosome."

He was being modest, of course. Noticing the link between the mutant chromosome and one uncommon leukemia was due to keen perception, not just chance. Nowell and his research partner had been readied for the find, trained by the practice of paying attention and an eagerness to explore. Their discovery was yet more proof of Pasteur's famous dictum: "In the fields of observation, chance favors only the prepared mind."

In the same way, Barnett Rosenberg, working at Michigan State University, was well prepared to understand the significance of the elongated *E. coli* in the electrification experiments described in the previous chapter. His recognition that something in the medium was preventing the bacteria from dividing led him to the discovery that a familiar metal compound, cisplatin, was a potent killer of cancer cells.

Still, a certain amount of luck was involved in both of these now-legendary discoveries. We are lucky, strange as it might seem, that these revelations occurred in the early 1960s, and not today. We are lucky that these brilliant scientific "noticers" got noticed.

That any voice, no matter how clear and compelling, is able to emerge from the crowd is at least partly a matter of chance. Not every talented musician on the subway gets a recording contract; not every "revolutionary" painter ends up in the Louvre. The world of science is no different. But in a few specific and critical ways, the culture of cancer science has grown progressively *less* hospitable to new voices and ideas over the past four decades.

It isn't that the research community, in the past, was less hostile or brutal to members who challenged the doctrines of the times. The realm of science has forever been rough-and-tumble—a place often ferocious, if not merely inhospitable, to new ideas. Francis Peyton Rous, in the first decade of the twentieth century, and Howard Martin Temin, a half century later, were ostracized and bullied for their then–radical notions. Temin's heresy, for one, had been to challenge what was known as the Central Dogma of genetics—the tenet that biological information traveled in one, and only one, direction: a stretch of DNA molecule (a gene) was transcribed into RNA, which was then translated into whatever protein the gene specified. Temin had theorized, in 1964, that certain tumor viruses—RNA viruses—like the one that Rous had discovered nearly a half century earlier, broke this inviolable rule. For that ultimately correct assertion, Temin was forced to spend a decade in the academic "wilderness." Reviewers at the top journals found any fault they could with his work so as to reject his manuscripts. Many fellow virologists scorned him; even friends kept their distance. As David Baltimore, a corecipient with Temin of the 1975 Nobel in medicine, would later attest, "Few have had to bear the silence of their colleagues for so long."

A similar treatment befell the late Judah Folkman, a gentle-voiced Boston surgeon who, in the 1960s, proposed that cancer tumors thrive in part from their ability to summon from the surrounding tissue an instant network of capillaries—an edge that gives their fast-dividing cells a constant supply of blood-borne oxygen and nutrients. The corollary to that, he surmised, was that there would likely be a complementary set of proteins that *blocks* this "angiogenesis." If so, that would offer a novel way to attack the disease.

Folkman was derided both for the idea and for his relentless attempts to prove it, with some critics advising postdoctoral students to stay away from his lab at Boston Children's lest their own careers be harmed. He, too, would be vindicated late in his career.

Science, without question, can be cruel. But more significant than what cancer investigators do to each other is what the system does to cancer investigators—to the ambitiousness of their thinking, to their risk-taking, to their willingness to pursue radical, as-yet-unsubstantiated notions. A 2008 report from the American Academy of Arts & Sciences, drafted by Nobel laureate Thomas Cech and twenty-one other prominent scientists, candidly revealed what they said had become "a troubling consensus" in the scientific community. "Many researchers," said the authors, "believe that federal agencies systematically shy away from high-risk projects. In the worst-case scenario, scientists stop even proposing such projects, leaving the agencies with nothing but more conservative proposals from which to choose." It is as though the cancer research community has inadvertently employed Folkman's own proposed therapy—anti-angiogenesis—on itself: squeezing off the lifeblood of new ideas to the point where progress has all but dried up. Young investigators, the risk-takers of yore, now stay away from the complex problems of cancer biology and resist the temptation to try an unconventional approach.

As described in the previous chapter, much of this change has been driven by the way we fund cancer research. But just as with cancer itself, the specific "mechanisms of action" in this growing problem are important to understand. And just as with the Philadelphia chromosome, the key mechanism here has a name. It is called the R01.

No one enters a life of medical research without at least a taste for risk-taking. The profession demands years of study and training, technical proficiency, and passion. And in exchange for this unending commitment, there is merely the remotest chance of real success, often so long in coming that only generations well into the future will comprehend the discovery's merit. The incentive that draws the young and ambitious into this field is not financial but the promise of doing good, of changing the world in some beneficial way.

That's what it is at bedtime, anyway—when the novice scientist sets his or her head down on the pillow and pushes the cares of the day away. In the morning, when the dream is suspended, a different motivation kicks in. Now, the aim quite often is not to do great science, but rather "good science"; now the primary incentive is getting published. There are lots of good reasons for wanting to put one's work into print, from the desire to share some hard-won insight to the hope of placing one's own stamp on an argument or idea. But for the new investigator, the primary reason for publishing, and of repeating the exercise as much as possible, is to get an R01.

An R01 is a government research grant—or technically speaking, one type of "research project grant" (RPG), discussed earlier. The NIH defines it as "an award made to support a discrete, specified, circumscribed project to be performed by the named investigator(s) in an area representing the investigator's specific interest and competencies, based on the mission of the NIH." The term has come to represent something else, however, over time. The R01 is the fundamental currency of the US research economy. "The R01 is the mother's milk of science," says one scientist. "Without it, you die."

The frenzied pursuit of R01s, however, is not strictly speaking about money—not for the desperate applicant, anyway. The cash, as much as $600,000 a year, as noted earlier, goes to the institution. The point of getting an R01 is to further a career. Winning a big award gives an applicant credibility at his or her institution. Over time, the more institutional credibility a scientist has, the better his or her chance of securing a tenure-track position, or another faculty promotion, or some other key role or appointment. The ability to bring in R01s can translate into better laboratory space, greater access to the modern machinery of science, or the opportunity to recruit the most sought-after postdoctoral fellows to the lab. And the more credible the scientist is, the more grant money comes his or her way. Ultimately, that will allow the investigator to do the unencumbered work he or she set out to do long before.

It is a long journey to get back to the point where the scientist hoped to be at the beginning. But these are the rules of the day job of science, and they are not new: publishing, grant-seeking, and institutional ladder-climbing have long been central to the profession of academic research (and scientists have forever griped about them).

This system, though, has evolved in dramatic ways since the days when Nowell and Folkman started out. The changes have been gradual, but accretive; and now, it seems to many, the gears and pulleys of the research enterprise are merely generating their own movement rather than churning out discovery. "There is no conversation that I have ever had about the grant system that doesn't have an incredible sense of consensus that it is not working," former NCI director Richard D. Klausner told the *New York Times* in 2009. "That is a terrible wasted opportunity for the scientists, patients, the nation, and the world." Or as Leonard Zwelling, professor of experimental therapeutics at the University of Texas/MD Anderson Cancer Center and the former vice president for research there, summed up to me, "I think the incentives are not aligned with the goals. If the goal is to cure cancer, you don't incentivize people to have little publications."

That is precisely what the R01 system encourages. To show how this happens to an actual aspiring scientist would, unfortunately, be to destroy his or her career. So let us follow the path of a composite budding researcher we'll call Alicia. As we saw earlier, the chances of an applicant's getting approved for an NCI research project grant are now at a record low (in 2011, the so-called success rate was just 11 percent). But only a fraction of those who win a grant are at the same stage of their career as Alicia. In 1980, more than a quarter of "principal investigators" (PIs) on NIH research projects were age thirty-six or younger. Today, the share is less than one in twenty. The odds are especially intimidating for Alicia, who is thirty-two.* But she has to try. Her career as a cancer scientist depends on getting not just one R01, but several.

Luckily for her, she has every making of a star. Brilliant and hardworking, she earned an undergraduate degree, summa cum laude, at a prestigious New England university, spent a year as a predoctoral student on a fellowship abroad, completed a well-regarded PhD program, and then a two-year training fellowship in molecular biology as she finished her dissertation. She worked for another three years as a postdoc under an established mentor ("Oscar"), getting rave reviews throughout. Now she is an assistant professor at a research university in California, in a department run by Oscar's old roommate at MIT.

The time has come, she knows, to try to secure a little bit of lab space for herself. It is not enough, however, to earn a spot on someone else's project grant (she has already done that). Alicia will have to be named principal investigator on her own. In the decades to follow, her success in winning grants will define her place in the hierarchy of her chosen field of study, which is still only loosely defined. She has been trying to learn as much as she can about the molecular biology of cancer in general. But that isn't exactly a smart strategy, her mentor tells her.

To apply for an R01 she needs a project, a focus of study that is "discrete, specified, circumscribed," as the NIH says. Oscar suggests something related to a protein called MYC (pronounced *Mick*), which is what he has been focused on for more than a decade; and Alicia did, after all, spend two of her three years with Oscar working on MYC-related

---

*According to the NIH Office of Extramural Research, a mere 0.8 percent of research project grants went to a principal investigator age thirty-two or younger in 2006. In 1980, the share was 7 percent.

research experiments. The choice is natural for another reason as well. The MYC protein, encoded by a gene called *myc* (or *c-myc*), does its work within the inner sanctum of the cell nucleus and seems to have a hand in every aspect of cellular life through its function as a "transcription factor"—one of a number of proteins that set in motion (or prevent) the copying of specific DNA sequences into their complementary strands of RNA, a step necessary for the expression of genes. Collectively, transcription factors thereby help determine which genes are turned on or off at any moment in a given cell.

Like other proteins central to cellular life, MYC plays a major (though, as yet, still unclear) role in carcinogenesis, its importance seen in the twenty-four thousand published scientific papers devoted to its workings. The protein MYC, in short, is a "hot topic."

There is a catch, of course. To have a chance at an R01 investigating some aspect of this protein, Alicia will need to have already published several MYC studies of her own. (Grant reviewers want to see "demonstrated expertise.") So far, she has six papers in all, just three of which focus on MYC. She needs more.

Her research cannot end up in print just anywhere. Alicia will need at least one standout paper to appear in a top-tier journal such as *Science, Nature,* or *Cell.* Most of the rest of her published studies will have to be in reputable second-tier journals, those that also publish work by the leaders in her particular field. The journal pecking order is well-known to seasoned investigators. But for the uninitiated, there is an ever-adjusting ranking system. The higher the "impact factor," the more "credible" the journal, and hence the more impressive the study published in it (and by extension, the researcher herself).

But getting published is only part of the battle. On more than a few of those papers, Alicia will have to be listed first in the stream of credited authors. A middling position in a parade of a dozen authors is a throwaway. (So much for collaboration.) While a first-author publication in a leading journal has never been easy to achieve, this, too, has gotten dramatically harder to get over the past four decades, as the number of scientists competing for each slot in the table of contents has rapidly grown.

In our scenario, though, Alicia does have an advantage over the competition. She is good enough (and lucky enough) to have published as first author in one of the premier journals during her postdoctoral stint. To win that prize, she had played some office politics, jockeying for position with her fellow labmates on work they had shared equally, begging the senior author—who, happily, was her own lab chief—to submit the paper.

Her real challenge now is not politicking but coming up with an original question she can answer quickly. Here, the complexities and vagaries of MYC biology will have to be teased into a clear narrative. She will have to start with a hypothesis and come up with a clever and definitive experiment to test it, finding an appropriate model system in which to prove or disprove her assertion. In this case, the broad subject of MYC is both fortunate and not. On the one hand, it is clearly relevant to the cancer process, and journals love to publish MYC papers. On the other hand, with twenty-four thousand studies flooding the literature, it is getting harder to find an aspect of the signaling pathway, numbingly complex as it is, that has not yet been cornered by someone else. The same issue faces those who toil in the cancer-gene realms of *ras* (46,000 published papers), *bcl-2* (39,000), TGF-ß (56,000), and so many other "signaling cascades."

Alicia, a few months back, briefly entertained the notion of switching her focus to another, less studied cancer-related gene or protein, but her mentor warned her away. Nothing is worse for an R01 applicant, he told her, than proposing to study something where she isn't demonstrably knowledgeable. Her publications are on MYC. To change her research focus now will push her first shot at an R01 back a few years—a move that will put her budding career in jeopardy.

Without knowing it, or choosing it, she has settled on her field of study for the next decade or longer.

At the advice of her mentor, she comes up with a MYC-focused research project that seems, as Oscar puts it, "doable." It is a spin on her old first-author experiments with him. There is nothing truly novel about it, she knows, but she can get some preliminary data quickly. (Another feature her mentor insists upon.) When she runs the idea by her department head, he thinks it has "merit."

A month earlier he had mentioned, almost offhandedly at a faculty reception, that he hoped she would start "swimming on her own" before too long. It wasn't a nasty comment—just frank. But it stuck with her.

Now, decided on her study question, she has to prepare the application itself. There is a simple rule in life: the level of a thing's difficulty is proportionate to the length of its instruction manual. The SF424(R&R) Application Guide—the manual for preparing and submitting grant proposals to agencies of the US Public Health Service—is 260 pages long. (That's two and a half times the size of the instruction booklet for the 1040 tax form.)

Once her SF424 application is complete, and she has filled out all the necessary PHS 398 components and supplements (more government forms), her proposal runs ninety-eight pages. Alicia has managed to get it done in six months, while fulfilling the rest of her research and teaching assignments.

The long, arduous process of getting funded is just beginning. Now, the rumble of paper-pushing machinery takes over—though blessedly, in this case, paper has been supplanted by the electronic page. That worthy innovation aside, the process is still a marvel of Rube Goldberg inefficiency:

Arriving first (1) at the NIH's Center for Scientific Review assignment office, Alicia's grant application is quickly assigned (2) to an NIH institute—in this case, to the National Cancer Institute, which forwards (3) it to the appropriate NCI program director. Meanwhile, it simultaneously makes (4) its way to one of 182 Scientific Review Groups, also called study sections, where, months later, up to eighteen leading researchers in the general field review (5a) the application, vote (5b) on its scientific merit, and assign (5c) it a score from one to nine (one being the unblemished best). Half of the applications get the dreaded NRFC—"not recommended for further consideration." Others go into a limbo called Deferral. The scientific review administrator (SRA) then averages (6) the scores from each reviewer for each applicant and converts that to a three-digit "priority score." In some funding institutes, for some types of awards, the priority scores of several rounds of review are then "percentiled" (7), or ordered in percentile rank from 1 to 100. (Higher-dollar grant applications also occasionally merit (8) a site visit from reviewers, which includes interviews with the principal investigator and an assessment of the lab facilities.) A summary statement of the SRG review is prepared (9) and sent back (10) to the would-be principal investigator for notification. Meanwhile, the summary statement, along with those for around 2,100 other grant applications in this cycle (there are three review cycles each year), is routed (11) to the eighteen–member National Cancer Advisory Board, accompanied (12) by a "Special Actions Booklet." The SAB includes additional information from the NCI program staff—calling attention to certain worthwhile applications, for instance. The NCAB then decides (13) how relevant the grant application is to the NCI's current needs and to the mission of the national cancer enterprise—which, in some cases, has little bearing on what the original grant solicitations (known as Requests for Application and Program Announcements) actually say the institute is looking for. It takes several more weeks for the grant to wind (14) its way back to the right program director at the NCI, who then takes the SRG scores and the NCAB verdicts and decides (15) which applications to accept for funding. But the machine cycle is not over yet. The NCI's central command first has to establish (16) a "payline" for research grants, based on the cancer institute's extramural research allotment for the year. Before that can happen, however, the budgeteers have to subtract (17) the prior years' financial commitments as well as any other directed funds for special programs the NCI or lawmakers have put in place. The previously funded grants are then accounted for on the outgoing side of the ledger. The rest is the payline. The 2011 payline for an NCI R01 (the payline varies depending on both the funding institute and the type of research project grant) is 10 percent, down sharply from its level a decade earlier. The low threshold has scientists in every field up in arms. Often, they yell (18) at the grants management specialists who are the unlucky go-betweens. The chief grants management officer, then, lines up (19) the grants by their now-reshuffled scores and checks off the winners until the payline is reached. The list of awarded grants now goes through (20) a "final review and negotiation"—a muddled process of in–house politicking, last-minute pleas and reversals—and then the congressional liaison is notified (21) of the real winners so that the appropriate congressman can, in turn, notify his constituents that a big chunk of taxpayer money is coming to the district. At long last, the award is issued (22), but not to the investigator herself. The check goes (23) instead to her institution, which takes at least a third (and often much more) of the taxpayer money for the "indirect costs" of keeping the university or research hospital going—which, in theory at least, provides a space in a laboratory for young investigators to gather the preliminary experimental data they need to apply for a research grant.

The whole process takes a year to complete. And nine of every ten applicants who fail or get deferred have little choice but to start all over again. Otherwise, eventually, they will be out of a job.

"It's not that the grants that are funded are bad or low-quality ideas," says John Ioannidis, a Stanford University professor of medicine and health research policy who is a prominent critic of the grants system. "They are no doubt decent and very good ideas. But it's extremely unlikely that they will be innovative and really change the paradigm. It's more of the same kind of low-risk research." Like an intellectual squeegee, the process rings out the last drops of outrageousness in an applicant's ideas, making sure that every concept to be explored has a long train of experimentation and theory to back it up.

The R01 tradition works well in some ways, says Ioannidis: "We know that the current system has managed to allocate resources and enabled probably a few million people in science to make a living." That gives it at least one advantage over any new research-funding system that has yet to be tried, he says. The long-enshrined peer-review process has also kept those ideas that Sam Donaldson referred to as flapping "a bedsheet at the aurora borealis" from gobbling up taxpayer money. But this insurance has come, says Ioannidis, at the cost of sacrificing what that public science funding, in theory, is most needed to support: the atom-splitter of an idea, that radical, counterintuitive notion that opens up a whole new way to attack the cancer problem.

That is the unmet need the grant system ought to serve, he says, "to really let people try high-risk ideas." Such investigations would inevitably have "a very high failure rate," he says, "but at least, even if one out of a thousand is successful, we may get something that is very important.

With the current running system, any seriously innovative idea has absolutely no chance. I'm not sure I have any seriously innovative ideas, but if I had one, I would not even dare submit it for peer review. It has no chance of surviving. Absolutely no chance. What I will send out for grant applications are ideas that are pretty much mediocre. If something is more than mediocre, I'm not going to ask to get funded because I know it's not going to get funded."

Stanford University biochemist Roger D. Kornberg, who was awarded the 2006 Nobel Prize in chemistry for his work elucidating the process by which DNA is transcribed into RNA, expressed the same sentiment to the *Washington Post* in 2007. "In the present climate especially, the funding decisions are ultraconservative," said Kornberg, whose father, Arthur, won the Nobel Prize in 1959 for his own insights into the transfer of genetic information. "If the work that you propose to do isn't virtually certain of success, then it won't be funded. And of course, the kind of work that we would most like to see take place, which is groundbreaking and innovative, lies at the other extreme." Kornberg said he is convinced that had he begun his own genetic studies now, rather than in the 1970s, he would stand little chance of getting funded.

Veteran cancer researcher Michael Sporn of Dartmouth concludes the same about his own work on the critical signaling network involving the molecule TGF-ß, much of it done decades ago at the National Cancer Institute—where, as an "intramural" researcher, he was fortunate not to have to apply for extramural grants like the R01. Over the past forty years, as a peer-reviewer for many NIH funding cycles, he has seen a transformation in mind-set that has left him despairing. "If you propose something totally new, without any preliminary data," he says, "you are laughed out of the study section, or, as they euphemistically call it, 'triaged.' The study section basically insists that you already have shown the results of the experiments before you even propose them." And "God forbid," adds Sporn, that a young investigator has a promising biological question to pursue, but "needs some time to make some observations before spelling out every last detail" of a study project. Both the grants process and the culture surrounding it are designed, he says, to make that impossible. "It is a totally destructive system."

There is a language that preserves this order, say those who sit on the inside. Older, familiar ideas are *supportable* in the argot of the grants realm; new ones are, potentially, a waste of funding assets. *Too ambitious. Interesting notion—but come back when you've done some more backup experimentation.*

Inside the study section, two or three reviewers—usually with some familiarity in the applicant's field of specialty, but not always—do a preliminary evaluation of the grant, each writing up a summation to deliver to the entire committee. Then the group begins nipping away. With these knives, points (or fractions of points) are *added*, not subtracted. Scores begin at the purity of 1.0 and then acquire demerits. Reviewers often start not with the idea, but with the applicant herself: *Middle-author type. Not really a leader in her field.* Or: *Up-and-comer—but a little loose with experimental protocol. Needs to do the work.* (Or a mortal blow, in the case of older applicants: *Never heard of him.*)

The study-section members parse the applicant's publication list, penalizing her for a lackluster curriculum vitae, or a letter of recommendation that seems to fall short in enthusiasm or sincerity. As for the idea itself, demerits are assessed for a dearth of preliminary data, among other things. With even the tiniest imperfections liable to sink a grant request, a desperate young applicant must stick to the straight and narrow.

More established investigators—those with credibility and a proven track record—can sometimes get modest funding to pursue the odd theory or a risky line of research as long as they serve on the right committees and continue to publish in the top journals. But some well-known achievers also feel the pressure to cast their research nets near to the shore. That even goes for somebody such as Josh Fidler, the long-serving (but now retired) chair of the department of cancer biology at the University of Texas and MD Anderson Cancer Center, and a beloved figure in the field.

"Look, look, look," shouts the Israeli-born, Oklahoma-schooled Texan, stabbing the air with his pointer finger, a trademark gesture. "The review committee consists of your peers. And I will tell you that if I wrote what I *really* wanted to do, I doubt that there would be more than two people on a study section that would agree to such a broad concept.

They're more comfortable with the focused: Here is the antibody I will use. And here, blah, blah. And then I get the money.

"You have a review committee, and you're going to talk about going to Mars? They're going to laugh at you. Somebody has to talk about going to Mars, for God's sake, if we'll ever do it!" That, however, is not the way to get funded.

Fidler, as it happens, did end up going to "Mars," at least in the cosmology of cancer science, as one of the earliest researchers to map the terrain of metastasis, one of biology's most otherworldly processes. It was Fidler and colleagues who, upon rediscovering the 1889 writings of a young British surgeon, figured out that the success of metastasis is as much determined by the colonized tissue ("the soil") as it is by the spreading tumor cell ("the seed"). Going to Mars today would be far more difficult. Junior researchers are taught by the R01 process not to try.

The latest generation of cancer leaders, though better trained and more technologically sophisticated than their predecessors, are shying away from novel research paths and are reluctant to explore the complex, overlapping systems that make cancer what it is. What the R01 engine churns out is a plethora of information and data and experimental results—an incomprehensible amount of the stuff in tens of thousands of academic papers each year. "It's all about getting reproducible data," MIT's Robert Weinberg told me in 2004. "But just because data is reproducible doesn't mean it's meaningful. The accumulation of data gives people the illusion they've done something meaningful."

And the accumulation has indeed been of staggering proportions. The forty-year war on cancer has, arguably, resulted in the grandest cataloging exercise in the history of science. At the venerable summer symposium at New York's Cold Spring Harbor in 2005, Sir David Lane offered a telling assessment of this exercise. The acclaimed biologist, who had shared in the 1979 discovery of the most famous cancer-related gene, *p53*, did his own estimate of what the then thirty-eight thousand papers devoted to *p53* had cost:

> If we calculate that the scientific funding required to produce the aver-
> age paper is $100,000 (I suspect quite a conservative estimate), then

academic *p53* research has consumed $3,800,000,000, and 75 million human cases of cancer with *p53* mutations have occurred since its discovery. Yet our certain knowledge of the *p53* system is surprisingly incomplete, and internationally, we still have neither effective *p53*-based therapies nor diagnostics in approved clinical use except in the People's Republic of China.

Eight years have passed since Lane's calculation, and already the math seems outdated. Now there are sixty-five thousand *p53* papers in the literature—bringing the bill to $6.5 billion. And still no therapies have emerged.

As a rule, the cryptic and brief disclosure that is returned to the investigator midway through the grants process—the "pink sheet"—does not fully explain why an R01 has been rejected. Often, though, four words, *proposal not hypothesis-driven,* will appear. This is the criticism that snuffs out more grant applications than any other. It is the catchall of kill-alls for the R01.

The Central Dogma of science has never truly been the doctrine that Howard Temin disproved decades ago (that genetic information moves in only one direction, from DNA to RNA to protein). The real Central Dogma is that all good science emanates from a worthy and testable hypothesis. Nearly every announcement of a government-grant offering now comes with the admonition that reviewers will be looking for strictly "hypothesis-driven" proposals. Editorial watchdogs at the best academic journals routinely toss out prospective manuscripts that seem to fall short of the threshold.

As eternal laws of nature go, however, this one seems to have sprouted up recently. Prior to the late 1990s, the term *hypothesis-driven* was rarely seen in the scientific literature.* Throughout the 1980s and during most

---

*The term may or may not have been coined, early in 1974, by a doctoral student at MIT's artificial intelligence lab; he had used it, perhaps tellingly, in reference to a new visual decision–making platform for computers, not humans.

of the decade that followed, the expression popped up in a mere handful of academic papers. Then—*boom!*—it was the golden rule.

The dramatic speed with which the phrase was absorbed into the scientific lexicon can plainly be seen in the pages of *Nature,* one of the preeminent scholarly journals in the world. From the magazine's founding in 1869 through the end of 1994, the descriptor *hypothesis-driven* never once appeared; in the years since then, the term can be found in more than seventy articles. Virtually overnight, the words became insider code for *a certain kind of research.*

In actual practice, however, the path to discovery is often not much of a path at all. Good, solid science is just as likely to swerve from chance observation to a question, to still more questions, and not arrive at a hypothesis until long after the information–gathering is done. Discovery has often leaped from the wreckage of experimental error. Or it has emerged from the melee of random thought. Good science follows hunches and instinct and serendipity as often as it does any best-laid plan. Good science is sometimes "ignorance-driven," to use the phrase of Sir John Sulston, the Cambridge geneticist who shared the Nobel Prize in medicine in 2002.

Hypotheses and rigorous experiments follow in due course much of the time. But more important than any postulate is the scientist's ability to *wonder*—to ask inspired questions and draw tenuous connections from far-flung clues. And still more critical than that is his or her willingness to pursue the mystery, by whatever means, to wherever it might possibly go. "My first studies of the worm lineage didn't require me to ask a question (other than 'What happens next?')," Sulston wrote in his memoir.

Throughout the history of science it has not been the isolated hypothesis that has changed the world, but rather the person tenaciously following, exploring, proving, and expounding upon it. So one straightforward way to fix the system, says Stanford's Ioannidis is to "fund people, not projects." The NCI spent $2 billion on five thousand extramural research projects in 2010. For the same money, it could award $100,000 annually to each of twenty thousand researchers, letting them follow whatever "What happens next?" questions as they arise. Instead of spending half their year writing, revising, and reviewing grant applications, investigators could spend that "lost" time investigating.

If such an idea sounds radical, it is what several funding groups do now. The prestigious MacArthur Fellows Program, for example, gives $500,000 unrestricted grants, popularly known as genius awards, to twenty to thirty individuals a year, based upon peer assessments of their exceptional creativity and promise for achievement. Recipients neither apply for the grant nor are required to say what they'll do with the money once they've won.

But, says Ioannidis, we might do just as well with a grant allocation process that does not even bother judging the merit of applicants. Doling out smaller grants at random, he says, might actually produce better results than we are producing now because it would inevitably funnel more research funds to younger, "unproven" investigators and to those with unconventional backgrounds or ideas. For the same money the NCI currently spends on funding research-project grants, it could award, by lottery, $50,000 a year to each of forty thousand scientists. (As it is, Ioannidis points out in a 2011 *Nature* paper, "the imperfections of peer review mean that as many as one-third of current grants are effectively being awarded at random.")

Another option is to bypass the entire direct-granting system and give the money directly to universities and research institutions, who could then make their own determinations about whom to fund. This would free investigators from spending time on grant-writing (or serving on grant review committees), remove the role of grant portfolio size from promotion decisions at universities, take away the disincentives for collaborations, and undo the need to devise an experimental project with broad appeal to a risk-averse study section. It is also, frankly, far more likely that a department chair will know better than any panel of reviewers who his or her most creative thinkers are. After all, this is the kind of determination managers at private companies make every day. Somehow, Silicon Valley has managed to produce innovation after innovation without study sections, scoffs Andy Grove, the celebrated former CEO of chip-maker Intel whose insights on management are the stuff of legend.

If the people funding our cancer research were the ones funding our first boatbuilders, Grove told me, no one would ever have sailed an ocean. "We'd still be studying the basic equations of flow dynamics," he said.

All of the funding options above, writes Ioannidis, "could be achieved—either through small, progressive steps, or through more extensive changes to the system." The key is to find a way to let scientists return to asking provocative questions, and chasing the answers wherever they lead—the way Peter Nowell and Josh Fidler and Judah Folkman did.

In a 2005 conversation I had with Folkman, he recalled his own experience chairing an NIH study section. Over two to three days, the review group would sit in judgment of some 120 grant proposals. "Every time one didn't have a hypothesis," Folkman remembered, "they would throw it out. 'It's not hypothesis-driven research,' they'd say. 'This is pseudoscience.'" But "every once in a while, there were these brilliant experimental things that didn't have any hypothesis, and [the review panel] turned them down. . . . So one time I came to the meeting, and I brought in the papers from six Nobel Prize winners with no hypotheses—starting with [Wilhelm Röntgen's discovery of] X-rays, going to Fleming's penicillin, then to [Banting and] the discovery of insulin, and so on. There was no hypothesis to any of those. Those were totally accidental. I said, 'You would have denied a grant to all these people.' I put the papers up on the wall and I said, 'We've got to be careful to ensure that there are alternate pathways to get to a good scientific thing, that there's not just one rigid way.'"

Folkman, who died in 2008, never fit the profile of a bench scientist either. He was a surgeon—a biological plumber, cutting out some pipes and welding others together. As with Röntgen's chasing an unexpected shimmer of light into the discovery of X-rays and Alexander Fleming's glancing at a mold-spotted petri dish and following it all the way to penicillin, Folkman had noticed and pursued oddities since his earliest days.

As a young surgeon in Boston, he'd had to operate on some very large pelvic and abdominal tumors, and it could easily take him many hours to stop the bleeding. The blood vessels would be only the width of a hair, but they would be coming from 360 degrees, as if they were parasitizing the vessels from the intestines, kidneys, and spleen.

Sometimes—it was always frightening when it happened—one of these tumors would rupture, and the patient would bleed ferociously, bringing a sudden drop in blood pressure. As the blood pressure fell, all the other organs would turn white. Even the kidney, an organ of blood vessels essentially, would blanch. The tumor, however, would be bright red and hot.

"Your hands feel it, okay?" Folkman recalled during another long interview in his Boston lab. "Now you finally get it out and everything's quiet, and you've stanched all the blood. And you've worked for hours. There are just so many blood vessels. And then you hand this tumor to the pathologist. And it's a white ball. It's actually chalk white. Bloodless. Because you've cut off all the blood supply. And the pathologist takes it and says, 'What's this theory you're talking about? I don't see any blood vessels.'

"The reason that angiogenesis research began in a surgeon's lab was because surgeons were the only ones who saw it live."

Folkman paused for a moment in the telling. He had remarkably soft features—a face that hardly looked weathered or tired or beaten by decades' worth of disbelief and sniping from colleagues.

"Everybody asks me, 'How could you keep going with all this criticism for so many years?' And I say, 'Because I saw it. I saw it personally.'"

Chapter 11

Deadly Caution

> Such risk aversion is a cultural rather than an individual characteristic. It is not the result of individually made conscious decisions; it is a consequence of the way the culture works. Most of the managers who are affected by it are unaware of such a cultural influence.
>
> —Russell L. Ackoff (1919–2009),
> pioneer systems theorist and management scientist,
> Wharton School, University of Pennsylvania,
> "A Major Mistake That Managers Make," 2006

Somewhere in the icy North Atlantic, on May 20, 1747, a naval surgeon serving on the fifty-gun HMS *Salisbury* rounded up twelve British sailors dying of scurvy—"all in general had putrid gums, the spots and lassitude, with weakness of their knees"—and divided them into six groups of two. For the next few weeks, the surgeon, James Lind, administered a different treatment to each. To the first pair of sailors, Lind gave a quart of cider a day. To the second, he dispensed twenty-five drops of elixir of vitriol (an aromatic tonic of sulfuric acid), "three times a day upon an empty stomach." His third group of patients received regular spoonfuls of vinegar; the next (and sickest of the bunch) were flushed with plain seawater; and each of the fifth pair got two oranges and a lemon daily. The final and least fortunate cohort were forced to consume a paste of garlic, mustard seed, dried radish root, balsam-pine resin, and gum myrrh—spooned into "the bigness of a nutmeg" (a nutmeg-size dose)—three times daily.

"The consequence" of this small-scale experiment, wrote Lind a few years later:

> was that the most sudden and visible good effects were perceived from the use of oranges and lemons; one of those who had taken them, being at the end of six days fit for duty. The spots were not indeed at that time quite off his body, nor his gums sound; but without any other medicine than a gargle for his mouth, he became quite healthy before we came into Plymouth, which was on the 16th of June. The other was the best recovered of any in his condition; and being now pretty well, was appointed to attend the rest of the sick.

This was the first modern clinical trial, a landmark that would place its Scottish-born investigator in the annals of medical history and save untold thousands of mariners from scurvy. The "plague of the sea," to that point, was thought to have killed more British sailors than naval battles and shipwrecks put together, and Lind's winning protocol suggested an easy cure. As important as that result was, however, many historians of medicine today are more apt to celebrate not the outcome of Lind's study, but its design. "Some 250 years later," notes the James Lind Alliance, a British group of clinical trials aficionados, the surgeon's "scientific approach is still regarded as the best (and perhaps the only dependable) means of enhancing understanding about the effects of treatments."

Lind's seaborne trial was, first of all, "prospective"—the conditions had been arranged prior to the start of the study and followed dutifully to the end. It was also rigorously "controlled": patients were sequestered in a makeshift sick bay in the forehold of the ship and, except for the six unique therapies being tested, fed a common diet of gruel and the occasional mutton broth. The study's six experimental arms, moreover, were (but for the pair given only seawater) evenly matched in the extent of their disease. In other words, the comparison was "unbiased."

And yet, of all the qualities that mark James Lind's experiment on the *Salisbury* as "good, medical science," there is one that is nearly always forgotten: it was *fast*. The whole trial answered six treatment questions and took less than a month to complete.

Today, testing a single new drug in human beings requires an average of just over six years. That is the "clinical development phase," from the drug's first evaluation in humans to the submission of a New Drug Application (NDA) to the FDA. Cancer drugs generally take longer: nearly eight years on average. But even that time frame does not reflect the true length of the testing period, because on either side of this phase are two additional stretches of examination and analysis: the preclinical stage (lasting on average about four years for cancer drugs) and the US approval phase, when the FDA reviews the evidence from clinical trials and decides whether to let the drug out on the market (1.3 years). All told, for those rare cancer drugs that make it through the process, it takes an average of roughly thirteen years to bring a candidate molecule to the clinic, according to Joseph DiMasi at Tufts University's Center for the Study of Drug Development and Henry Grabowski, a Duke University economist, who are considered by many to be the leading authorities on the process.

How Lind's one-month shipboard study evolved into the modern thirteen–year vetting is a complicated tale. At its heart, unfortunately, is one more reason why we are losing the war on cancer. As with our system of funding basic research, the modern clinical research effort is governed by a profound, and often paralyzing, fear of risk. That mind-set has resulted in a string of costly, unintended consequences: slowing the rate of development of new cancer therapies, pushing the price of drugs that do get approved to unaffordable levels, discouraging innovation, and ultimately harming patients.

What makes this problem so hard to fix (or even recognize as a "problem" in the first place) is that the fear that underlies the lengthy drug-testing process is both appropriate and understandable: FDA regulators worry that patients might be injured or killed by a therapy that is not properly vetted.* From that reasonable concern, a cycle of actions follows. Drug developers worry about anything that might cause regulators to worry, fearing any apparent loosening of the rigid testing protocols that the FDA demands. And because this lengthy testing is largely what has driven the cost of drug development (and the cost of failure) to such astronomical heights, drug companies are left with another nagging anxiety: betting on the wrong investigative agents. Which pushes them from the outset to narrow down their lead candidates to mostly what has worked before.

Whether publicly or privately owned, pharmaceutical companies and biotech firms—*sponsors,* in the language of the realm—appropriately worry about earning a profit on their hundreds of millions of dollars in investment. They fear anything that might shorten the period when they can market, free from the competition of cheaper generic versions, any drug that makes it through the vetting.† Firms fear rivals' piggybacking on their development efforts, so they patent aggressively and defensively and keep a tight lid on any data generated, and knowledge acquired, from the process. They dread anything that might contaminate their *labels* (drug-safety profiles), which makes it nearly impossible to combine multiple experimental agents in any clinical trial. Sponsors are so guarded about the perceived effectiveness of their drugs in clinical testing that they exclude patients who are unlikely to respond, and those who are too sick, and those with *comorbidities* (that is, patients with additional ailments), and those who have already gone through many other treatments, which includes most of the population living with cancer, and cer-

---

*In recent years, American consumer advocates and political leaders have, if anything, demanded more rigorous vetting of drugs before they are allowed onto the market, as well as heightened vigilance from the FDA once the medicines have been approved. This has been the case particularly since 2004, when drugmaker Merck withdrew its painkiller Vioxx after reports linking the drug with an increase in fatal heart attacks. That episode followed well-publicized withdrawals of the drugs Baycol (2001), Propulsid (2000), and the combination diet medicine known as fen–phen (1997).

†The longer the approval process, the shorter the *period of exclusivity,* which is the span between the FDA's marketing approval of the drug and the end of the molecule's term of patent; patent protection, as a rule, expires twenty years after filing.

tainly those who are seeking to join a clinical trial. (This makes any study data unlikely to reflect outcomes in the real world.)

Medicare, hoping to combat already skyrocketing costs, and private health insurers, fearing the erosion of profit margins, limit their formularies (lists of covered medicines and procedures) to "clinically accepted" therapies, which in theory reflects the practices of oncologists themselves—who mostly prescribe for their patients what is already on the list, which gives sponsors a single, overarching goal: getting on the list.

"That element of risk, and risk management, permeates the entire drug development scene," says Rick Pazdur, who as director of the FDA's Office of Hematology and Oncology Products is the agency's chief gatekeeper for new cancer therapies. "There's tremendous pressure on the sponsor to get the drug approved. . . . The bottom line is, if you do not have an approved drug, you don't have anything. The approval of the drug will make [for] widespread access to the patient, it will cause further investment in the drug, but that drug approval is a very important aspect because it gives life to a drug as a commercially viable entity."

The pharmaceutical business model that arises out of this necessity is not surprising. As the Government Accountability Office reported to Congress in 2006, companies are driven "to produce drugs that require little risk-taking but still offer the potential for high revenues . . . a strategy [that] has created an emphasis on producing 'me too' drugs." Such drugs, which have a similar chemical structure to, or which follow the same mechanism of action as, a drug already on the market, are obviously safer and cheaper to develop because they are following a trail that has already been blazed. That doesn't make them bad. (A tweak in formulation can sometimes improve the response in one group of patients or another.) But at the same time, it is unlikely that the "next" in a long line of me-toos is going to produce the treatment breakthrough that so many patients desperately await.

"With all of the hype, and with all the publicity and promise regarding drugs and new mechanisms," says Pazdur, "I am somewhat disappointed by the types of drugs that are coming to the agency. There's a lot of money being spent on me-too drugs and minor, minor advances."

Even many of the newer "targeted" cancer agents, he says, are often only "kissing cousins" of one another. "Here again, a lot of this is risk reduction. This whole idea of risk, it permeates through the oncology field." And it has led, he says, to a state where the new drugs that do emerge have "this relatively meager degree of efficacy."

Indeed, the problem runs deeper than that. The once-unstoppable global pharmaceutical engine that produced nearly one thousand novel drugs (known as new molecular entities, or NMEs) between 1940 and 1975*—including the bulk of cancer chemotherapies that are still in use today—can today barely reach idling speed. The decline in new-drug output in the decades since then has been so dismally consistent that, as four London–based analysts concluded in a widely read 2012 academic paper, pharmaceutical productivity seems to be governed by an economic principle opposite to Moore's Law, the famous dictum that appears to predict the remarkable efficiency gains of computer processors from year to year. "The number of new drugs approved per billion US dollars spent on research and development," calculated Jack Scannell and three colleagues, "has halved roughly every nine years since 1950, falling around eighty-fold in inflation–adjusted terms."

US drug officials (and even some top executives in the pharmaceutical industry) have been remarkably candid about the decline. "It is no exaggeration to say that the industry is in crisis," Janet Woodcock, director of the Center for Drug Evaluation and Research at the FDA, who oversees all US drug regulation, told a congressional committee in 2011. "There is a severe productivity problem worldwide in drug development, in which an ever-increasing R&D investment is producing ever-fewer new drugs. It is incredibly frustrating to see the explosion in biomedical knowledge and, at the same time, to watch the struggles and repeated failures of drug-development programs that try to utilize this knowledge."

There is no shortage of explanations for these serial failures. Drug companies argue that patent lives are too brief, leaving little time for earning back their investment on each approved drug, which they say discourages risk-taking and innovation. Many blame the FDA, saying regulators

*More than six hundred of which were developed in the United States.

raise the approval bar too high and take too much time to approve drugs when they do. Woodcock says the FDA "can't approve drugs that don't come in the door," and "the scientific challenge . . . is the major challenge that we face." Medical researchers say the most obvious of "druggable targets" have already been exploited and blame pharmaceutical companies for being interested only in the biggest disease markets, where a successful drug can bring in over a billion dollars in annual sales. All these explanations, though, have their root in the cultural mind-set—the paralysis of caution—that reigns over the nation's clinical research enterprise.

Jonathan Baron, a professor of psychology at the University of Pennsylvania, sees it as the inevitable consequence of "omission bias": the seemingly natural predisposition to think that a harm of action is worse than one caused by inaction. "It's how we think about cause and effect," Baron explains. Most of us think of causality the way it works in a pinball machine: "The pin pushes the ball, the ball hits the thing, the light goes on. There's a physical law connecting each cause with its effect." The other, if less instinctive, way to think about causality, says Baron, is the way it is reflected in tort law, "where the question is not 'Did you cause this physically?' but 'Did it depend on your behavior?' So, they use this phrase *but for*—but for your action or but for your inaction, this harm would not have occurred." While we may be predisposed to think of cause and effect only in the physical sense, he says, the behavioral framework better reflects the true impact of both our actions and inactions.

In the war on cancer, the consequences of omission bias are immense. To see its profound real-world effects, one has only to look at the centerpiece of America's drug-development enterprise, the clinical trial. Or simply at how long it takes to open one.

In what he calls his "previous" professional life, David Dilts studied die sets. Dilts, a professor of health care management at Oregon Health & Science University and director of strategy alignment at Knight Cancer Institute, in Portland, was a systems engineer who focused on computer-integrated manufacturing processes. He had worked on systems engineering for the Trident II ballistic missile for the Pentagon and written a book on "shop-floor control," but mostly he had studied car companies.

In the 1990s, says Dilts, "One of the problems at General Motors and all the US car industry was they accepted the time it takes to set up a machine was a given and that you couldn't change it." To stamp out the body of a car, companies use a die set. "Think of it as a bunch of cookie cutters." So when a carmaker wants to go from making one model of vehicle to another, it needs to remove one die set from the line and replace it with another. At US manufacturing plants, that process took anywhere from twenty-four to forty-eight hours. Everyone in the industry, says Dilts, accepted that "this was just the time it took.

"But all the Japanese manufacturers said, 'No, no, no, we don't accept that assumption,' " he says. Instead, they focused on the setup until they understood where nearly every second of time went. "Honda can now do it in three minutes.

"The setup time was insane. But there are all kinds of ramifications for that. If it takes you twenty-four to forty-eight hours to change a die set, that means you've got to run a whole batch of cars to spread that fixed cost. Honda, every three minutes, hell, let's just change our cars."

Then, in 2004, Dilts began looking into cancer clinical trials, "and I discovered that no one had ever looked at setup." Dilts was then a professor of engineering at Vanderbilt University (with a dual professorship at the university's Owen Graduate School of Management) when Alan Sandler, an oncologist at the Vanderbilt-Ingram Cancer Center, suggested they apply for an NIH grant to study just that. Trial recruitment is a major problem: only between 3 and 5 percent of adult cancer patients who are eligible for a study actually enroll in one, a meager participation rate that the National Cancer Institute has been concerned about for decades. When the NIH turned them down, Dilts turned to Sandler and said, "Let's do it anyway."

Dilts and Sandler began to record the discrete steps involved in setting up clinical trials at multiple cancer centers around the country. Before a new drug can be marketed, the drug's sponsor must prove the safety and effectiveness of its candidate molecules in a series of phased trials. Phase

I studies check the safety of the agent by raising its dosage incrementally in human volunteers and determining the maximum dose that can be tolerated. Phase II trials test the drug's effectiveness in a small group of patients. For those relatively few agents that survive the first two stages, Phase III follows. Far larger and lengthier than either of the previous studies, Phase III studies typically carry the extra safeguards of being randomized and blinded.* Their aim is to compare the effectiveness of the experimental drug to that of a standard therapy for the disease in hundreds or even thousands of willing patients.

But in the last of these categories, cancer drug-testing differs sharply from other therapeutic areas. Pharmaceutical companies are not the only ones, for instance, to initiate drug trials. Nearly as many Phase III studies are sponsored by the National Cancer Institute. These, in turn, are run by one or more of twelve "cooperative groups," essentially loose confederations of physician–researchers at hundreds of institutions around the country.† Dilts and Sandler began by focusing on what it took to set up a Phase III trial with the oldest of these groups, Cancer and Leukemia Group B (CALGB), founded in 1956.

Just printing out what they discovered, however, turned out to be a challenge. The pair had trouble finding a Kinko's in Nashville that could do it. The "process map" recording the steps was thirty-five feet long by five feet wide and would have been longer had each step not been marked in a tiny, eight-point font. When Dilts and his colleagues

---

*When trials are compared to something with a known effect, as in placebo or long-practiced "standard" therapy, they are said to be controlled. Most late-stage cancer trials (Phases II and III) are randomized as well: Patients are evenly "stratified" into populations on the basis of factors such as age, gender, and extent of disease, and then randomly assigned to different treatment arms of the study (or to a control group)—the point being to create equally distributed cohorts. Often, major drug-efficacy trials are also "blinded" to prevent bias from slipping in. In a double-blind study, neither patients nor investigators know at the outset who is getting the experimental drug and who is not.

†The reason for these NCI-sanctioned trials has to do with the nature of cancer therapy. In the vast majority of cases, a patient's treatment will involve multiple drugs (either in "cocktail" form or in close sequential order), often in conjunction with a different mode of treatment, such as surgery and/or radiation. Combination therapy has been the rule in cancer for decades. So the purpose of a cooperative group trial is to test one such combination of approved therapies against another, usually the standard protocol at the time.

began to unfurl the thick Mylar roll in a hotel meeting room in Chicago, where CALGB's oncologist leaders had gathered, the hotel staff would not let them. (There was no way to mount the map on the wall without blocking the exit doors.) Dilts, the systems engineer, had examined every Phase III study that the three-thousand-member CALGB had activated between 2002 and 2005. He then isolated each work step, decision point, manager sign–off, and processing loop (back-and-forths between, say, various committees or between cancer centers and the NCI), calculating a median time consumed by each item, based on the actual records. To "set the die" for the typical CALGB Phase III required 370 distinct processes, the Dilts team found, including 317 work steps and 42 decision points, requiring a median 784 days from concept approval to "activation." That was before a single patient was enrolled in the study. It took, for example, 193 days to develop the "concept" for the trial, then another 16 days to review it, then 2 more to vote on it, then an additional 7 to approve it, and then 126 days more to review it again. The actual protocol took sixteen months to develop and another nine months to review. (One of the shorter major steps, interestingly, was the review by the FDA, which took but 100 days.)

"So we're describing the process map to people and they're just aghast," says Dilts. The different sections are colored, so you can see which pieces of the effort consume how much time. And then, says Dilts:

> I tell the group, "I just want to let you know that once you've approved a study, there is no stopping point in your process." And there was this stunned silence. Once the executive committee says we're going to go forward with the study, even if it takes another two years, there is no way that you can stop it. And this one guy said, "You mean, this is like throwing a boulder off a cliff?" And I said, "Exactly. That's exactly what it is."

Within each trial phase is similar "process." Some of it, of course, protects patients or serves another legitimate need; much of it does not. Before an "investigational new drug" (IND) can be tested in patients, for example, a trial sponsor must get the preapproval of not just one "institutional review board" (IRB), but those at every hospital or research center where the studies are to take place. A third of the hours devoted to running a modern trial are now devoted to filling out forms, submissions to IRBs, and other paperwork. Even the number of medical-testing procedures performed per clinical trial—bloodwork, X-rays and scans, pain and functional assessments—have been growing, though few can say precisely why. The number of procedures performed per trial during the years 2004–7, according to an analysis by the Tufts Center for the Study of Drug Development, was roughly 50 percent higher than in the years 2000–2003. And along with the extra testing has come extra record-keeping.

In every trial stage, and between each stage, is delay. The delay is invariably not the fault of any one individual. (Everyone who sets up a clinical trial or joins it *wants* the study to move forward.) The delay is embedded in the culture—born of a rational caution, evolving into the seemingly benign forms of inertia, bureaucracy, and indecision, and often bringing the entire process to a standstill. An astounding 40 percent of NCI-sponsored Phase III clinical trials take so long to get going that they are never completed, a 2010 report from the Institute of Medicine found, leaving the treatment questions that launched these vast human experiments unanswered and the patients who bravely volunteered for them in limbo. It is "a terrible waste of human and financial resources," said John Mendelsohn, the former president of the University of Texas MD Anderson Cancer Center, who led the IOM's investigation.

For an NCI cooperative group, it is no more expensive to run a trial that fails to reach its testing goal (the "end point") than one that does. No profit is at risk. Nor, generally, is there much urgency to the therapeutic question being asked, many oncologists agree. "I do think that some of the effort, particularly in clinical trials, tends to be trivial," says Irv Krakoff, a pioneering oncologist who long presided over the chemotherapy program at New York's Memorial Hospital and the Sloan–Kettering Institute. "I have a personal bias against the cooperative groups, which I believe are devoted to getting significant answers to insignificant questions."

For an industry-sponsored trial, however, there is, at the least, an immense financial cost to failure. A high-profile drug candidate that fails to earn FDA approval can cost a company several hundred million dollars and often sinks the company's share price. (It is telling that news of such events is carried in the business sections of the big dailies.) Even in the latest stage of the process—the FDA review—after all the phased human trials and preclinical tests have been completed, some one in five candidate drugs do not succeed. Of this group, most cannot show they are any better than the older and generally cheaper medicines in use. This inability to show that a new agent will *"actually benefit people,"* said the FDA in a 2004 report, "is the source of innumerable failures late in product development."

Attrition rates in new-drug development are now significantly worse than they were in the mid-1990s, and even worse than in the 1980s. According to one analysis, 79 percent of cancer drugs entering Phase II trials do not succeed; and of those that do go on to be tested in Phase III, 65 percent fail to meet their end points. Such late-stage losses accelerate the vicious cycle described earlier because drug developers are increasingly, said the FDA, "forced to use the profits from a decreasing number of successful products to subsidize a growing number of expensive failures." Each misplaced investment has an opportunity cost, and over the past three decades that cost has soared. So much so that it has led to a radical change in corporate behavior. Just as with many a stressed organism, the survival strategy for drug firms has evolved.

In most cases, it not only makes little sense, from a business perspective, to pursue novel chemical entities—the compounds many call "first-in-class"—it can often be smart to stay out of the discovery business altogether. The big pharma companies now either "in-license" other firms' compounds after they have navigated through a couple of treacherous clinical phases or, increasingly, they seek to expand the use of products in their own portfolios that are already approved. Drug discovery today, especially in oncology, is rarely about finding and bringing novel compounds to market; it is about increasing the number of maladies for which an already approved drug can be prescribed.

Even this least risky of paths requires a heavy investment of resources. Resetting a formulary is possible only after changing (or expanding) the standard of care for a given disease, which means convincing the specialists in that field of the usefulness of the sponsor's drug, which means setting up additional human trials to prove it. For a therapy that is already FDA approved, a sponsor can restart the vetting in Phase II or Phase III (saving years and tens of millions of dollars). But the task still requires recruiting willing patients by the hundreds into each new clinical trial.

Or make that 1,067 separate trials, in the case of the drug Avastin.*

Avastin—researchers prefer to use its clinical name, bevacizumab—is a biological compound: a humanlike antibody designed to home in on a growth factor called VEGF and prevent it from signaling. Secreted by many cancer cells in high levels, VEGF instructs certain other cells in the body to form blood vessels, a mechanism that lets tumors secure the blood-borne oxygen and nutrients they need to thrive and grow. The strategy, as discussed previously, was actually conceived decades ago, springing out of the work of Judah Folkman. Avastin, made by Genentech, part of the Swiss pharmaceutical giant Roche, is the first FDA-approved medicine aimed specifically at thwarting tumor angiogenesis.

It earned its first US approval in 2004, after a Phase III study in metastatic colorectal cancer showed that the antibody, in combination with a standard regimen of drugs, extended patient survival by an average of 4.6 months. As for metastatic breast cancer, for which Avastin also gained an "accelerated approval," the compound does not keep patients alive any longer than the standard therapy, at least according to Genentech's pivotal trial.†

The antibody, at a treatment cost that can run $90,000 a year (with

*Such was the number of Avastin–related studies listed on the US government's clinicaltrials .gov website in late 2010.

†In early 2008, the FDA okayed the marketing of Avastin for a type of metastatic breast cancer (HER2-negative), overruling its own expert advisory panel, which recommended against approval, citing the therapy's apparent lack of efficacy. Then, in December 2010, the FDA reversed itself, announcing its intention to rescind approval for Avastin in the treatment of breast cancer after further studies suggested that the antibody is not "safe and effective for that use." Genentech challenged that decision, but in June 2011, the FDA formally revoked Avastin's approval in this setting. "Avastin used for metastatic breast cancer has not been shown to provide a benefit, in terms of delay in the growth of tumors, that would justify its serious and potentially life-threatening risks," said the FDA in announcing the decision. "Nor is there evidence that use of Avastin will either help women with breast cancer live longer or improve their quality of life."

potential serious side effects), has also earned nods from the FDA for use against non–small-cell lung cancer, renal cell cancer, and recurrent glioblastoma multiforme, a form of brain cancer.

Avastin, it seems, has charted a new kind of path into the realm of cancer blockbuster: though unlikely to change the long-term prognosis for more than a handful of patients, it has nonetheless managed to rack up an extraordinary $6.3 billion in global revenue in the year 2010 alone. Of this money, roughly a billion dollars in annual sales came from treating women with metastatic breast cancer—a condition for which, the FDA now admits, Avastin doesn't work.

The strategy of doubling, tripling, and quadrupling down on a barely effective cancer drug has not just been the apparent approach of Genentech and its parent, Roche. Every pharmaceutical and biotech company understands this dynamic. The only barrier to the strategy, apart from the huge start-up costs for any Phase III study, is getting the patients. Trial sponsors need plenty of them.

To have a drug comparison with enough "statistical power" to be credible to FDA reviewers, a sponsor needs the participation of hundreds, or often thousands, of willing patients—enough to create substantial and evenly matched populations for each arm of the study. Ironically, the sizes of these trials are generally inverse to the anticipated effectiveness of the new agents. Unlike James Lind's scurvy trial, where the effect of a few pieces of citrus was abundantly clear from the swift recoveries of two patients, the results of virtually every Phase III cancer study today are determined not by *noticing* the differences between groups, but by *parsing* them. Tiny variances in treatment outcome are detected only with the help of sophisticated statistical tools. The purported benefits of one drug (or drug combination) over another is often so minuscule that they can be seen only by aggregating the results from several trials into a *meta-analysis*.

Yet, such an analysis rarely offers a definitive answer either. It is by no means uncommon for two meta-analyses, examining the same therapeutic question, to disagree fundamentally in interpreting the underlying data. To cite one striking example: fifty-one separate clinical trials, involving 13,611 patients, conducted between 1993 and 2007, could not settle upon an answer as to whether a commonly prescribed class of anemia-fighting drugs called erythropoiesis-stimulating agents (ESAs) are appropriate to use in cancer patients, the large share of whom suffer from anemia.* (Five distinct meta-analyses, conducted between 2002 and 2007, likewise ended up with five variations of an answer, none of them conclusive one way or another.)

Dozens upon dozens of such long-running back-and-forths clog the medical literature. Two meta-analyses of nine studies of 2,581 individuals spread over thirteen years, for instance, still could not establish with confidence whether giving patients a standard regimen of chemo or doing nothing at all is likelier to keep Stage II colon cancer patients alive longer.

To arrive at such inconclusions, of course, the clinical trials process requires the willing participation of more and more cancer patients each year. And to make the notion even stranger, drug companies need so many patients to volunteer, in part, because they want *fewer*. Trial sponsors do not want just anybody with lung cancer for their lung cancer trials. They want patients who are most likely to show a response to the tested agent, and least likely to have an adverse "event." So they set up parameters, called protocol inclusion and exclusion criteria, that lessen the apparent risk—and end up barring many of the patients for whom the drug is ostensibly designed. Both sets of criteria vary from study to study, but the effect of the rules is to sharply limit the participation of individuals over the age of sixty-five (who make up some 60 percent of actual cancer patients in the United States) and to exclude those who would, conceivably, be the most eager to try a novel, last-ditch treatment approach (i.e., those with advanced disease).

The extent to which trial sponsors can use such criteria to goose trial results is disturbing, as Adriana Petryna, a professor of anthropology at the University of Pennsylvania, discovered in 2007. Petryna interviewed the chief scientific officer of a firm that manages trials for various sponsors. The clinical researcher told Petryna, "In my recruitment strategy, I can use subject inclusion criteria that are so selective that I can 'engineer

---

*The concern, raised by some studies, is that the drugs increase the risk of dangerous blood clots and death to a point that might outweigh their benefit in combating anemia.

out' the possibility of adverse events being seen. Or, I can demonstrate that my new drug is better by 'engineering up' a side effect in another drug (by doubling its dose, for example)."

In theory, even with such protocol limitations, it ought to be easy to stock the massive clinical trials pool with willing patients. After all, every year in the United States more than one and a half million people are diagnosed with cancer, fully a third of them with malignancies that have dismal five-year survival rates. In theory, patients should be knocking down the walls to bust into the latest clinical trials. But they are not. As noted earlier, fewer than 5 percent of adult cancer patients in the United States are currently enrolled in a clinical study.

Drug companies have undertaken the controversial practice of paying doctors for each patient they bring to a trial. Even so, the enrollment rate has not risen.

Sponsors have begun outsourcing the recruitment of patients—and the actual running of the trials, in many cases—to groups called contract research organizations (CROs). To an increasing degree, these private companies are now "offshoring" their clients' trials to countries in Eastern Europe and other parts of the world where recruitment is much easier. (A recent study in the *New England Journal of Medicine* found that roughly a third of the more than five hundred trials sponsored by the twenty largest American pharmaceutical companies in 2007 were conducted solely outside the United States.)

In the United States, however, patients are still not coming.

Some in the cancer research community have been complaining about this low enrollment for decades. They have been complaining that patients are not made aware of the value of clinical trials, that they have incorrect perceptions about the quality of treatment, and that they have been guided away from trials by their private oncologists, who are reluctant to give up their patients to an unknown doctor in a faraway clinic.

Each of these reasons plays a part, certainly. But mostly, patients stay away for the same reason the trial statisticians insist on highly "powering" the studies. They stay away for the same reason that clinical trial end points—the measures by which the competing regimens are to be compared—now focus on measures such as "time-to-progression" and "objective response rates" instead of actual "survival." They stay away for the same reason that stage-specific survival rates for the majority of cancer sites and subtypes have barely improved over the past several decades: because the new therapies, mostly, do not work.

That is the theory the FDA's own cancer czar, Rick Pazdur, put forth to me during an interview in 2004: "When you talk to people, has anybody ever told you that one of the reasons that cancer patients might not go on clinical trials is that they might consider the drugs *poor*? When you see blockbuster drugs or drugs that are unique, frequently we have no problems in patient accrual. However, if it is a me-too drug or a drug that appears to have very meager activity and really offers very little advance, perhaps that could be an explanation why people may be somewhat reluctant to go on clinical trials.

"Study accrual is part of a very complex issue," said Pazdur. "Nevertheless, as a community of oncology, we have to take a look at ourselves in the mirror sometimes. Some people don't like to hear that."

Cancer patients are not naïve. When there is the chance of testing a potentially prognosis-altering treatment, many patients race to join the study. Before the first Phase I trial for STI571 (what would later be called Gleevec) was even formally announced, scores of patients were clamoring for a spot. "I had medical oncologists calling me up," Pazdur recalls, "I had patients lined up here ready for this drug."

Patients *know*, even if the cancer war's leaders pretend not to. Their lives depend upon it.

The modern clinical trials system has severely hampered "innovation," wasted precious time, and stranded tens of thousands of patients in unfinished studies. But perhaps more damning is what this labyrinthine answer-seeking process has *not* revealed: no one knows which compounds might have worked under the right circumstances but were eliminated from consideration prematurely. No one knows which shards of therapeutic magic are resting in otherwise lackluster trials.

To comprehend the depth of the problem, it helps to return to that remarkable 2003 study by Pazdur and FDA colleagues. The study authors had gone back thirteen years from the end of 2002 and examined the stated reasons for every US approval for a cancer indication during that time. Three-quarters of those approvals happened for a reason other than that the drugs improved patient survival.

If all those compounds did not extend the lives of cancer patients, clinical trials had taken many, many years to make that failure clear.

But more damning was what the FDA's approval process *didn't* tell us about those drugs. It didn't tell us whether any of them might have been more effective if used in combination with other agents or drug regimens, or under different dosing schedules, or if used on patients in an earlier stage of disease, when the mutation burden was not so high (antiangiogenesis therapies might have fallen into this category).

Either way, the sacred, untouchable system for evidence-based medicine has failed to help us understand what actually worked and why—and what didn't work and why. In the ever-cautious purge of soft science, of ever-lurking bias, of self-delusion, we have thrown away precious knowledge, irretrievable time, and no small amount of public investment.

Medicine is an art, not a blind science. Its practice is to move from one educated guess to the next. But somehow, the modern clinical trial has eliminated that hallmark of medicine—the educated guess; it has been cloaked in statistical jargon, schooled in paralyzing regulation, and turned into a figure that no longer resembles its progenitor at all. The clinical trial now struts around as a pretender to certainty, and something great has been lost in the process.

We have forgotten why James Lind turned to the structure of the clinical trial in the first place: to *learn.*

The solution is not to throw out the clinical trial, but rather to redefine it. We must replace the current model with one that allows investigators to learn as they go along, just as physicians learn continually in their medical practices. One that lets investigators build on the information living in the patients in front of them, ask new questions, and follow leads. One that encourages clinical researchers to draw from their experience and to use their wits, to learn as they go. One that employs smaller, quicker studies, rather than the "Big Box" Phase IIIs of today. One that is dynamic and allows for course changes when necessary. One that uses multiple arms, in groups with just a few patients, to gauge bigger deviations from the average more quickly. One that reflects the real patient populations of the drugs being tested.

The good news is, this radical new paradigm is uncannily like the old paradigm. Not Lind's grand experiment on the HMS *Salisbury*—but rather the one that saved the life of young Brian Quinlan. It is time for the clinical research community to learn from its greatest success: the victory over childhood leukemia.

Chapter 12

Zero to Ninety

The problem of the patient is a pressing one, and research dare
not remain unnecessarily long in the ivory tower.

—Sidney Farber,
"Advances in Chemotherapy of Cancer in Man," 1956

In the history of cancer treatment, there is no more epic reversal of
fortune than that for patients with acute lymphocytic leukemia (ALL).
And as great, epic stories tend to be, this one is instructive, too.

How this achievement was accomplished offers lessons aplenty: how
an almost incidental observation about the role of an ordinary vitamin
could be transfigured, in a few lightning strokes, into the extraordinary;
how a dead-wrong theory could be flipped on its head into the right one;
how a string of "ineffective" single agents could be strung together into
a cure few thought possible—and how all of this could happen with a
nimbleness, speed, and collective sense of urgency that is, frankly, un-
imaginable today.

Likewise, in the story of ALL is a reminder of the inseparability of
rescue from risk, of the uncomfortably thin line between progress and
recklessness.

Within the tale is also a model for small-scale community science—
an intimate, rapid-fire exchange of ideas. So it was in the early days of

chemotherapy experimentation for acute leukemia: the knowledge and clues derived from each clinical study were factored into the trials that followed—not after years of delay, but rather after months, weeks, or even days.

The mantra in the cancer fight then was to embrace risk, not to fear it—to hurry up and try something, even if that meant there would be terrible misfires. Arguably, it was this cultural imperative, as much as any one or two discoveries, that drove the turnaround in the outlook not only for ALL, but for the entire spectrum of childhood malignancies. And if that drive was felt anywhere, it was in the heart and head of a Boston doctor named Sidney Farber.

Over six feet tall with serious, dark eyes, thick eyebrows and mustache, Farber had come to Boston's Children's Hospital right after graduating from Harvard Medical School in 1927, settling in the pathology lab. The job was at least one step removed from patient care. Pathologists spend their days attached to the ocular of a microscope, peering at cells on a rectangular wedge of glass, not examining or tending to the sick. Farber, though, considered the divide between lab and patient bedside an artificial one, a view that became even clearer to him as he turned his attention to childhood leukemia.

In some ways, it was a surprising choice for a research focus. Cancer was a clinical backwater back then, and acute leukemia seemed to offer particularly hopeless odds. A serious moral debate played out in the medical literature of the day on whether true compassion lay in treating a child for the illness or in treating the pain as best one could and letting the child die peacefully.

Farber could not imagine the latter. First of all, there was generally no "peace" to die in. The ravages of the disease, particularly in its final throes, were horrible. Three- and four-year-olds would hemorrhage—sometimes in massive profusions, sometimes by the continuous oozing of blood—into their gastrointestinal tract, into their skull, or from their skin. Their bones would ache as if they were being crushed, or the children would succumb to massive infections. Such outcomes were tied to the underlying biology of the disease. Leukemia starts when one type of white blood cell transforms into a mutant that won't stop growing. But before long, it affects every blood cell. The body's blood-making machinery collapses on itself.

By the late 1940s, doctors at Children's Hospital were trying a number of approaches to help their young patients. They injected them with high doses of the new antibiotics, developed during the recently ended world war. They tried blood transfusions and ionizing radiation. Infrequently, a child would achieve a partial remission, but the cancer would soon recur.

Farber turned his attention to the problem of anemia in leukemic children. In 1926, another Boston physician and Harvard professor, George Minot, had cured pernicious anemia in patients by feeding them liver. As a student and a young doctor, Farber had avidly listened to Minot's lectures on diseases of the blood. Minot was masterful at linking the realms of pathology (the study of disease on a cellular level) with physiology, clinical medicine, and nutrition. As Farber would later write of Minot, "His liver treatment of pernicious anemia fired the imagination of all who heard him to a consideration of the role of nutrition in other incurable diseases of unknown etiology."

Minot had set the stage. Soon other scientists isolated the nutritional deficiencies that lay at the heart of many types of anemia. The problem, it then seemed clear, was a lack of a particular B vitamin—either B_{12} or folic acid, depending on the anemia. Reports began to circulate that folic acid, or folate, was some kind of supernutrient. In January of 1945, researchers at Mt. Sinai published in *Science* their finding that breast tumors in mice, injected with folic acid, disappeared. The cancer vanished, they claimed, in thirty-eight of eighty-nine tumorous mice—to the point where the scientists had pronounced thirty-three of the animals "healed." In the sixty mice of the control group, by contrast, no tumor had disappeared and most grew worse.

After isolating the factor from chick livers, the Lederle Lab in Pearl River, New York, had managed to synthesize the compound, calling it pteroylglutamic acid. The lab's scientific director, Yellapragada SubbaRow, was a preternaturally brilliant chemist who had earned a PhD in tropical medicine in India before coming to the United States to pursue a second doctorate from Harvard Medical School in biochemistry. Without even a small fellowship to support him, he had to work nights as an orderly in one of the Harvard teaching hospitals. But his rise at Harvard was swift. After graduating in 1927, he was offered a teaching position and, before long, was named an associate professor of biochemistry at the medical school. By 1940 he was directing research and development at Lederle, probing the secrets of the new miracle vitamin.

Farber wrote SubbaRow and asked if the lab might send a small quantity of folic acid to Boston. Within weeks, Farber and Louis Diamond, the chief of hematology at Children's Hospital, were injecting the substance into eleven children with incurable leukemia.

The disease didn't regress at all. Indeed, the exact opposite happened. Farber observed what he called an "acceleration phenomenon," in which the leukemic blasts began proliferating faster. At first, he wondered if this acceleration might not be a good thing in disguise—priming the fast-dividing cells for treatment with radiation or with nitrogen mustard, a compound whose cancer-killing potential had been discovered, with equal serendipity, only a few years earlier. (That drug was closely related to the sulfur mustard used as a poison gas during the First World War.)

But then, after corresponding with SubbaRow about the results, something clicked in both men's minds. If folate was making the leukemic cells grow faster, then perhaps a "folate antagonist" might make them grow slower or halt the growth altogether. No such compound existed, unfortunately, so it would have to be created. The aim was to concoct a nutritionally *inactive* compound that looked enough like the B vitamin that it could take its place in the cell's "diet," so to speak. Biochemists call such molecules antimetabolites because they interfere with metabolites— the normal products of human metabolism or other molecules involved in it.

SubbaRow began work on synthesizing compounds that might fit the bill. Farber and his colleagues in the clinic tried one of them, aminopterin, in sixteen dying children. In November of 1947, ten of the children achieved "impressive remissions," said Farber, "characterized by a return almost to a normal state in some and to a state almost indistinguishable from normal in others."

As much as the results were encouraging, however, they were horrifying. Aminopterin was as toxic as it was effective. The children's stomachs would burn, their mouths would fill with ulcers, and their windpipes would go raw. It damaged their intestinal linings, caused severe diarrhea, and actually increased the level of gastric bleeding that made leukemia so deadly in the first place. These effects would cease only when the drug was withheld. Worse, even if the doctor continued treatment with the drug—and the children weathered the pain and bleeding—the remissions didn't stick.

Rather than be disheartened, Farber was quietly, resolutely encouraged. In a terrible, inescapably terminal cancer, temporary remissions were a glorious "proof of principle" that this revolutionary type of treatment, *chemotherapy,* could work. When the results were published the following year in the *New England Journal of Medicine,* the news caused a stir in the research community. Many simply did not believe Farber—at least not until others had repeated his results. What was needed, Farber knew, was another antifolate, one that was an equal or better inhibitor of the vitamin, but that wasn't nearly as toxic.

That drug would come soon enough in the form of methotrexate. An analog of folate nearly identical to aminopterin, methotrexate was far more tolerable. Once again, remissions did not last long, but patients were clearly responding to the drug. What was more, methotrexate was starting to show encouraging activity (though rarely curative) in a range of "solid" tumors, including those of the breast, bladder, and bone. It didn't exactly matter that doctors were not sure how it worked. (Not until 1958, a decade after the antifolates' debut in Boston, did researchers isolate the critical enzyme that methotrexate and its fellow impostors clamp on to, thereby disrupting DNA synthesis.)

Farber's approach to clinical investigation had speed and urgency, but little formality. He and his clinic director, Dr. Rudy Toch, oversaw the treatment of each new patient, recalled Donald Pinkel, a fellow pioneer in the antileukemia effort, who as a young doctor worked in Farber's lab. "They were resistant to the use of standardized, written treatment protocols," wrote Pinkel, "pointing out that each child was different and each ALL or other cancer was different. Therefore, drug dosage, combination, and sequence must be individualized and integrated into the child's total treatment."

Farber called the concept "total care." While the scientific goals of any study were important, he believed, the personalized care of the cancer patient was more so. "The evaluation of a chemical compound for anticancer effect," said Farber, had to be based upon some understanding of the natural history and biologic behavior the disease. And as with any scientific inquiry, it required "precise definition of criteria used in formulating conclusions concerning response or efficacy of treatment." But Farber was adamant that "research standards dare not be the primary consideration" in any therapy experiment "set up in the wards and clinics of the hospital."

For Pinkel, who would go on to make his own important discoveries in leukemia treatment at St. Jude Children's Research Hospital in Memphis, the Farber way was ultimately hard to accept. "While I appreciated the need for customizing care to the person," he wrote, "I thought it necessary to establish well designed and conscientiously followed written protocols in order to ask key questions and obtain reliable answers. Scientifically valid new information is essential to progress. As valuable my experience, as generous was Dr. Farber, and as well the children were being treated, I needed to move on to a more scientific research approach to childhood ALL."

Overall, though, speed ruled the day, as the 1950s and 1960s brought with them a frenzy of discovery in cancer science—science that straddled the worlds of the basic chemist, biologist, and clinic doctor. An amazing twenty-eight major drugs came to the cancer clinic during those two decades, many of them as accidental discoveries. Clinicians were so excited about the new drugs that they published their preliminary findings right away, often with the promise "Further details will be given later."

One of the swiftest to be developed was 6-mercaptopurine (6-MP). Like Farber's antifolates, 6-MP was another type of antimetabolite. George Hitchings of the Wellcome Research Laboratories, in Tuckahoe, New York, had reasoned that it should be possible to stop the growth of any rapidly dividing cell, whether bacterial or that in a human tumor, by blocking its ability to synthesize essential nucleic acids (such as DNA). One possible way to achieve that, he thought, was by attacking their building blocks, their purine and pyrimidine bases. By 1951, Hitchings and colleague Gertrude Elion had synthesized more than one hundred so-called antipurines, testing them against a bacterial screen. The most potent cell-killer was a molecule that differed from the DNA component guanine by a single atom.*

After some brief animal toxicology studies, recalled Elion in her 1988 Nobel Prize lecture, oncologist Joe Burchenal at the Sloan–Kettering Institute, brought 6-MP "rapidly to clinical trial" in children with acute leukemia. At the start of the 1950s, the median life expectancy for such children was between three and four months; only 30 percent lived as long as a year. Said Elion, "The findings that 6-MP could produce complete remissions of acute leukemia in these children, although most of them relapsed at various intervals thereafter, led the Food and Drug Administration to approve the drug for this use in 1953, a little more than two years after its synthesis."

Along with 6-MP came 5-fluorouracil (5-FU), cyclophosphamide (Cytoxan), vincristine, vinblastine, prednisone, procarbazine, cytarabine (Ara-C), actinomycin D, daunorubicin, doxorubicin (Doxil), and asparaginase. The rationale behind each, simply, was to kill dividing cells. Some of the drugs, like 6-MP, interfered with DNA synthesis by attacking its building blocks; some damaged cells' vulnerable genetic material directly; some prevented a step crucial for cell division. These were the "principles of action." It could be years, as with methotrexate, and sometimes decades, before researchers figured out the "mechanism of action" of any of these compounds—exactly what happened on a molecular level once the agent entered the body. All that mattered at the time was that they had some effect in slowing cancer's march.

Despite the glimmer of hope these drugs offered children with leukemia in the 1950s, none offered a cure. A child would receive the best drug available, and when it stopped having an effect on the transformed blast cells, a second one would be given, and then a third. This "sequential" strategy, as it was known, extended the patient's life in monthly increments. As late as 1960, the cure rate for ALL remained near zero. Half of children diagnosed with the disease died within a year; the other half

---

*The oxygen atom at the 6-position of guanine was replaced by sulfur.

remained in remission a little longer. Hardly anyone survived to adult-hood.

The reason was drug resistance. Among the tens of billions of cancer cells circulating in the blood, some would inevitably survive the chemical onslaught and evolve mechanisms to flush the toxins out right away.

At the start of the 1960s, a man named Howard Earle Skipper, at the Southern Research Institute, was trying to understand why. Skipper had grown up in Florida and worked on his father's cattle ranch as a boy. He had gone to the University of Florida on an athletic scholarship, was captain of the swim team and a champion diver, before he turned his attention to science. He earned his doctorate in biochemistry and nutrition at the same university and then, in 1946, set up a research program in cancer chemotherapy at the Southern Research Institute, based at the University of Alabama. There, he and his team turned out scores of scientific treatises on cancer that became known, simply, as "Skipper Booklets."

Skipper's experiments, often on a mouse model of cancer called L1210, typically focused on quantifying some aspect of the cancer process. In biology, as Joe Hin Tjio had discovered in the case of human chromosomes, the straightforward act of *counting* could reveal something that others had overlooked. Such was the case with Skipper's studies on the "kinetics" of cancer cell growth. With colleagues Frank Schabel and William Wilcox, he determined that a given dosage of a chemotherapy drug killed a relatively consistent *fraction* of cells in a malignant-cell population, as opposed to an absolute number. All that was needed was for a single leukemic cell to survive, and the doubling would start anew, and the disease would return with a vengeance. One survivor. That was all it took.

As trivial as it might seem, the simple observation, in 1961, that some cells are resistant and others are not would have more direct impact on cancer treatment than any discovery up until then. While Skipper and his colleagues were studying the phenomenon in mice, another set of researchers was thinking about its implications in human beings.

The key revelation came at the National Cancer Institute's Clinical

Research Center—in a conversation between two men who could not have been more different, but who just happened to have nearly identical names: Emil Frei III, known to everyone as Tom, and Emil J. Freireich, known as Jay. Tom had gotten to the NCI six months before Jay. And Jay, when he arrived, thought it was an elaborate practical joke when Tom told him his name. As Tom put it, "Some people thought we were only one person who didn't know how to spell."

Jay, the son of Hungarian immigrants, was combative, fearless, and passionate about everything. "I have never seen Freireich in a moderate mood," joked Frei at a symposium honoring his friend. "I have never heard him described as 'easy to get along with.' Most of us try to avoid confrontation; Jay revels in it, across the board, from science to politics to sports."

One summer afternoon in 1961, Tom and Jay were deep in discussion when one of them expounded on the implications of drug resistance in leukemia. "I thought I formulated it first; Jay thinks he did," said Tom. In either case, a burst of optimism energized both men. Selective drug resistance meant that tumor cells, though descended from the same wayward ancestor, were different from one another. Or to use the term that would soon become part of the cancer lexicon, the cells were *heterogeneous*. Some readily sucked up methotrexate, others did not. That, in turn, meant that doctors needed to view one patient's leukemia as *multiple* diseases. And to hit those multiple targets at the same time, from different angles, one needed to use multiple drugs in combination. To be most effective, each of the drugs had to focus on a different metabolic pathway or strike at a different point in the cell cycle.

The thinking was not unique. Infectious disease specialists treating tuberculosis had learned this approach. To keep the bacterium from mutating, they needed to use several antibiotics in conjunction. But in cancer, in 1961, the idea was radical.

Less than a year later, Tom and Jay put it to the test. First came the VAMP program, which combined *v*incristine, methotrexate (*a*methopterin), *m*ercaptopurine (6-MP), and *p*rednisone. The drugs were given for two weeks and then suspended for two weeks; the cycle repeated six times. It was brutal, but for the first time there were longer-term survivors—at least one in ten children. Then came BIKE, and then POMP, and soon a host of other four-letter treatments.

Not everyone was wowed by the results of this "shotgun" approach. One group of Boston doctors, including the leukemia pioneer William Dameshek, scoffed in a journal editorial that "not only may this method be considered unscientific, but the initial toxic reaction may be lethal, particularly in adults."

They were wrong. The programs were deeply rooted in science—science conducted both in laboratories and hospital wards. And the combinations became slightly more effective and slightly less brutal. Scores of clinical trials were done, trying to determine which cocktail was most effective at prolonging life. The improvements in survival for children with leukemia were still incremental, however, measurable in weeks or months.

Then another problem was discovered. Patients who went into remission would often see the leukemia return venomously in their brains or spinal cord. Most of the drugs being tested did not cross the blood-brain barrier,* so malignant cells could find sanctuary in the central nervous system. In almost every case, they did.

Donald Pinkel, then director of St. Jude in Memphis, used high-dose radiation on the patients' heads and spines to prevent relapse. By 1971 five-year survival rates approached 35 percent.

Jay Freireich would push hard to give children transfusions of platelets to stem the hemorrhaging. The view went against the prevailing wisdom at the time: many thought it would be a waste to give precious blood to dying patients. But the salvage worked dramatically. St. Jude and other centers also practiced what they called "supportive care," which involved everything from aggressively fighting infections to making sure the kids were eating well.

By 1975, five-year survival was 53 percent; and by the end of the decade, 67 percent.

---

*The blood-brain barrier is not an anatomical wall, but rather a phalanx of tightly woven endothelial cells and protein complexes that restrict certain substances from passing from the circulating blood to the central nervous system (the brain and spinal cord).

The achievement—long before the age of molecular biology, before the oncogene hypothesis, before the big machines and bigger money had transformed the research enterprise—was stunning. The turnaround in survival for children with Wilms' tumor, a kidney cancer, was nearly as spectacular as that for ALL. At the start of the 1960s, the five-year survival rate was 33 percent; by the end of the 1970s, it was 79 percent. Over these same two decades, the proportion of children with Hodgkin's disease living at least five years rose from 52 percent to 83 percent. For children with neuroblastoma and cancers of the bones and joints, the same rate more than doubled. Overall, more than two-thirds of children diagnosed with cancer in 1960 were dead five years later (with most dying within a year). Nearly two-thirds of children diagnosed in 1979, by comparison, would still be alive five years later.

Treatments for all these cancers have gotten better in the years since 1979, though this improvement has come with more intense therapy. Protocols for ALL, in particular, have gotten dramatically longer and more aggressive, extending from six months to three years. Beginning in the 1990s, molecular analysis of tumor cells helped identify which patients were likely to respond well to treatment and which were not. Doctors could then tailor drug regimens to the individual patient. "Nonresponders" and relapsing patients are today being caught much earlier, when they might be saved. Stem cell transfusions have gotten more effective and less risky as doctors have found ways to prevent rejection and deadly "host versus graft" disease.

Progress, happily, has not stopped there. Medical oncologists are now trying to determine if they can begin to scale back the toxic therapy in children who are likely to respond well and early so as to lessen the already high risk of secondary cancers later in adult life. Doctors have already limited the practice of radiating the children's still-growing skulls.

On a trip to St. Jude I stood beside the oncologist Ching-Hon Pui as children pulled upon the hem of his white smock and shouted playfully for attention. Pui, one of the top leukemia specialists in the world, turned about to greet them, just as playfully, as he told me about the effect of radiation therapy on the central nervous system in a child.

The change in gait was often subtle, but Pui could always notice it.

"I can spot these kids one hundred yards away," he said. "I know this is a survivor of leukemia."

When I heard the comment, standing with the good doctor in a swarm of running, laughing children—a typical St. Jude's mayhem—I felt a chill.

The story of ALL can be read as a reminder of what is possible, and as a reminder of how much further we have to go.

Chapter 13

Fossils

Four stories up from the ground, in a pink-granite and brownstone fortress on Manhattan's Upper West Side, is the dinosaur wing of the American Museum of Natural History. Stand for even a moment within reach of the ferocious *T. rex,* or the paired skeletons of duck-billed Anatotitans, or the crouching triceratops with its jutting horns and mighty fanlike frill, and you will witness an improbable feat of science: ancient and lifeless bones springing to life.

That the bones are here at all is improbable in itself. Many were found more than a century ago, when self-trained paleontologists began foraging through sandstone quarries in the American West, scouring dried riverbeds in Texas, padding across deserts on five continents, and sending back remnants of creatures that had lain in the earth for up to 200 million years.

Often, these fossils were mere fragments (or fragments of fragments): pieces from ribs, sections of limb bones. Nearly all had to be carefully extracted from the crusty earth and rock or pried out of muddy, gluelike shale—tasks that would have seemed impossible with the primitive gear the adventurers lugged along. Somehow, they managed. A wheelbarrow would be jury-rigged out of some old hardware found near a digging site; a crane would be conjured from rusted farm machinery.

In such creative ways the dinosaur hunters moved hundreds of thousands of fossilized specimens across continents and oceans, then fit them together as though piecing together a jigsaw puzzle. When they were missing pieces, as they always were, the investigators imagined where the unknown, unfound parts might fit and created plaster molds to go in their stead. In other words, they guessed.

Throughout the museum's fourth floor are large rectangular signs that call attention to this uncertainty. "This evidence amounts to only a tiny fraction of information about what the living animals were really like," reads one. "The overwhelming absence of explicit data makes the many questions that these intriguing animals arouse difficult to answer" goes another.

But then, from the start, the aim of the dinosaur hunters was far more modest than achieving certainty: their goal was simply to put a working draft of prehistory on public view. In that, they transformed a worldwide scattering of debris into one of the most extraordinary narratives ever told. What came out of these barely funded, century-old explorations— what emerged from all this intuition and guesswork and imagining—was discovery. From tens of thousands of bits and pieces of mud-caked data came an understanding, even if only a fledgling one, of life millions of years before mankind's first steps on earth.

This, indeed, is the way cancer research is supposed to work. Like the study of dinosaurs, the study of cancer centers on fossils: in this case, the preserved remnants of tumors and malignant blood cells. Just as the early dinosaur hunters did with their museum mountings a century ago, so, too, do cancer scientists aim to reconstruct—from the molecular data stored in hundreds of millions of animal and human tissue specimens— authentic "living" models of the disease process: ones that might, with any luck, reveal hidden vulnerabilities in this otherwise indomitable predator.

That's the idea: oncology as paleontology.

To that end, cancer researchers would seem to have an advantage over the dinosaur hunters: it's much easier to find and retrieve specimens of cancer today than it was, in the early twentieth century, to discover and carry home the giant pelvic bone of a ceratopsian. Cancer fossils are recovered every time a patient undergoes a biopsy or other surgery. They are gathered and filed away even during many diagnostic tests.

Multiply these events by a million and a half—the number of Americans told they have an invasive cancer each year—and it is obvious that there is a huge inventory of such specimens stored throughout the country. A 1999 RAND Corporation study done at the request of a presidential commission estimated that US repositories were then holding more than 176 million "cases" of human tissue—including blood, saliva, urine, bone marrow, cell lines, extracted DNA, and samples from every organ of the body—and that this number was growing by some 20 million per year. Even this figure does not fully represent the total because initial cases (those from an individual patient) are typically carved up into multiple segments or slices, preserved, and often doled out to different researchers, hospitals, or storage facilities.

By many estimates the total number of specimens has likely grown to some 400 million today. The number archived around the world is well over a billion. Not all of these specimens are from cancer patients. But probably hundreds of millions of them are. Which brings up what might seem an odd problem indeed: the overwhelming majority of cancer investigators in the United States who study human tissue can't seem to find any. Or, at least, any worth having.

Somehow, the cancer hunters of the early twenty-first century are being stymied at the starting point of their research expeditions: they can't get their hands on the fossils that abound all around them.

I first heard of the tissue "shortage" in 2004, while reporting an article for *Fortune* magazine. But I did not comprehend the depth of the problem, nor its consequences, until the following year, when I served on an advisory board for a research group studying prostate cancer at the University of California, San Francisco.

The group, led by a pair of seasoned investigators at UCSF, one of the premier medical research institutions in the world, had won a big-dollar grant from the NCI called a SPORE (Specialized Program of Research Excellence). The grants are prestigious and hard to get. The institutions that get them are generally like UCSF: big, plugged-in, well funded, and attached to a leading cancer hospital.

Major centers, the thinking goes, are more likely than smaller institutions to have the wherewithal—the expertise, equipment, technical support, access to patients—to "enable the rapid and efficient movement of basic scientific findings into clinical settings." Or, to translate the NCI jargon into laymen's terms, to turn a promising discovery into an actual treatment.

In keeping with this apparent sense of urgency, recipients of SPOREs "are *required* to reach a human end-point [to either be helping actual patients or, at least, being tested in a clinical trial] within the 5-year funding period." Few SPORE grant recipients, in reality, come anywhere close to meeting this obligation. But in March 2005, when the UCSF group met with its outside advisers for an annual progress review, the mood was mostly optimistic. The investigators had cobbled together several worthy study projects focused on a relentless form of advanced disease called hormone-refractory prostate cancer. Three of the ideas involved potential therapies; one was a proposal for a prognostic test.

The last of these, if proven valid, would have the biggest impact on patients. From a quick examination of a panel of some three dozen genes in the cells of a new patient's tissue specimen, the UCSF collaborators hoped to determine the likelihood that the person's cancer would return.

Doctors, as it is, make guesses about their patients' long-term prognoses based on various clinical facts (including the level of prostate-specific antigen [PSA] measured in the blood, the size and grade of the tumor, whether any tissue in the vicinity of the gland has been invaded, whether nearby lymph nodes show evidence of the disease). But such predictions are only middling in their accuracy and are therefore of little help to patients agonizing over what to do next: whether to opt for more aggressive treatment right away (which might well be debilitating) or wait it out and risk a deadly recurrence in a few years.

If the UCSF group could improve upon this guesswork with a simple gene-based test, tens of thousands of men would benefit each year in the

United States alone, and many more around the world. This was precisely the sort of research project that SPORE was designed to speed along: to bring a potentially lifesaving idea to a quick "proof of principle" test.

And UCSF seemed the ideal place to try. To provide the critical research specimens for this and the other projects in the SPORE, the collaborators had carved out their own team within a team, known in the jargon of the realm as a *tissue core*. Leading this cadre was a practicing pathologist who also taught at the medical school. Working alongside him was a *core manager*, with ten years' experience in tissue collection and banking. Their two assistants, between them, had seven years of on–the-job training.

Money from the generous government award had been set aside to pay for a new freezer for storing the project's specimens (it could chill to −80 Celsius); but the big expense would be the "high throughput" machine capable of scanning the slides of stained specimens ($200,000). As for other essential tools of the trade—the "tissue processor and embedding station," microarray, photomicroscope, mass spectrometer, flow cytometry machine, and a sophisticated meat slicer called a laser capture microdissection apparatus—the SPORE team had been promised full access to the resources of the main tissue lab at the UCSF cancer center.

With such advanced technology in their grasp, investigators would, in theory, be able to probe the molecular secrets of human cells in a variety of tissue-sample types—those, for example, that had been flash frozen just after being removed from a patient on the operating table, or those that have been preserved by traditional means. The latter specimens are first "fixed" in a solution called formalin—which keeps the cells and their biochemical reactions in suspended animation—and then embedded in waxy glass blocks. (The technique, believe it or not, is a hundred years old.) As for the proposed gene-marker panel, the UCSF group had all the resources necessary to test it.

Everything, it seemed, but the specimens themselves.

UCSF's central tissue bank had archived over a thousand prostate cancer samples over the previous eight years, a resource that in theory was to be shared with not only the projects of the SPORE grant, but with dozens of other ongoing research studies as well. But even among the specimens that were available for use in the biomarker study, many were not a good fit for one reason or another. The number that were both available *and* appropriate to the study was simply too small to give the researchers what they needed—or, at least, needed if any of their eventual findings were to be considered anything besides the results of chance. Vetting a biomarker test—confirming its predictiveness, making sure its mistakes ("false positives" and "false negatives") are few—generally requires hundreds or even thousands of samples. The SPORE investigators, by the spring of 2005, had looked at twenty-seven.* The tissue core, for its part, had been trying for months to get workable specimens from other hospitals and labs, but this was seldom easy.

By the close of our review meeting, it was becoming clear that none of the great science discussed that day would amount to much. The researchers were brilliant, passionate, and well trained. Their idea had the potential to help thousands of cancer patients. None of that mattered.

Even more disturbing was what this implied about the rest of the multibillion–dollar cancer research enterprise: If these guys couldn't get the specimens they needed, who could?

As it turns out, hardly anybody. Those who have good samples, for the most part, rarely lend them out. Those who don't can try begging them off colleagues at other research institutions—or more rarely, buying them from a commercial biobank. (Typically, about 6 percent of an investigator's samples comes from such places; another 4 percent is borrowed from nonprofit repositories.) Roughly one in a hundred specimens comes from tissue providers of various sorts outside the United States.

Finding the samples, however, is no guarantee that one can use them. Sometimes the specimens are too small, or the amount of dead tissue too high, or the condition of the cells too poor for the planned analysis to be done.

---

*Nearly five years later, in January 2010, the project's principal investigator and colleagues published an update on the recurrence-predicting assay (called GEMCaP) in a leading journal. By then, they'd managed to test the gene panel on thirty cases of prostate cancer and twenty-four controls. The results, said an accompanying editorial, were perhaps a little promising—but remained inconclusive "due to sample size concerns."

Or, quite often the tissue itself is fine—but the way it has been prepared and stored on the slide proves limiting. Chemical fixing, the strategy hospitals have been using for a century to archive pathology specimens, was ideal when researchers were only interested in how the tissue looked under the microscope. In the age of molecular study, though, formalin fixing has proven an obstacle: the process can change the molecular dynamics of human cells in untold ways. Flash freezing, the most common alternative method, preserves the DNA, but the necessary thawing can alter proteins in ways that are not always apparent. What occurs during the minutes or hours after a tumor is removed from the body and before it is preserved by one technique or another is a concern as well.

Just as Judah Folkman marveled at how dramatic the difference was between the steaming, blood-drenched tumors he held in his hands during surgery and the chalk-white masses the pathologists would see an hour or two later, so, too, the molecular profiles of individual cells can be transformed during this time. Cut off from the circulation, in the sudden life-and-death gasp of ischemia, it is no wonder that cells change what they say to each other: proteins undergo rapid changes in signaling; the expressions of some genes change as well. The longer this interim is, the more dramatic such changes are.

But researchers fortunate enough to get the tissue months or years later are unlikely to have any idea how long this time to fixation was. Nor are they likely to know what specific techniques (beyond the obvious) were used to prep the specimen. Nor will they be aware, in most cases, of what type of anesthesia was used in surgery. (That can alter the tissue, too.) All of this, in the words of one NCI report, makes it "difficult for scientists to compare or pool genomic and proteomic [protein profile] results from biospecimens across institutions."

Sometimes, the problem doesn't concern the tumor specimen at all, but rather what is not sent with it: a matched "control" from, say, nearby healthy tissue or the blood. The researcher won't have a normal template of DNA with which to compare the malignant set. Occasionally, important clinical data, such as the age and gender of the patient, along with the what, where, and when of the disease, will be missing or incorrect.

The stage or type of cancer can be badly misclassified, or there won't be any follow-up on whether the patient's disease returned and, if so, how long he or she survived.

Frequently, a sample is fine but lacks patient authorization to use it for a specific research study, or such permission isn't wholly clear from a consent form signed years earlier. (In one 2008 study, more than five thousand patients with advanced colorectal cancer were given a therapy directed against a known cancer protein called EGFR. But when investigators later wanted to see if mutations in a related gene [*kras*] were potentially affecting the outcome of treatment, many were told by their own institutions that they couldn't do the test—even on specimens the patients had already given them—because the original "informed consent" forms had not explicitly authorized it.)

Such frustrations are now a routine part of cancer science. By far, though, the most common specimen problem is the one that flummoxed the SPORE researchers in San Francisco: not being able to get enough of them.

When the National Cancer Institute surveyed more than seven hundred researchers on the topic in the summer of 2008, 70 percent said that, regardless of the quality of specimens, they found it "very or somewhat difficult" to acquire the tissue they needed for their projects.

This difficulty is a huge obstacle to progress in the cancer fight. And ever since the National Dialogue on Cancer, a forward-thinking group of advocates, scientists, and political figures, now known by the name C-Change, brought a flush of attention to the issue in a March 2002 forum, it has been at or near the top of the cancer leadership's Fix-It list.

A 2010 report from the NCI spells it out in blunt language:

> The lack of standard and uniform operating procedures for . . . biospecimens has resulted in a critical shortage of these important resources. Many potentially high-impact research initiatives and cancer diagnostic and therapeutic development efforts are being significantly hindered by the limited quantity and quality of biospecimens. In fact, studies have shown that cancer researchers restrict the scope and question

the validity of their work because of the uncertain quality of the biospecimens available to them.

The last of these lines is so remarkable that it bears repeating: the tissue problem is not only limiting what can be learned in the molecular age, it is leading cancer researchers to *question the validity* of the work they've already done.

What is more shocking is that the NCI has had a workable solution to the problem for years.

After the study on tissue repositories by the President's National Bioethics Advisory Commission in 1999, after the National Dialogue on Cancer's report on the subject a few years later, the NCI commissioned its own study. What came out of this study, in 2003, was a plan—a dense 175-page blueprint for a National Biospecimen Network.

Its premise was smart and obvious: to create a standard set of procedures for collecting and analyzing human–tissue specimens as well as a nationwide system for storing and distributing them. Plenty of tissue banks were in existence already. As far back as 1987, the NCI had partnered with five research centers to form its Cooperative Human Tissue Network; over the years, several other small-scale partnerships had sprung up to share specimens in one type of cancer or another. None, however, could provide enough quality tissue to do even a single definitive biomarker study. And without a slew of such markers available—without reliable, easy-to-spot beacons that could alert to the presence of a stealthily developing tumor within—there was no chance of reducing the cancer burden.

What was needed, said the NBN's framers, was a system that could provide genuine critical mass, one that would let researchers everywhere search through a database with records of tens of millions of quality samples. When scientists found what they were looking for, they could either request the needed tissue or, better yet, retrieve the molecular data from within. In the molecular age of cancer study, after all, it is the "digital" fingerprints of the cells within the physical specimen that matter: millions of data points regarding such things as gene expression, DNA mutation, and protein signaling.

The idea got enough traction at the NCI for the director to organize a "coordinating committee" in 2004. A year later, an official bureaucratic outpost—the grandly named Office of Biorepositories and Biospecimen Research—was set up to put the plan in motion. A series of workshops and meetings were then held to hammer out details and get "buy in" from the myriad "stakeholders" in the process—from surgeons and pathologists on the front end of the tissue chain to hospital archivists, researchers, and drug developers down the line.

I got the chance to be a fly on the wall at one of the first of these NCI symposiums, in the fall of 2005, and even a fly on the wall could not help but be impressed at the sophistication and comprehensiveness of the discourse. Crammed into the session were expert talks on the nuances of biospecimen collection, processing, and dissemination. Other speakers covered the complexities of bioinformatics, the science of turning the molecular signals of living cells into digital information that can then be stored and shared. Experts from Singapore, Austria, Great Britain, Australia, Iceland, and Japan spoke on the need to harmonize tissue-banking practices around the globe—and on the challenges that went with that, from concerns over patient privacy to intellectual property. (One key question was, who would *own* a medical discovery derived from the study of a patient's tissue?)

By 2009, the annual symposium had lengthened to three days instead of one and was held in a slightly bigger conference room in the basement of a slightly bigger Marriott. The presentations were a bit longer and more data-laden this time around, the break-time snacks a trifle nicer. The expert talks, however, seemed to tread upon the same muddy ground and get stuck on the same sticking points as those on the 2005 lineup.

Four years had passed between these meetings, six since the NIH had laid out its "blueprint" for a National Biospecimen Network, many more years had come and gone since rank-and-file cancer researchers had begun to recognize the seriousness of the "tissue issue." But whenever one started the clock, it was clear that the worthy idea had gotten little closer to becoming real.

In the world outside the cancer realm, networks for sharing anything and everything—networks achieving true critical mass—were springing up as quickly and colorfully as wildflowers.

In 1996, two Canadian couples cataloged the holdings of four small independent bookstores in Victoria, British Columbia, into an online database—allowing readers anywhere to browse through these largely obscure, out-of-print collections and make purchases online. Within four years the company, called AbeBooks—the initial letters stood for "Automatic Book Exchange"—had linked together the inventories of sixty-three hundred bookstores around the world, transforming thousands of once-inaccessible collections into a vast searchable network of 23 million volumes. (Four years.)

On Labor Day weekend in 1995 a moonlighting computer programmer, Pierre Omidyar, tested his new Internet-based marketplace by auctioning off a broken laser pointer to bidders who happened upon his website. (It fetched $14.83.) Four years later, Omidyar's marketplace—known as eBay—had 10 million registered users around the world and was connecting sellers and buyers in nearly half a million auctions per day.

In six years of workshops, symposia, and summits; of working groups, coordinating committees, and panels; of think-tank reports and concept grants—the would-be developers of the government's National Biospecimen Network were still discussing "best practices."

It is, perhaps, easy to think that there is something about human tissue that inherently conflicts with the power laws of network sharing. It is easy to think that the thicket of complex issues surrounding the process is too thorny to sort out, or that the technical requirements are too great to master. It is easy to think that a lack of government funding has been the limiting factor. But then, it is only easy to think such things if one does not know about the thriving biobanking networks in Iceland, the United Kingdom, Finland, Japan, and Estonia. (All these countries have made the idea work.)

It is only easy to see the NCI's effort as being effective, indeed, if one has never had the chance to meet Kathy Giusti.

———

Almost from the minute she was diagnosed with multiple myeloma, Kathy Giusti understood what she was up against. In truth, she had understood some two weeks before the diagnosis. That was when she had found the note from her husband, Paul, on the kitchen table. It was around Christmas 1995, and Kathy, then a thirty-seven-year-old executive at the pharmaceutical firm Searle, had just returned to her suburban Chicago home from an exhausting business trip. The note, sitting on the kitchen table, in Paul's scribbled handwriting, said simply, "Dr. called. Needs to see both of us in office." But that was the moment. That was when she knew.

"I said to my husband, 'How long has that been sitting there? That obviously means that something is horribly wrong,'" Kathy recalled during a conversation in 2007. "My dad was a doctor. You never say, 'We need to see both of you,' unless there's something horribly wrong."

She and Paul had been trying, without luck, to have another baby. Nicole, their daughter, was eighteen months old, and Kathy was eager for her to have a sibling—someone for her to be as close to as Kathy was with her twin sister, Karen. But before Kathy could get the green light from her insurance company to see a fertility specialist, she had to be screened by her primary care physician and take a few routine blood tests.

She had been feeling run–down and had lost a little weight, but she had chalked up the symptoms to her recent business trip abroad. As director of worldwide operations for Searle's fleet of arthritis drugs, she was traveling much of the time. Exhaustion came with the job.

It was not until the next evening, when Kathy was driving home from work, that she and her internist spoke. "We didn't have cell phones then," she recalls with a laugh. "He called me on my car phone! And I kept saying, 'You need to tell me. You need to tell me.' And he goes, 'Well, you have cancer. And it's a tough one.' And I just kept driving."

Early the next morning, Kathy, Paul, and baby Nicole went to a nearby Borders bookstore to learn everything they could about the strangely named cancer the doctor had said she had. ("This was all pre-Internet, of course.") They sat on the floor surrounded by medical textbooks, scouring the indexes for any mention of *multiple myeloma*, a malignancy that develops in a particular form of white blood cell, called a plasma cell, found in the bone marrow. "And I'm looking at Paul and saying, 'This is horrible.'" She cataloged into memory the somewhat sketchy parameters that seemed to mark each stage of the disease; she filed every known treatment option and complication, every test she would likely take, into her brain. She now understood the meaning of a low reading of hemoglobin in the blood and a high measure of total protein. She knew how unlikely it was that a white woman in her thirties would get the disease. (The typical patient profile is old, male, and African–American.) She knew the officially recorded odds of surviving five years (then, about one in three) and the chances of beating the disease altogether (zero).

By the time she and Paul sat down with the doctor, says Kathy, "I knew exactly what I was getting myself into."

That wasn't quite the case.

She had bravely come to terms with the awful prognosis. And perhaps, at least in broad, black-and-white brushstrokes, she understood what sort of treatment awaited her. None of what she'd read in the textbooks, however, had prepared her for the revelation that there was no ongoing, coordinated effort to cure the disease. She simply assumed that such a program had long been under way. But among the scattering of myeloma researchers and medical specialists around the world, there was no single unified, managed effort to gather and share information; no evident plan of attack in place at all, Kathy began to learn. It was shocking enough to learn such a thing as a patient—but in the eyes of a businesswoman, it was no less than blasphemy.

"Almost immediately after the formal diagnosis," says Kathy,

I was getting first, second, third, fourth, fifth opinions about what to do. Myeloma was such an unknown disease back in '96. So I'd tell one doctor at the University of Chicago that I was going to the Fred Hutchinson Cancer Center to see Bill Bensinger [a top myeloma researcher], and they'd say, "Oh, could you take notes and send it to me?" Everywhere I went I was the person getting the data together . . . there was no place where they were *working together.* It was so obvious that no collaboration was going on in the field whatsoever.

Within just a few months of receiving her diagnosis, before she had even settled on a course of treatment, Kathy set her mind to changing that culture. Everyone who knew Kathy knew that she would.

As toddlers, twin sisters Kathy and Karen would babble all night to each other. Their mother had the good idea to put the two cribs on either side of the room. But, says Karen, the younger of the pair by seven minutes, "It took only one night for Kathy to figure out that if she jumped in the crib just right, it would move just a little bit to one side. So she kept doing it until we were, once more, right next to each other, gabbing non-stop as before."

Growing up in Blue Bell, Pennsylvania, just off the Philadelphia Main Line, blond and blue-eyed Kathy was welcomed in by the popular group of girls in elementary school. But one morning, Karen remembers, Kathy woke up and said casually, "I don't feel like doing the whole popular-girl thing." That day, after school, she formed her own group of not-quite-so-popular kids.

Kathy's first job out of college was at Merck, doing sales and marketing for an antibiotic drug and a hepatitis vaccine. She left for Harvard Business School in 1983 and when she graduated two years later, took a job at Gillette, but soon ended up in a top marketing position at the pharmaceutical company Searle. Just months on the job, she cornered the chief operating officer and told him she wanted to be president of the company some day. "It was classic Kathy," says Karen.

Multiple myeloma changed none of that determination. Eager to continue trying for another baby, Kathy underwent in vitro fertilization treatments in the weeks after the diagnosis. Her doctors were nearly apoplectic: "Are you insane? You have a fatal disease!" she remembers one shouting. Kathy's response, as always, was unrelenting: "I will die anyway. Why not give my little girl what I think she needs before I go?"

Her twin, an attorney who spent many years working for media giant Time, Inc., making sure that the often provocative writers for *Sports Illustrated* didn't step over the legal line, has an expert ear for the artistry of blunt talk. Kathy is a master, says Karen with untempered admiration: "She *always* cuts to the chase. She *never* minces words. My sister says exactly what she's thinking. When we were little, her family nickname was Razor-tongue."

Not long after the diagnosis, and with Karen's help, Kathy started a community fund to raise money for multiple myeloma research. In their first fund-raising event, in October 1997, they pulled in nearly half a million dollars in contributions. It was a massive success. Kathy wanted to take steps to ensure that the money would be best spent.

By then, months of in vitro fertilization efforts had worked: a baby boy, David, had been born five months earlier. Kathy was now caring for her infant son and Nicole, who was almost three. On top of that, the Giustis had just moved from Illinois to Connecticut (in part to be nearer to Karen, who had settled in Greenwich). Paul had sold his company and taken another job; Kathy had left Searle. Now, in between doctor visits and trips ferrying her toddler to and from preschool, she plotted how to turn the community trust fund into a foundation that would both raise money and funnel it toward the development of new treatments.

The first, modest step was to bring together a handful of top myeloma researchers and executives from several pharmaceutical companies and biotech firms for a conversation. At the first of these meetings, Kathy recalls, "I was sitting there in disbelief that these guys had never talked to each other. . . . There were then no drugs for multiple myeloma. None of the academics knew anybody [on the drug-development side], let alone how to work with them. They were hopeless at it. So over time, we ended up doing a lot of these roundtables, just to bring these different worlds together. You'd think that was simple. There was nothing complex about it. Any moron could do it."

Kathy even bought a how-to guide for moderators at the bookstore, and opened up one of the meetings with a "leader's question": "We will be successful in our effort if we do *what?*"

There was a pause, as the dozen or so people gathered looked around to see who would answer first. "And then one of the industry guys said, 'If you give us tissue in which we can validate a drug.'" He snickered at what he must have thought was a throwaway line—an obvious impossibility.

But that was it. Like the hand-scribbled note Kathy had found on the kitchen table a couple of years earlier, the one that said the doctor wanted to see her. The words shot right through her:

> I didn't realize at the time that every academic center had its own tissue bank. I didn't know until 2002 that they were hoarding tissue. I didn't know the crappy quality of the tissue they had in their freezers. But I can tell you, I knew the importance of it. I was always giving bone marrow at Dana Farber, as was my sister. Because we are identical twins, this was a great resource for looking at genomic issues. And as they would fill these huge tubes of marrow . . . I would notice the techs standing right outside the door. It hit me then how fresh this needed to be; how fragile these myeloma cells are. You can't kill them in the body, ironically, but they die right away outside of it. I had seen this all, personally, as a patient. And now I was hearing it at a [foundation] roundtable. I realized right away that we had to get tissue. And I realized that industry was not going to believe in us, or bother with this [uncommon] disease, until we started showing them we could bank tissue—and prove that we could help them get clinical trials done faster. And so I decided to do the tissue banking first.

Her fellow board members at the foundation "freaked" when Kathy suggested that the group begin collecting tissue and recruiting clinical trials for testing new drugs, fearing that the foundation could be sued into oblivion if anything went wrong. So Kathy did an end run around the dissenters and formed a second entity, the Multiple Myeloma Research Consortium. The foundation board had been right about one thing: it took forever to find an insurance company willing to provide liability coverage for the consortium and its directors and officers. As for the other bureaucratic and legal tangles, they were so impenetrable that even negotiating a membership agreement with the initial four research centers consumed a full year. And this, in turn, was possible only because Kathy agreed to take on all of the critical tasks.

Her new organization, MMRC, would find and maintain the storage facility, set up the standard operating procedures, put together the information–technology systems that could process and store the huge volume of molecular data, connect a fast-growing network of myeloma patients with the research centers, and pay for it all. Each member institution would get access to the "whole" of the tissue resource, as needed. In exchange, they agreed to send in any new specimens collected (though, in truth, it would be only a portion of them), and follow the rules.

Not that their end of the process was easy. The consortium worked out some fifty separate laboratory and logistical procedures, all of which required rigorous compliance. When a patient's marrow was drawn at one of the MMRC sites, "the pull" (the tube of marrow) was collected in a specially designed kit, bar-coded, paired with consent forms, case reports, and matching peripheral blood, packed in liquid nitrogen, and sent overnight to a facility in Scottsdale, Arizona, where slides were made and key genomic data was extracted.

By January of 2007, the consortium had ramped up to thirteen member research institutions and had collected and networked a thousand fragile blocks of fresh tissue from myeloma patients, linked with complete clinical and molecular reports. By the start of 2011, the MMRC's stash of pristine samples had grown nearly three times. The tissue had, all the while, been used to screen antibodies, test tumor vaccines, and identify new potential targets for drugs. So precious was the resource and the consortium around it that they had brought a frenzy of new scientists and drug developers to focus on multiple myeloma—a cancer that until Kathy Giusti was diagnosed with it had been much a research hinterland.

When I ask Giusti, petite and elegant in a wide-lapeled suit, about the moment she realized that none of this infrastructure existed prior to her building it, she is blunt:

> Isn't it scary? I sat in wonder the first time it hit me: "You mean all those times I gave a bone marrow in the hospital it's just been sitting in a freezer? When a drug developer could have had access to that tissue and validated a possible lifesaving drug?" It's insane. If patients knew that, they'd be in an uproar right now. They'd be furious.

What makes the failure to achieve a national cancerwide tissue network so noteworthy is that such a resource requires "building" very little. There is no Hoover Dam to construct, no requirement for any next-generation Buck Rogers technology. Integrating the software can be complex, but the programs themselves are off-the-shelf. As pieces of infrastructure go, the costs for building and maintaining a National Biospecimen Network are minuscule.

A network, after all—whether it be for exchanging rare books or basement "collectibles" or human tissue specimens—is not, at its core, a piece of machinery, high-tech or otherwise. The Internet is not, fundamentally, the servers, routers, and pipes that compose its fiber-optic skeleton; the global system for air traffic control is not the sum of its radars, radios, and transponders. At its heart, a network is an *agreement.* Simply that. It is an agreement among many to use a shared set of protocols and language. What makes any such system viable to begin with are its conventions and standards.

Yet cancer researchers have not found common ground on any system, technological platform, or even vocabulary. This disarray has led to an inability to achieve critical mass in many areas of cancer science. It has hampered the ability to forge collaborations across borders and scientific disciplines.

"The great thing about standards in cancer research is that there are so many good ones to choose from," jokes David Agus, a leading oncologist and professor at the Keck School of Medicine in Los Angeles. "We've got good standards for genomics, and proteomics, and clinical trials for data annotation. The problem is we've got so many of them. And so one of the tasks going forward is to develop a taskmaster. The hope is we can reach a conditional standard to which we can all adapt."

Consider, for example, the sophisticated machines at the heart of today's cancer research effort: the sensitive instruments known as "microarrays," designed to measure (among other things) which of thousands of genes in a given sample of cellular DNA are turned "on" or "off" in the cells of a cancerous tissue. Page through any leading cancer journal and you are almost certain to see a multitude of smears in red and green, luminous Rothko-like patterns that purport to reveal the gene expression "signatures" of malignant diseases.

Essential to the modern treatment paradigm is that physicians will have the ability to read the genetic signatures of their patients' cancers. After all, there's no point in developing precision–targeted drugs if doctors can't identify those same targets in their patients. That would be like building a sophisticated telephone system in which no one knew what anyone else's phone number was.

For the Gleevec model to have even a prayer of working, physicians would have to be able to molecularly subtype, or "oncotype," tumors with extraordinary accuracy. (Just as knowing nine digits of a ten–digit phone number is not sufficient, it's of little use to know only part of a tumor's molecular signature.) But a lack of common industry standards, says Agus, who is also director of USC's Norris Westside Cancer Center as well as the Center for Applied Molecular Medicine, a laboratory focused on fulfilling the promise of personalized medicine, makes the already formidable scientific challenge harder still. The molecular signals of such tissue are read differently by different types of microarrays, he explains, because each brand of these expensive instruments uses its own proprietary algorithm to "normalize" their readings; that is, to separate the so-called noise in gene expression from a bonafide signal. Every chip reader is "a black box," says Agus. "You don't know how those samples are being normalized. You don't know how that data is being changed before it goes onto your individual spreadsheet. They're not reproducible [from one system to the next]."

The situation is worse on the proteomic side, in the study of the protein profiles of cancer cells. "We still have marked differences in technologies, and these technologies are not comparable," Agus says. "There is no reference standard to compare the different methodologies for mass spectroscopy [a protein analysis tool], and again, you've got proprietary software in each of the mass-spectroscopy machines that modulate the data. And clearly on the clinical trials side, it's been most evident over multiple decades that we have no standardization of common data elements."

Likewise, there are no standard practices when it comes to measuring many critically important antibodies—markers, for example, that can identify the estrogen receptor (ER) or HER2 protein in breast cancer cells, or a telltale growth receptor (EGFR) in lung cancer cells.

"We all call things by different terms," says Agus. "And so because of that, there can be no national databases of results, outcomes, or comparability between clinical trials."

The inability to establish a set of standards, to find a common language for cancer research and medicine, says something important about our National Cancer Program. There is none. The global corps of medical oncologists and scientists who study this disease, who have aggregated into powerful guilds (some with memberships that soar above twenty thousand) and who gather at several hundreds of conferences each year, seldom work in any truly collaborative way. Theirs is neither a self-managed community of professionals nor a top-down–managed corporate enterprise.

The war on cancer is tens of thousands of individual research wars— not one unified quest.

This is not the way it has to be. There is, indeed, a worthy model for cancer research that can serve as a guidepost for the future, a template for team discovery that teaches everything there is to teach about the power of collaborative science. The surprise, perhaps, is where and when this model is to be found: half a world away and half a century ago.

Chapter 14

The One-Eyed Surgeon

The boy's name was Africa. He was five years old. And he was terrified. The surgeon at Mulago Hospital peered inside the child's wide-open mouth, trying not to show his surprise. But he had never seen anything like it. The boy's jaws were swollen with what appeared to be four equally spaced tumors. There was a mass in his upper jaw on the left side and a parallel one on the right. The lower jaw, the mandible, was a distinct bone from the maxilla. It was unlikely that the cancer would have spread there so quickly—like a forest blaze jumping over a fire wall. But here, too, were growths on both sides of the boy's face. The tumors had uprooted his teeth from their moorings. They were halfway out of his mouth.

Surgery was impossible. The cancer was too deep and too widespread to cut out. So after the examination, the surgeon, Denis Parsons Burkitt, took out his camera and photographed the child several times. There was little else to do. The boy named Africa would die within days or maybe weeks, Burkitt knew.

The year was 1957. Burkitt had been in Uganda for ten years, based for most of that time in Kampala, the rolling hill city of the old Buganda kingdom that was now the capital of the British colony. Though he ran one of Mulago Hospital's three surgical wards, he was not, by his own account, a great surgeon. He was a decent one, a "bush surgeon," as he'd say.

He would have had more time for artistry, perhaps, were it not for the numbers. There were so many patients to see—and so few physicians, let alone surgeons—that it was difficult to spend much time on any of them. That many of the sick and dying were children made the task that much harder. Parents would bring their young into the Mulago, or to the clinics in outlying villages, with limbs that were bent from polio, gouged from animal bites, ulcerated with infection, congenitally malformed, or wilted from hunger. The list went on. Kwashiorkor, a miserable condition caused by malnutrition, was especially prevalent. Due to a lack of protein and calories in the diet, kwashiorkor would leave a toddler's body emaciated, his skin tinted red, and his stomach distended on the way to starvation. The name meant "the one who was left behind," and its effects were most often seen in children who had been weaned from their mother's breasts too soon, thanks to the arrival of an infant sibling. Burkitt's colleague at the Mulago, Hugh Trowell, had discovered a humble remedy for the condition in skim milk, but still the cases kept coming.

The region seemed to have no end of plagues—malaria, sleeping sickness, yellow fever, o'nyong-nyong fever, chikungunya fever, dengue fever, hemorrhagic fever, yaws. The last, a highly contagious bacterial infection that deforms a child's bones, joints, and skin, affected some 80 percent of the local population, according to Burkitt's estimate. That, too, could be treated—with penicillin, though laying hands upon any wasn't always easy. More gory still was the illness caused by a parasite called bilharzia, a flatworm larva that harbored itself in a freshwater snail. It was everywhere a person might bathe or swim. Victoria Nyanza, Africa's largest lake, which spread across the boundaries of three countries, was a hotbed for the parasite. The larvae could enter human skin in less than a minute after contact.

In Burkitt's first eighteen months in Uganda, he had been stationed in the northern town of Lira, in charge of a hundred-bed hospital and responsible for a district spanning seven thousand square miles with a quarter million inhabitants. By the end of the first year, he had tallied up more than six hundred surgeries. Many were performed at what the Colonial Medical Service grandly called "sub-dispensaries." Burkitt would visit two of these outlying huts per week. He'd spend hours alone on flat, dusty stretches in his brakeless Ford pickup, roll to a stop by a village clinic, clean up, and perform an operation. He sterilized surgical instruments over a portable gas stove. A hanging oil lamp gave him his only light. Many times, Burkitt would have to administer the anesthesia on top of everything else.

The Mulago Hospital in Kampala was modern by comparison. The main building was a modest, two-story pavilion with an elegant, miniature domed clock tower. Bundled around the main building were the wards and various clinics, a number of white, one-story structures with polished concrete floors and corrugated-iron roofs. Inside and out, camped on benches or waiting noiselessly on the neatly mowed grass, were patients.

The pace would have been grueling enough for a young doctor, fresh out of medical school. Burkitt was forty-six. He had three daughters, ages three, seven, and nine. His wife, Olive, had been in and out of good health. And then, of course, was the matter of Burkitt's strange occupational handicap. The surgeon was missing an eye.

At the age of eleven, standing in the driveway outside his preparatory school near Enniskillen in Northern Ireland, Burkitt had been caught between two warring factions of boys. In the melee, someone threw a rock that hit his eyeglasses, shattering a lens into his right eye. Three attempts to remove the shards proved hopeless. His damaged eye was replaced with a ball made of glass.

It had not been easy convincing the British Colonial Service that it should give a one-eyed surgeon a try. But Burkitt had been relentless.

His depth perception had suffered as the result of the accident. That was true. But then, the loss had amplified his vision in a different way. There was no explaining it: with his lone eye, the Irishman saw things that others missed.

Fifty miles from the Mulago was the district hospital in Jinja—a town on the banks of Lake Victoria. Here, some said, is the mythical source of the Nile, where one of the river's mighty arms begins its four-thousand-mile stretch from equatorial Africa to the Mediterranean Sea. Burkitt was in Jinja, giving rounds to a handful of medical students, when he turned his only eye to an open window. On the grass outside the hospital was a little boy sitting with his mother. The boy's jaws were badly swollen, as if the bottom of his face had been stretched out like a balloon.

Burkitt ran out to see him. He was the second child Burkitt had seen in weeks with the same bizarre tumors—could that be coincidence? Was it a new form of cancer? Was it something else? The doctor urged the boy and his mother to accompany him in his truck to Mulago Hospital. There, he examined the child, finding still more growths in his abdomen. Burkitt took several photographs, as he always did, and developed them in his bathtub at home.

His daughters would sometimes sneak into the bathroom to see what Daddy was "cooking" in the tub. This time they saw the black-and-white images floating eerily in the water and stared at the little Ugandan boy's contorted face. It didn't look real, they thought.

Within days, though, the child was dead, just like the boy before him. His parents brought an armload of flowers to their lifeless son and carried the body home. Burkitt could not get the image of his swollen face, or that of the boy named Africa, out of his head. The strangeness and ferocity of the tumors stuck with him during hospital rounds. He had trouble sleeping at night.

During one of those restless nights, Burkitt resolved to solve the mystery. And the mission he and colleagues from around the world were about to undertake would prove to be one of the greatest, and most heroic, accomplishments in the history of cancer research.

By any stretch of the imagination, the middle-aged man from Enniskillen was no revolutionary. Denis Burkitt was methodical, efficient—and down–to-the-penny frugal. That had become an ongoing joke among family and friends. Burkitt despised waste so much, his daughter Cassy liked to say, that when he'd draw a hot bath for himself, he'd fill the tub an inch high.

Standing ramrod straight even in the wilting heat of Uganda, the bush doctor carried himself like a colonel in the cavalry. He had served as an officer (earning the rank of captain) during the Second World War, but the erect posture was more a reflection of his own moral register than of any wartime training. A devout Christian and teetotaler, he saw himself as a missionary in Africa at least as much as an employee of the British government.

His father had been a warden in the Church of Ireland, his uncle a brimstone missionary and doctor in Kenya, their father before them a Presbyterian minister. And Burkitt himself looked eminently like a Sunday school teacher. His mouth was a thin, flat line; his receding hair was parted neatly on the right side of his head, leaving open a pale expanse of forehead. High on the bridge of his nose were the eyeglasses—thick, black, horn–rimmed frames that appeared to dissolve at the bottom, leaving the top of the frames to serve as the man's eyebrows.

The sober image would have remained intact were it not for Burkitt's voice. Somehow, emerging from this resolute face of propriety came an easily excitable, high-pitched voice, bathed from top to bottom in Irish lilt. Burkitt could be such a fast talker that it was often hard to understand what he was saying, and hard not to be interested anyway. It was, in short, charming.

He was also smart enough to use it, asking everybody in sight if they had seen a tumor like the ones in the two boys. The question, in some ways, defied logic. If anyone had ever witnessed such massive, lightning-fast growths, surely he or she would have called attention to them. A giant protrusion in anyone's face—let alone in a child's—wasn't the kind of thing a doctor could ignore. Certainly a parent could not.

But what if the tumors manifested in a different way . . . or in another, less obvious place in the body? Burkitt checked the Mulago's archives for records of odd cancers of the head, and then for childhood malignancies of any type. A surprising number of jaw tumors were, in fact, recorded in the hospital's files. In every case, the boy or girl had died.

A few postmortem exams had been done, with complete annotations and photographs. The pathologist in each case had labeled the malignancy "small round-cell sarcoma." *Sarcoma* was a general term for any cancer in the body's connective or supportive tissues—cartilage, fat, muscle, blood vessels, and bone.*

Just as with the little boy from Jinja, nearly all of those with jaw cancers also had tumors in the abdomen or elsewhere. The pathology reports classified the cancers based on where the "primary" tumor seemed to have sprouted—though, for the most part, the pathologist had simply guessed: If a tumor was in the eye, it was called a "retinoblastoma"; the kidney, a "Wilms' tumor"; and so on. But the descriptions of what the diseased tissue looked like under the microscope were strikingly similar. "Small, round cells," the reports all said.

The Irish surgeon paid a visit to a pair of pathologists, Jack Davies and Greg O'Conor, who taught in the medical school at the nearby university. Drawn in by Burkitt's excitable pitch, the two pulled 106 slides of cancerous tissue they had collected over the years from African children. Amazingly, under the microscope, the cells on most of the slides looked strikingly similar. It didn't matter whether the tumors had been found in the jaw, in the abdomen, or somewhere else—the look of the cells was nearly identical. What's more, suggested Davies and O'Conor, this cancer was not a sarcoma at all. Nor was it a carcinoma, a solid tumor—the kind that began its destruction in the cellular linings of the lung, colon, breast, prostate, and virtually every other organ of the body.

This was a cancer of lymph tissue.

The distinction was important. Just as there was a network of vessels circulating oxygen–rich blood through the body, a second elaborately constructed system brought infection–fighting cells to wherever they were needed. White blood cells called lymphocytes traveled slowly through thin lymph vessels and gathered in honeycombed nodes situated in the neck, abdomen, groin, and dozens of other strategic locales. There, microorganisms and other infectious agents were enveloped and destroyed by

---

*Cancers of the bone were typically considered their own subset of malignancy, called osteosarcoma.

immune cells, while other lymphocytes made antibodies to recognize the same species of invader the next time around. Organs such as the spleen and tonsils were also part of this still-mysterious anti-infection apparatus, though it was not yet certain what roles they played.

Not only were any of these "lymphoid" cells vulnerable to transforming into cancer, once transformed they could easily spread to far-flung organs of the body by way of this extensive network of vessels.

In other words, lymphomas could travel quickly, seeding invasive colonies throughout the body.

But was this incredibly aggressive lymphoma a new disease? Did it come out of nowhere? The surgeon thought of a good place to check. Mengo Hospital stood on the outskirts of Kampala. Opened in 1897 by a British missionary named Albert Cook, it was one of East Africa's busiest hospitals, and its archive of patient records was impressive. Burkitt sifted through the cancer cases and found a number that resembled this strange lymphoma. Cook himself had drawn sketches of the jaw tumors in his notebooks, though he, too, had called them sarcomas. He had even penned an article in 1901 for the *Journal of Tropical Medicine* in which he'd written, "Sarcomas are common in Africa, particularly sarcomas of the jaw."

The cancer wasn't new. That much was clear.

Just as important, Burkitt was discovering something key about *who* was getting the disease. Now, with scores of case records from Mulago and Mengo Hospitals, along with the reports from other nearby hospitals, he separated the patients by age. He put the three-year-olds into one column, the four-year-olds in another, and so on. The distribution seemed meaningful, though he had yet to figure out why. No one younger than two was affected. The cancers, which began striking at age three, built to a peak at ages four through seven and then dropped off. None of the patients was older than ten. Boys appeared to get the disease twice as often as girls.

He was looking for whatever patterns he could find—where the children came from, what schools they went to, what other illnesses they might have had. To do that, though, he needed to survey more hospitals and clinics. Already it seemed as if this type of lymphoma was the most common form of cancer in Ugandan children, though until now, no one had recognized it as a single disease. Maybe that was the case on the rest of the continent as well.

The following February, Burkitt presented his findings to a group of East African surgeons meeting in Kampala. Then he sent off a paper entitled "A Sarcoma Involving the Jaws in African Children" to the *British Journal of Surgery.* The article got no reaction.

George Oettlé was the director of the Cancer Research Unit at South Africa's national cancer center. At thirty-six, he was already making a name for himself in research circles. He had been invited to speak at conferences in England, Japan, the Soviet Union, and the United States, and now he was visiting tiny Kampala. Burkitt led his guest into the children's ward to see a boy freshly diagnosed with the terrifying lymphoma. Burkitt then showed Oettlé photo after photo of protruded jaws, describing how the tumors would nearly always be found in organs throughout the body as well.

Oettlé cut him off. "This tumor does not occur in South Africa," he said with certainty.

Burkitt pondered the statement for a while, then was struck by a question: If the cancer was common in Uganda, but didn't exist at all in South Africa, where did it stop?

Surely the geographic distribution of the tumor would give some clue as to what was causing it—and, he hoped, a way to stop it.

As it happened, Burkitt already had some experience studying the link between disease and place. In this case, though, it had been accidental. Within months of his arrival in Uganda, working among the Langi tribe in the north, Burkitt found himself performing scores of minor surgeries on men and boys who were suffering from painfully enlarged testes. Fluid had built up in their testicular sacs—in some cases, as much as a gallon— the result of a condition called hydrocele. Burkitt noticed that in the eastern part of the district, the ailment was quite common; in many villages, as much as a third of the male population were infected. In the west, the infection rate was about 1 percent. (The culprit turned out to be a microscopic parasitic worm that is transmitted by mosquito bite. Burkitt's finding helped lay the groundwork for the discovery.) He submitted his observations to the venerable British medical journal *The Lancet*, the first of some three hundred-seventy papers and books he would publish during his lifetime.

Could the strange, ferocious lymphoma also have a geographical component? If Oettlé was right, Burkitt would have to find the lymphoma's "edge"; that is, where it stopped. Burkitt had a simple notion as to how to find it: He would ask around. His plan was to send out a questionnaire about the jaw lymphoma to hospitals all across Africa. He printed up twelve hundred flyers with black-and-white photographs of three afflicted children—a three-year-old boy with a tumor in every quadrant of his jaw, a six-year-old with his upper jaw and eye swollen beyond recognition, and a four-year-old whose mouth could no longer close—accompanied by a handful of straightforward queries, such as "Do you see this jaw tumor?" "Do you see this tumor in other sites?" "How long have you worked at this hospital?" He spent weeks compiling the addresses of hospitals and clinics all across Africa. To cover the cost of the printing and postage, Burkitt applied for his first-ever government grant—and received fifteen pounds (then, about forty dollars) from the British Medical Research Council.

Over the next three years, some four hundred responses trickled in. With each confirmed sighting of the aggressive lymphoma, Burkitt put a colored pushpin into one or more of the three maps hanging on his office wall. The first was a map of Uganda, the second of East Africa, and the third of the continent as a whole. "We couldn't afford fourpence each [eleven cents] for mapping pins," Burkitt told one of his biographers, Bernard Glemser, "so I painted the heads of drawing pins myself in different colors to distinguish the different tumors." He noted on the maps whether there was just one recognized case of the disease or a number of cases.

Another clear pattern was emerging. The lymphomas were occurring in a belt across sub-Saharan Africa, from Senegal on the Atlantic coast through Cameroon and the Congo, all the way to Kenya on the Indian Ocean. The upper limit of the belt was a line somewhere between fifteen and eighteen degrees north of the equator. The bottom edge was harder to see. On the eastern end of the continent, for example, the path snaked southward, moving from Uganda to Tanzania (then Tanganyika),

Malawi, and Mozambique. Yet, in Southwest Africa, there weren't any of the strange lymphomas to speak of. In all, the "lymphoma belt" ranged through some thirty countries.

The almost ridiculously straightforward research technique of sending out a questionnaire had yielded a bonanza of epidemiological information. While the emerging geographic pattern of the disease was just that—a *pattern,* not an answer as to why the pattern existed—it represented a leap forward in knowledge about a common childhood cancer that, only four years before, no one knew existed.

The patterns and far-flung connections, however, were just beginning to come into sight.

Tony Epstein ran a lab at the Bland-Sutton Institute, a research facility attached to Middlesex Hospital in central London. He had heard of Burkitt. Every few years, the self-proclaimed "bush surgeon" from Uganda would emerge from the wild to give a lecture to Middlesex medical students, typically on exotica such as elephantiasis or the grotesquely enlarged testicular sacs of men with hydroceles.

It was March 1961 and Burkitt had just given a lecture at London's Royal College of Surgeons. It had been in a massive hall, big enough to seat a thousand. Twelve people had shown up. Burkitt had made a joke of it, but it was embarrassing nonetheless. He was to give a second speech, which had been billed as a "combined medical and surgical staff meeting" in the Courtauld Lecture Theatre. Its title: "The Commonest Children's Cancer in Tropical Africa. A Hitherto Unrecognized Syndrome." Tony Epstein wasn't sure why at the time, but he decided to attend.

Epstein had listened to the fast-talking presenter for barely ten minutes when he was struck by the importance of Burkitt's findings. Epstein had been studying tumor viruses at the Bland-Sutton. The apparently rigid geographical distribution of the African lymphoma suggested that an infectious agent might be at work.

Indeed, it had already been shown that viruses had played a role in transmitting a few cancers from one animal to another. In 1908, a pair of Danes, Vilhelm Ellermann and Oluf Bang, had devised an experiment to demonstrate how a healthy chicken could get leukemia from the filtered blood of a chicken with leukemia. Three years later, Peyton Rous of the Rockefeller Institute showed that even if the tumor from a cancer-ridden fowl was ground into a pulp (so that no malignant cells could possibly remain), and the resultant extract was then injected into a second animal, the cancer would be conveyed. The implicit conclusion was that only something *sub*microscopic—smaller even than a bacterium—could be the culprit.

In 1956, Epstein himself, with the help of an electron microscope, had managed to see and describe individual particles of the "agent" Rous had discovered forty-five years earlier, and which had become known as Rous sarcoma virus, or RSV.* The viral particles were a mere seventy millimicrons in size, or seventy millionths of a millimeter. Experiments similar to Peyton Rous's had revealed connections—again, seemingly causative ones—between viruses and breast cancer in mice (passed along through mother's milk), fibromas in cottontail rabbits, and kidney cancer in North American leopard frogs. But thus far, no one had found a virus linked definitively to cancer in humans.

That gap had cast a shadow of doubt over the field. For every researcher pursuing the virus connection, there were others who scoffed at the notion that viruses, bacteria, parasitic worms, or some other mysterious germ could play much part in cancer development. After all, despite the seeming presence of cancer clusters and even pronounced geographical patterns, cancer did not act like a communicable or infectious disease. There were no cancer "outbreaks" as there were with cholera or trypanosomiasis or polio. Even in cases of the brutal African lymphoma that Burkitt had come to London to discuss, it was remarkable if more than

---

*In the mid-1970s, RSV would star in one of the landmark discoveries of cancer research. Studying this same virus, Michael Bishop, Harold Varmus, and colleagues at the University of California, San Francisco, would reveal how malignant transformation is initiated by mutations in certain *normal* genes called proto-oncogenes, which when functioning properly regulate the cell cycle or another essential aspect of cell life. (Proto-oncogenes, when altered or rearranged in the wrong ways, became *oncogenes*, in the new parlance.) The Bishop-Varmus model, which would later earn the pair the Nobel Prize, unified then–competing views of carcinogenesis by showing how everything from DNA-purloining viruses to toxic chemicals in the environment to inherited gene irregularities to mere accidents of mitosis might lead to the oncogenes that ultimately "drive" cancer.

one person in a village came down with the disease. Caretakers didn't get it. Brothers and sisters who slept, played, and ate alongside the patient didn't get it. What kind of infectious agent worked like that?

In truth, most of those who supported the virus-link theory did not believe that viruses transmitted cancer like a traditional infection. Rather, in some way not yet understood, the ultratiny pathogen was able to transform a cell (or maybe cells) in a way that pushed it down the road to malignancy. Many questions remained to be answered.

After the speech, Epstein approached Burkitt and invited him to tea. Between sips, the young virologist asked if it would be possible for Burkitt to send some tumor samples from his lymphoma patients to London? The request was by no means trivial. Burkitt would have to freeze a substantial portion of the tumors he biopsied from his next several lymphoma patients, vacuum-pack them in special vials, and transport them to the Kampala airport in a freezer chest for the long flight to London. Burkitt happily agreed.

Three years later, out of cell cultures made from Burkitt's tumor samples, Epstein and two colleagues, Bert Achong and Yvonne Barr, would discover a virus—the Epstein–Barr virus—that would command the world's attention. Finding that virus, a globally ubiquitous member of the herpes family, would prove to be one of the most important medical discoveries of the era.

It would also help solve one of the key mysteries of the African lymphoma.

Just as Burkitt had arrived in London, the March/April issue of the American journal *Cancer* was reaching mailboxes in the States. Prominent in the issue was a second article by Burkitt on the fast-growing tumor, jointly written with Greg O'Conor, his fellow ex-pat in Uganda, who had been studying the cellular pathology of the disease. O'Conor detailed the characteristics that made this disease distinct from other, more familiar lymphomas in the West. Under the microscope, the cells, fixed in place by formalin, seemed to paint the image of a "starry sky." *Burkitt's lymphoma,* as it began to be called, was suddenly the talk of oncology labs everywhere.

Burkitt didn't mind the flurry of attention. It came in handy for the next phase of his research. While the questionnaire had been helpful—the responses had led, after all, to the mosaic of colored pushpins on Burkitt's wall—plenty of unexplained gaps remained on the maps. Epidemiology was too difficult to conduct by postal carrier. Doctors might remember the more striking cancer cases, particularly the prominent tumors of the jaw, and might even take time to respond to a faraway researcher they'd never met. But as Burkitt's own experience had shown, it was easy to miss the more subtle connections between things. Albert Cook, after all, had recorded, in 1901, that sarcomas of the jaw were particularly common in Africa, and Burkitt had spent a decade in Africa without "noticing" one of them.

As biographer Glemser writes, "What occurred to Denis Burkitt was no sudden vision, no sudden flash of inspiration, nothing as dramatic as Sir Isaac Newton's apple falling in the orchard. After ten years, so he says, he woke up to something that had been there all along."

As self-effacing as he was about his own powers of detection and deduction, Burkitt had limitless faith in the abilities of others to remember crucial details. He knew that when confronted in person, doctors and nurses and mission workers could conjure up long-buried observations that mattered. The trick was getting to talk to them in person. Burkitt had the answer in his head, long before he'd figured out how to do it. His plan was do a "geographical biopsy" of Africa; instead of sampling tissues and examining them under a microscope, he would sample memories and investigate the connections between them.

Once again, he needed a team.

Ted Williams did not want to go. Williams, the director of a mission hospital in northeastern Uganda, had been planning to take a long-awaited leave to England with his wife. As nicely and firmly as he could, he told Burkitt no. Nicely and firmly, the Irishman urged him to put off the vacation a while longer and, instead, join him on an epidemiological excursion across half the African continent.

Williams was not only one of Burkitt's closest friends, he had a rare skill for a mission doctor: He was a gifted mechanic. In Burkitt's estimation, his friend "could change a big end bearing while you were having a cup of coffee." As it happened, in the summer of 1961, a fellow missionary fleeing the civil war in the Congo crossed the border into Uganda with a 1953 thirty-five-horsepower Ford Jubilee station wagon, its chassis worn thin by forty-five thousand miles of mud and dust. It was the perfect vehicle on which to test Williams's skills.

Burkitt had secured another grant from the Medical Research Council—this one, a lavish 250 pounds—which he used to purchase the Ford. Williams went straight to work on the automobile, tying two spare tires to the roof, reinforcing the floorboards with a steel plate, installing a secret circuit breaker for the ignition, and throwing as many spare parts and medical supplies into the rear bin as it could hold.

The two left Kampala at 9:15 in the morning on October 7, 1961, for their ten–week journey to Johannesburg and back. They would pick up the third man on the expedition, a Canadian missionary named Cliff Nelson, in Tanzania. Burkitt had spent months contacting hospitals all along the route, specifying the date and estimated hour they would arrive. In all, the team would cover ten thousand miles, through often endless stretches of sun–scorched bush, visiting fifty-six hospitals and mission stations in twelve countries. At each stop, Burkitt, then fifty years old, would tirelessly display his grim photographs of protruding jaws, interview doctors and administrators, and check the hospital records, if possible, for tumors that might fit the description. He'd walk the wards, peppering the handful of clinical staff with questions, then record the responses in his scientific journal. The key was discovering where the patients had lived before they trekked to the hospital, which was often hundreds of miles from their homes.

During the "safari," the researchers would uncover more than two hundred recorded cases of probable Burkitt's lymphoma that had eluded the questionnaires. More compelling than the numbers, once again, was the pattern. On the shores of Lake Tanganyika, in Kigoma, evidence suggested that the tumor was common. North of the lake, near the mountainous border with Burundi, there was no sign of the disease.

Near the town of Tunduma, they veered off the path to visit a mission hospital run by an Irish doctor who was well over eighty years old. ("A very wide-awake lady," Burkitt noted in his journal.) She recalled one child with the tumor who had come from the upper part of the Luangwa River valley, many miles away.

In northern Zambia, the cancer was either rarely or never seen. The Karonga hospital in Malawi, on the other hand, had admitted five patients in the prior six months. From Karonga to the town of Livingstonia, on the Malawi plateau, the road climbed treacherously up a mountainside, making 22 hairpin turns (Burkitt nervously counted each along with 112 lesser "bends") at such a steep gradient the station wagon could barely manage it. On the other side of the mountain was a hospital, a mission station of the Church of Scotland. No one there recalled seeing the lymphoma. In coastal Mozambique, the jaw tumor was well-known; a few miles inland, it had never been seen—and then, in a hospital in Lourenço Marques, on the Indian Ocean near Swaziland, there had been forty documented cases. A pathologist at the hospital, working with a local museum curator, had even thought to make plaster head casts of the children. Burkitt, tireless as ever, carted the lot up to the roof and photographed them.

Most of the journey was spent on the less exciting, more exhausting task of getting from one stop to the next. The drives, at thirty-five miles per hour, often seemed interminable. The trio could easily travel fifty miles or more without seeing another vehicle. On some stretches, rolling down the windows could be a choking hazard, as clouds of dust would fill the car. Not opening them was a baking hazard, with temperatures in the tin can easily soaring above ninety degrees. Whenever the engine boiled, Ted Williams would run out, pour in water, and hope for the best.

To pass time, they sang songs and Bible hymns at the top of their voices and exchanged exotic tales of doctoring. And, naturally, they talked for hours and hours about the lymphoma and its undeciphered code. Burkitt, reflecting upon the journey years later, could not remember who first brought up the possibility that altitude might play a role, but that he was sure the revelation would never have occurred had they been flying from one hospital to the next. It was the dividend of "unhurried discussions," as the surgeon put it. "I would almost certainly have missed the point had I traveled alone."

By the time they had trundled back to Kampala, Burkitt and his colleagues were sure they'd found their "edge." The divide between those who were getting the disease and those who were not was less an outline of geography than topography. It was as if there were an unseen and slowly sinking rope from the equator south to the tip of Africa. Between the equator and a latitude of eight degrees (about the middle of Lake Tanganyika), the tumor was absent in villages that were higher than five thousand feet above sea level. The farther away from the equator, the lower the cutoff point. In Zimbabwe, the tumor did not show up at altitudes above three thousand feet; in Swaziland, never above one thousand feet.

But what did altitude have to do with cancer?

Alexander Haddow worked at the East African Virus Research Institute in Entebbe, not far from Kampala's Mulago Hospital. Like virtually every other doctor in Uganda (and many others throughout the world), Haddow was captivated by what was now being billed in newspaper articles as "the Long Safari." An entomologist by training, he looked at Burkitt's maps, now thick with colored pins, and came up with a different conclusion. There were two limiting factors in this brutal lymphoma, and both were only tangentially related to altitude, he believed. The cancer, it now appeared, was contingent on both temperature and rainfall.

Later safaris to the mountain–rimmed countries of Rwanda and Burundi, and then to Nigeria, and then to West Africa, confirmed Haddow's theory. If one highlighted a map of Africa showing only those areas where the temperature rarely fell below sixty degrees Fahrenheit and annual rainfall exceeded twenty inches a year, it would look virtually identical to Burkitt's array of colored pins. What was more, said Haddow, it would resemble a map of insect-borne disease in general. He recalled a map in an old entomology textbook showing the distribution of outbreaks of sleeping sickness over earlier decades. The plagues had been transmitted by the bloodsucking tsetse fly. The distribution was nearly identical to that for Burkitt's lymphoma.

Another colleague, pathologist Jack Davies, whose slides of childhood cancers Burkitt had first examined years before, suggested a different airborne nemesis: the *Anopheles* mosquito, which also thrived in warm, moist climes. Just maybe, the cancer had some relation to the mosquito's infamous payload in most of equatorial Africa, a single-celled organism called *Plasmodium falciparum*. This microscopic invader was responsible for a disease that sickened and killed millions of people in sub-Saharan Africa every year—malaria.

Once suggested, the connection seemed obvious. Parallels between the prevalence of malaria and Burkitt's lymphoma were uncanny. A map of one was a map of the other, down to the marshes and river valleys. Nevertheless, it was hard to see how even this compelling link was anything more than circumstantial. What did a parasitic infection of red blood cells have to do with a cancer in the lymphocyte, a type of white blood cell?

In the early 1960s, cultivating human cells outside the human body wasn't easy, especially a lineage of cells that would thrive in perpetuity. The feat had been managed for the first time in 1951, when a Johns Hopkins researcher named George Gey created the first human cell line from the aggressive cervical tumor of a thirty-one-year-old Baltimore woman named Henrietta Lacks, who died that same year.

To keep a cancer cell and its progeny alive *in vitro* (literally, "in glass"), one had to create exactly the right growth medium (usually a mixture of animal serum—the yellowish remains of blood after the actual blood cells and fibrin had been centrifuged out), with exactly the right nutrients, salt content, and acidic balance. One had to maintain the ideal mixture of oxygen and carbon dioxide and keep it at precisely the right temperature. One had to be vigilant in making sure that bacteria, which typically have a doubling rate some forty times higher than that of human cells, did not contaminate the batch—that external viruses, yeasts, and molds were not inadvertently introduced, something that was all but inevitable with time and human handling. One had to make sure that the cells were properly "passaged," or split off, every few days so that the continuously dividing "clones" did not squeeze one another to death in the glass tomb of a petri dish. After all, immortality, even for an immortalized cancer cell, was an unnatural state.

After first going through twenty-four of the tumor samples that Burkitt had sent and faithfully kept sending, Tony Epstein and his colleagues got lucky. At long last, three of Burkitt's lymphoma cell lines emerged. Epstein had less luck, even with the aid of a rare electron microscope, in isolating and studying the herpeslike virus particle he had glimpsed in 1961. It was now 1964, and he needed help.

Gertrude and Werner Henle were waiting to provide it. The German-born Henles had emigrated to the United States during the Nazi era and were now ensconced at Children's Hospital in Philadelphia. They were already world-renowned virologists by the time Epstein wrote a letter offering to send his precious cell lines across the Atlantic in exchange for their eyes and expertise.

The Henles were more eager to study Burkitt's lymphoma than Epstein could have guessed. A year earlier, the chief surgeon of Children's Hospital, C. Everett Koop, had gone to Africa and met personally with Burkitt. He had come away wowed by the Irishman's investigation. Upon his return, Koop went straight to the Henles' lab and told them about the fine-combed epidemiological work Burkitt's team had done. "Henles," he said, "if you want to work on a human tumor that is likely to be virus-induced, Burkitt's tumor is it."

The Henles also had trouble isolating the virus in the cell lines—but they came up with another idea. If there was a virus in the Burkitt's tumors, then surely there would be specific antibodies to it in the blood. And to find those, they sent in another type of antibody targeted to home in on any human antibody. This batch was traced with a dye that would fluoresce (glow in apple-green color) when stimulated by the light of the microscope. It was like sending the hounds to sniff out the fox and then finding the dogs by listening for their howls and barks.

Just three years after Burkitt's team returned from its journey to the southern reaches of the African continent, the Henles in Philadelphia were finding antibodies to Epstein's herpesvirus, in huge concentrations, in 98 percent of African lymphoma cases. In remote Papua New Guinea, a second region where both malaria and this fast-growing cancer were found together, EBV was omnipresent as well. Blood samples from these lymphoma patients showed a tremendous antibody response to a specific protein in the herpesvirus. More telling, virus particles were consistently found in the nuclei of the tumor cells themselves—and importantly, each cell in the tumor appeared to have an identical copy of the virus, as if one infected progenitor cell had taken over the mass with photocopies of itself. This, at long last, was as close to proof as there was of the link between a virus and a human cancer.

Years later, when Epstein published a textbook on the virus that bore his name, the first illustration would be of the flyer of Burkitt's 1961 lecture at Middlesex. For some reason, on the day of the talk, Epstein had plucked the announcement off the wall and saved it.

Still, even as tantalizing clues were emerging, the mystery remained far from being solved. For one thing, the Henles weren't just finding the Epstein–Barr virus in lymphoma patients, they were finding it in almost everyone they tested. The tiny virus now appeared to be ubiquitous. Which brought up a nagging question of mathematics: If malaria infected millions upon millions of people, primarily in Africa, Latin America, and Southeast Asia, and Epstein–Barr virus was present in billions of people (more than 90 percent of adults worldwide, regardless of race or place of birth, carry antibodies to the virus), why on earth were cases of this lymphoma still relatively infrequent, countable in the hundreds? Though the cancer was now the most common diagnosis of childhood malignancy in Africa—accounting for one in five cancers in Uganda, one in four in Nigeria, four of every ten in Malawi—it was still an oddity. Cancer was rare in Africa compared with the West. The sad fact was that most people in Africa did not live long enough to worry about it.

There were plenty of additional questions to answer. To begin with, assuming that two distinct infectious agents—one a parasitic protozoan, the other a near-universal virus—were involved in the development of Burkitt's lymphoma, how did they conspire to initiate a malignant transformation of cells? Was yet another type of virus involved as well? Was there a contributing factor in diet or the surrounding environment? Was there an inherited gene that made some children susceptible to the disease? Was there a reason, beyond sheer coincidence, for the consistent age pattern among the children who developed this cancer? Did it matter when the malaria or EBV infection began?

None of the riddles was trivial. Burkitt's lymphoma remained dizzying in its complexity. By early 1966, however, the widespread expectation was that the mystery would soon be solved. Burkitt's strange tumor had become a celebrity in the cancer world, as scores of medical scientists rushed to study the disease. Many were drawn to the cancer's tantalizing link with a virus, the first to be demonstrated.

By this time, the Henles had definitively tagged EBV, found in the remotest tribes of the earth, to its own common *non*malignant disease—infectious mononucleosis, which shared some interesting traits with lymphomas, and particularly with Hodgkin's disease. Could "mono," the infamous "kissing disease" of high school and college campuses everywhere, be somehow related to this African lymphoma?

It was Epstein, however, who pointed out why Burkitt's tumor was so fascinating to so many. It was, quite possibly, the Rosetta stone for cancer as a whole.

In the early nineteenth century, linguists from Great Britain and France were able to parse the hieroglyphic decree of a boy pharaoh from the second century BC by first translating the other two scripts on the same black granite slab. Understanding of the language written on the bottom of the stone (ancient Greek) led to a slow translation of the text chiseled above it (Demotic Egyptian), which led to the deciphering of the sacred picture-writing of the pharaoh's priests at the top of the stone.

Burkitt's lymphoma offered the same challenge—and promise. If researchers working together could make sense of the mechanism by which the two suspected pathogens—malaria and EBV—could transform a single healthy lymphocyte into a relentless invader, the world might get closer to understanding how other cancers are initiated. And that, in turn, meant being closer to the goal of either preventing cancer in the first place, or curing it.

Back at Mulago Hospital, Burkitt couldn't stand the thought that he could be doing something useful and wasn't. After days in the operating room or the wards, Burkitt would often head to his hospital workshop, where he would build makeshift limbs to replace the ones he occasionally had to amputate. He'd fashion them out of plastic piping and whatever industrial supplies he could find. He would make crutches, calipers, and leg braces out of iron rods, stray hardware, and broom handles. They weren't pretty. But waiting around for a cosmetically appealing limb that wasn't ever likely to come was foolish. Young lives would be ruined in the wait. As with much in sub-Saharan Africa, the good was of far more use than the perfect.

In the same way, in the midst of his surgical duties at the hospital and his epidemiological work on the new lymphoma, Burkitt sought to treat the stream of swollen-faced children who were now coming to his clinic. Several years earlier, in 1960, Joe Burchenal, a Sloan–Kettering physician known for his efforts in the relatively young art of chemotherapy, had visited the Mulago Hospital. He had recommended that Burkitt try a drug called methotrexate, which blocked folic acid, a B vitamin, needed for DNA synthesis. The ability to copy DNA was necessary to cell division—and if cells could not divide, the thinking went, they could not amass into destructive tumors. (The failure to divide would trigger them to self-destruct.) Of course, healthy cells needed to divide as well, and blocking folate would kill them, too. The drug's potential in Burkitt's lymphoma, Burchenal surmised, was that the tumor cells were dividing so rapidly that they'd be knocked out in much greater proportion—or at least at a quicker rate than the critically important cells of the liver, brain, and other vital organs.

Sidney Farber had used this same strategy to achieve temporary remissions in children with acute lymphocytic leukemia in the late 1940s. Roy Hertz and Min Chiu Li at the NCI had followed the same approach in 1958 to cure—actually *cure*—patients of choriocarcinoma, a rare, fast-growing solid tumor.

Burkitt did not have time to set up a proper clinical trial. Children were dying in six to twelve weeks after getting the lymphoma. He begged some methotrexate pills off the local distributor of the American manufacturer and gave them to a child in the manner and dosage Burchenal had suggested. The drug dramatically shrank the boy's tumors for a time. Then the cancer returned. Burkitt tried the drug in several other dying children. In some of his young patients, the tumors returned; in others, miraculously, they disappeared.

Next, the doctor tried cyclophosphamide, another poison that interfered with cell division. (He begged and borrowed for that drug as well.) He knew there wasn't much science to his treatment "protocols," but cyclophosphamide seemed to work. Dozens of children were living instead of dying.

Soon other physicians and researchers—Peter Clifford in Nairobi, Eva and George Klein at the Karolinska Institute in Sweden—were advancing the clinical treatment of Burkitt's lymphoma. By 1966, the cure rate was up to 20 percent. The pace of progress seemed astounding, given how few chemotherapy treatments were effective in other cancers.

In one gathering of international researchers in Kampala that Joe Burchenal had organized, Burkitt showed large photographs of several children, their faces distorted with tumors, eyes bulging out of their sockets, teeth thrust from their mouths. Then, after the lecture, Burkitt brought the children out, twenty-three of them, all symptom-free—all of them looking like healthy children again. Eva Klein thought it the most moving thing she'd ever seen.

In the nine years since this disease had first been recognized, an extraordinary amount had been accomplished. A unique cancer had been diagnosed, its morphological signature verified, its all-too-vulnerable quarry identified, its occurrence plotted in two far-flung continents, its association with two pathogens (one of them also newly discovered) made clear, and a swift and certain death sentence commuted to something more hopeful. The what, who, when, and where had all been answered—all that remained were the how and why.

But Denis Burkitt's journey to discovery is more than a remarkable feat of medical sleuthing. It is also an archetype, in many ways, for how to do cancer research today. In its simplest form the model is to let scientists follow questions wherever they might lead, to let them *learn* as they go. Our current research-funding system, as argued previously, demands that investigators formulate discrete hypotheses related to discrete biological mechanisms, to choose experimental systems in which to test these hypotheses, and to spend half the year applying for a research grant (prospectively laying out the details of such hypotheses and experiments) that, if granted, will allow them to do the experiments in the other half of the year.

Burkitt had no hypothesis to explain the strange African tumor—not at first, certainly. He had no experimental system but for a sprawling continent to explore. He had no preset protocols to follow but for the mandate to ask questions ("Where is the geographical 'edge' of the disease's reach?" "What does altitude have to do with it?") There was no way to know what questions would arise from the data or from the insights of others. Burkitt, luckily, was not constrained by the rules of NIH funding to outline the specifics of his investigation ahead of time. He had the freedom to change directions whenever newly uncovered research data presented a new path.

A second lesson of the Burkitt model is that some mysteries in cancer—maybe even most of them—are best solved through genuine collaborations. In the case of the African lymphoma, doctors and scientists working in several nations, in disciplines ranging from virology to entomology, led by a one-eyed missionary doctor with a fistful of pushpins, exchanged their insights and experience with hummingbird speed. Burkitt enlisted the help of missionary doctors and nurses throughout Africa, of chemotherapists and drug manufacturers in the United States, of every physician who happened onto the grounds of the Mulago Hospital in Kampala. He freely shared tumor samples as others shared data and information with him. It was, perhaps, the single best example of spontaneous international cooperation in medical history.

The R01 system of research funding, by contrast, encourages investigators to carve out their own scientific niche, to become expert in it, and not to share "ownership" of any theory or idea. Our current system is designed not to solve problems, but to produce studies. It is the reason, as noted earlier, we have spent $6.5 billion on sixty-five thousand academic papers detailing the molecular circuitry and apparent function of the *p53* gene and its protein product—and yet, in the words of biologist Sir David Lane, the gene's codiscoverer, still have a "surprisingly incomplete" understanding of its workings and no effective *p53*-based therapies or diagnostic tools to speak of.

Third, the Burkitt model breaks the myth that great cancer science need be expensive. Save for one electron microscope, no high-tech machines were used to solve the mystery of the African lymphoma. The amount spent for Burkitt's entire ten–thousand-mile safari was £650 (less than $1,800 at the time), which was a bit cheaper than expected because the three men had the good sense to sell the Ford Jubilee after the expedition and recoup half its cost. The discovery of the Philadelphia chromosome by Peter Nowell and David Hungerford, likewise, "evolved in a laboratory which cost five thousand dollars [$39,000 in 2012 dollars] annually to run, including technician," Nowell later recalled.

Certainly some types of biomedical research are more expensive than others. But, as shown previously, the high "cost" of much of what is studied in cancer today is driven largely by the demands of the institutions where that research is being done, not by the actual expense of what is being done. As the US Office of Technology Assessment told Congress more than two decades ago, the nation's medical research enterprise operates under a unique set of economic principles: "The rise in demand for funds from the research community . . . is due primarily to increased *spending* on research, and only secondarily to increases in the 'costs' of individual components of research budgets."

Fourth, the Burkitt model, as the Farber model before it, shows the need to act, not to wait endlessly for more study, when lives are at stake. It is the most controversial, and perhaps uncomfortable, of the lessons drawn from this story, and from the chapters leading up to it. Risk-taking is often dangerously close to recklessness; but then, progress is rarely achieved without it.

Somehow, the world has forgotten that, just as many have forgotten Denis Burkitt himself. Once one of the most celebrated figures in the cancer world, Burkitt is today little more than a footnote in medical textbooks, if he is mentioned at all.*

---

*When Burkitt is remembered, it is primarily for his pioneering work connecting the low-fiber diets of Western countries to their generally high rates of colon cancer and digestive disease—an epidemiological link he identified years after his discovery of the strange African lymphoma. Burkitt was also an early crusader for cancer prevention. Long before anyone else had heard of the importance of a high-fiber diet, Burkitt—the "Fiber Man"—had become a global evangelist for preventive nutrition.

We have *un*learned the lessons of his Long Safari and in the process, I believe, forgotten how to win the war on cancer.

Again, one has only to look at the case of Burkitt's lymphoma for a vivid example—though, in this case, the period covers the four decades that followed 1966. Disappointingly, medical science has yet to solve the mystery of the African jaw tumor or even come much closer than researchers were in the years immediately following Burkitt's famed expedition. While the cure rates of *treated* patients have indeed climbed over the past forty years, most families in sub-Saharan Africa cannot afford the cure. (The cost of the appropriate drug regimen in the Ivory Coast, for example, according to a 2001 study, was $2,800—three times the annual income of the average family there.) Likewise, there remains no way to prevent the disease nor identify which children may be at risk.

Somewhere between the time of the Long Safari and the not-too-distant past, somewhere between what could only ambiguously be called "then" and "now," the cancer research culture changed. As that culture became ever more shaped by the frenzy of grantsmanship, publication, and bureaucracy, as it became ever more fearful of risk-taking, it lost its collective sense of urgency to solve the cancer problem. We must find it again.

Part Four

The Way Forward

Chapter 15

Matterhorn

Rising 14,692 feet into the air, the Matterhorn cuts the sky like a stone arrowhead, a pyramid of rock so steep that even ice and snow lose their grip and tumble to the glaciers below. Jutting up from the border of Switzerland and Italy, the peak is a thousand feet lower than that of Mont Blanc, the tallest of the Alps, and lower even than several neighboring mountaintops. But for nearly eight decades following the ascent of Mont Blanc in 1786, the Matterhorn remained out of reach—the only peak in Europe that had never been summited.

One group after another had set off from the Valle d'Aosta in Italy and begun the arduous trek from the mountain's southwestern ridge. Almost accidentally, Edward Whymper of London, an artist and wood engraver by trade, found himself among them. Dispatched to Switzerland in 1860 with instructions from his publisher—"Draw me some Alps!"—Whymper had never before scaled a mountain. Within weeks of seeing the Matterhorn, he, too, felt compelled to try.

Six times over the next five years he began the ascent. Six times he was forced to turn back.

Then, in June 1865, Whymper, barely twenty-five years old, was struck by a hunch so irrational that he thought it had to be a revelation. In all the attempts to conquer the mountain, none had attacked from the northeast. The reason could not have been more obvious: viewed from the Swiss village of Zermatt, the Matterhorn was a towering, featureless wall of stone.

But what, the artist wondered, if its sheer face was an illusion: a trick of light and distance and even popular imagination?

The mere possibility was enough to push him to organize a seventh expedition—from the forbidding Swiss side. The Matterhorn fought back again. This time it would be an avalanche that turned the climbers away. "That awful mountain," the one that had stolen more lives than any other in Europe, could not be overcome, it seemed.

Whymper would not be dissuaded. Just a month later, at the crack of dawn on July 13, 1865, he and six others set out on yet one more unlikely journey from Zermatt. What they found, on this eighth attempt, would amaze even the unwavering believer: it was a hidden "staircase" of ridges leading them straight to the top.

The Matterhorn was theirs.

Elwood Jensen, who would later become a legendary figure in the field of cancer research, first heard the story of Edward Whymper in 1947, when studying in Switzerland on a Guggenheim fellowship. The tale, coupled with his own summit of the Matterhorn (following the same path of the English wood carver), changed his perspective on life, Jensen said. Indeed, it would be Whymper's law—to always look for an "alternative approach"—that would frame Jensen's long, extraordinary career in science, one that would earn him a Lasker Award, the science accolade many consider to be America's Nobel Prize.

Jensen died in December 2012 at the age of ninety-two. When I interviewed him in 2007, he was still spending most weekday mornings in his faculty office at the University of Cincinnati, sorting out the remaining mysteries of estrogen signaling, the area where he had made his indelible mark. Jensen had been the one who figured out *how* this hormone actually communicated its powerful, tissue-specific growth messages—a finding that would come as a complete surprise to experts in the field.

Through the late 1950s, the accepted wisdom was that estrogen (or its dominant form in humans: 17ß-estradiol) went through a series of bio-chemical changes when it entered its target—a cell in a mammary duct, for example. These oxidations and reductions, prodded along by waiting enzymes, ultimately resulted in the growth of the cell. (Or in the case of cancer, the runaway growth of the cell.) In the established view, estrogen was merely the first whispered phrase in an enzymatic game of telephone: it was *metabolized,* as scientists said—and the product at the end of the line was something altogether different.

Investigators from around the world had spent decades, to no avail, trying to map out the various chemical chain reactions that estrogen seemed to be initiating.

Jensen, for his part, thought of Edward Whymper. For any towering challenge, he now imagined, there was surely an alternative approach that no one had yet considered.

With that in mind, Jensen embarked on the estrogen hunt in an unusual fashion. Rather than ask, "What does the hormone do to the tissue?" he would ask, "What does the tissue do with the hormone?"

The first step in answering the question was not easy. It required finding a way to track estrogen. But Jensen and a postdoctoral student named Herbert Jacobson rigged up an apparatus to "tag" molecules of the hormone with tritium, a radioactive form of hydrogen gas. (Such tracers had been used before, but the duo came up with a few innovations.) Now, they discovered, they were able to detect the hormone in quantities as remote as a trillionth of a gram—and follow it wherever it went in the body.

When they injected the radiolabeled hormone into female rats, they found that in most of the animals' tissues (the liver, lung, skeletal muscle, kidney, and so on) estrogen was expelled almost as quickly as it came in; meanwhile, in the organs of the reproductive tract, the hormone aggregated and remained for some time. The real surprise, however, was *where* much of it was huddling: in the nuclei of the cells—the same vault where genes are kept.

Later experiments would reveal just what the hormone was doing there. Estrogen did not go through a biochemical alteration, as experts had long contended; instead, it bound to a uniquely matched partner—a *receptor*—that waited patiently for it in the nucleus (or in the cytoplasm nearby). Then, the two molecules, bound into a single complex, made their way to a specific region on the cell's winding, chromosome-sheltered genome to initiate the process of transcription. To turn a given gene "on," in other words.

The discovery, in 1958, opened a window into an entirely unknown mechanism by which cells translated signals (from either outside or within the cell) into genetic commands.

But then, it did well more than that. By the 1970s Jensen's revelation would lead to a new way of attacking and preventing cancer—in the case of breast cancer, for example, through drugs that block the estrogen receptor (and thus disable the "gas pedal" in the malignant cell). This is the rationale behind tamoxifen.

Jensen, again by following Whymper's law, would play an instrumental role in the development of this drug—offering the world a concrete, if imperfect, demonstration of how the "theory" of cancer chemoprevention might work in practice. And flawed as tamoxifen is, one thing is clear: no other therapy derived in the modern war on cancer has done as much to reduce the breast cancer burden.

In the course of writing this book I have thought again and again of Elwood Jensen, and of the sheer, spiking face of the Matterhorn, and of the English wood carver who reimagined this indomitable rock as a gently sloping hill disguised by sunlight and sky.

The preceding chapters are, each in its own way, reflections of such counterintuitive vision: stories of men and women who have found striking clarity in the muddle and misinformation around them.

By taking the time to do something simple—to *count*—Joe Hin Tjio and Frederick Hoffmann revealed the true number of things (chromosomes and cancer deaths, respectively) when respected colleagues did little but repeat the conventional wisdom. Judah Folkman and Mina Bissell each saw the dynamic, frenetic exchange of a cellular neighborhood when many around them could focus only on the mechanics of an individual cell. The one-eyed Denis Burkitt, somehow, "discovered" an endemic and horrific childhood cancer when an entire continent of witnesses could recall no more than a scattering of cases. Benno Schmidt, a financier without a shred of scientific training, could see—even forty years ago—the failure of an experiment that a nation of medical scientists can merely claim "needs more money to complete." And then there is the courageous, irrepressible Michael Sporn, who for three decades has pointed to the only viable (if still formidable) route to reducing the cancer burden, even as so many others seem to ignore the growing toll.

All are visionaries. The history of cancer science, as the pages above ought to make clear, is filled with such brave and expansive thinkers: Francis Peyton Rous, who showed a century ago that a virus could trigger cancer; Howard Martin Temin, who revealed an alternative path for the transcription of genes in certain viruses (including the very one Rous had discovered); Josh Fidler, who has spent half a lifetime proving that a tumor cell's environment (its "soil") is as critical to the process of metastasis as is the malignant cell (the "seed") itself. The list goes on longer than any one volume can catalog.

Which brings us to a paradox that has played throughout this book. We have no shortage of heroes in the cancer war. Even in the crush of a Byzantine research-funding system—one that represses originality, snuffs out the outrageous, and discourages risk-taking—brilliant scientists somehow manage to break free. Even in a "cancer culture" that rewards conformity, paradigm-shifting ideas emerge; and novel theories push the boundaries of knowledge ever further. As they always have.

With such ambition and fortitude, researchers have detailed the circuitry of human cells down to their tiniest and most intricate components, mapping with ever greater precision the complex chains of molecular signals that appear to turn healthy cells into malignant ones.

Yes, great science is being done on the cancer front and great scientists are doing it.

Yet the cancer burden continues to grow with abandon. To look at the crisis now—1.6 million new cases and some six hundred thousand deaths each year in the United States, many tens of billions of dollars spent on treatment and research with few life-prolonging therapies to show for the investment, the fastest-growing health threat in the developing world at a time when "standard" treatments (even in the developed world) remain unaffordable—is to see an apparently insurmountable challenge.

The biology of cancer remains, in many ways, a mystery. Treatment remains, in many ways, a guessing game. Early detection remains an empty talking point.

As an obstacle of *medical science*, indeed, the "cancer problem" has proven to be as impassable at the beginning of this century as it was at the beginning of the last.

Like the Matterhorn fifty years before that.

And so we return to Edward Whymper. It is time now to look with fresh eyes at this awful mountain. Heretical as it sounds, we must stop thinking of the cancer crisis as a problem of medical science—and reimagine it as a wholly different genus of problem: a *challenge of engineering*.

The transformation is not a semantic one. This change in perspective brings with it a dramatic change in approach: a new and risk-embracing path to the summit, new and unfamiliar milestones that must be reached along the way, new tools that must be forged, new collaborations to be put in place, new oversight, new accountability, new rules.

Sharply reducing the number of people getting, suffering from, and dying of the disease will be profoundly difficult even if we can pull off such a radical change in perspective. But Whymper's law, at least, offers authentic hope. Because when framed as a test of engineering, beating back the cancer threat ought to be no less achievable than so many other great feats of the past. Science determines the limits of the possible. Engineering lets us reach them.

The laws of gravity and motion are the stuff of high school science classes the world over. But only one nation in history has been able to land a spacecraft on the moon, let alone a man, let alone bring him back.

The elements that made these marvels possible—vision, planning, coordination, teamwork, and, most of all, *management*—seem almost trite in black and white. But this is what Mary Lasker was imagining when she called for a Moon Shot for Cancer. (And this is what the scientific and medical communities feared and fought.) The story that Lasker and others hoped President Nixon and Congress would tell was of a great quest of engineering: the brightest scientists and the most ambitious problem-solvers working in concert to achieve an urgent goal.

The presumed achievability of that goal was then, and remains, beside the point. The near-impossible missions that launched Apollo and split the atom share a common ancestry with engineering feats that seem more *this*-worldly in nature. The efforts that tunneled a roadway under Mont Blanc and a railway under the English Channel share the same DNA. So does the system of interstate highways that crisscross America and the mass of skyscrapers that crowd into a few square miles of granite on an island in New York Harbor—the tallest of them, at 102 stories, built in little more than a year. So do items a fraction of the size.

The first Intel microprocessor was introduced in November 1971, one month before the National Cancer Act was signed into law. It had twenty-three hundred transistors, a remarkable feat for the time. Engineers have since grown that number to 781 million—all squeezed together in near-impossible harmony onto a single silicon wafer and following some two million times as many instructions in the same split second.

Over the four-decade span of the modern war on cancer, the mere "ordinary" of technology has gone through one revolutionary transformation after the next, zooming from the humble eight-track cassette player to the iPhone. The era has witnessed the birth of the personal computer, the Internet, the cellular phone, the digital camera, the GPS navigator, WiFi, Google, Facebook, the iPad, and Skype—even as the mammogram has barely improved. It is not a failure of science that has held back the last.

So, too, the most famous achievement of modern biology—the decoding of the human genome—is in reality a feat of engineering. What this and every other of the marvels above have in common is that each began as a project: a project whose success depended, most of all, on how well it was—and, in many cases, continues to be—managed.

The more ambitious and complex the undertaking, the more intuitive and sophisticated and responsive the management must be. The notion that, somehow, projects of science are exempt from such coordination and goal-setting—that "good science," left to its own collegial ways, will "get there on its own"—is a myth.

And there is no more instructive lesson for this than the man–made miracle that was supposed to serve as the model for the cancer effort: few will remember, but the moon shot began in utter failure.

When we think of the race to the moon, we think of Apollo, the mission that landed Neil Armstrong and Edwin "Buzz" Aldrin onto the gray dust of the Sea of Tranquility. Not long before Apollo, though, was Ranger.

The idea of the Ranger mission, the initial phase of the space program, was straightforward in principle: to hurl a box of electronic sensors and cameras onto the moon, before attempting to do the same with a human being. Implicit in the mission was that it would teach NASA a few lessons about getting there, too.

The spacecraft was less a vehicle than a slender cone on a six-sided base, five feet across, stuffed with a dozen sensing gadgets: a solar-plasma detector and a device for measuring magnetic waves, a primitive-looking chamber that could detect ion discharges in space, another for cosmic rays. Underneath this skinny module was a bomb: a five-story, two-stage rocket with 360,000 pounds of thrust. It was an actual bomb, in fact. It was an ICBM, a ballistic missile whose original mission had been to carry nuclear warheads to other continents. Now it was being used to catapult a seven–hundred-pound sliver into space.

It was, that is, if the countdown could ever get to zero. The first attempt to blast off the ground came on July 28, 1961, three days past schedule. It was aborted due to various preflight warnings. So was the second. Twenty-eight minutes before the end of the third countdown, a power failure in the area blacked out Cape Canaveral. The fourth was scrapped when *Ranger*'s solar panels opened prematurely on the launchpad.

Finally, after another month of delay, came countdown number five. The Atlas rocket shot upward at dawn on August 22, but things quickly went wrong. Due to a faulty switch, the upper stage fizzled way too soon, leaving *Ranger 1* far from its target. The high point of its very elliptical orbit was supposed to have been 620,000 miles above the earth; *Ranger 1* got only to mile marker 313 before sliding back into the planet's atmosphere and frying to a crisp.

The launch of *Ranger 2*, three months later, was worse. Again, the second-stage Agena rocket misfired, leaving the spacecraft in an even lower, more precarious orbit. Ranger craft were supposed to survive for months, taking measurements of cosmic phenomena; this one lasted twenty hours before disintegrating.

Two months later went *Ranger 3*. This time, a single inverted sign in a line of computer code caused havoc, sending the craft in precisely the opposite direction of its intended flight path. Two days into the mission, the computer failed.

Ranger 4 had a little bit of luck, managing to crash-land on the far side of the moon: But the spacecraft could provide little data regarding any of the mission to mission control. Almost immediately after separating from its rocket, the module's onboard computer crashed. So did the internal clock, which allowed preordained commands to run in a choreographed sequence. The craft had become, as one NASA official put it, "an idiot with a radio signal."

Ranger 5 followed in October of 1962. Little more than an hour passed before the calamities began. Yet another faulty switch robbed the craft's solar panels of electrical power; then the battery drained; then the computer overheated; then more shorting; then the radio transmitter went dead. The gyroscope that kept the spacecraft in relative balance malfunctioned along with the rest, throwing the vehicle into a wild somersault and far off course. Adding to the frustrations were more failures at a pair of tracking stations on earth. Machines that were supposed to radio telemetry data to the spacecraft simply stopped working.

There could be little doubt about what was responsible for the Ranger fiasco. Three official investigations—one from NASA, one from Congress, and one from the Jet Propulsion Laboratory (JPL) in Pasadena, home of the brainy rocketeers who had pioneered many of the telemetry and guidance systems for the army's missile arsenal and who now ran Ranger—all came to the same damning conclusion: the problem was slack management. Even the review board from JPL was shocked by the glaring weaknesses in JPL's oversight and recommended sacking the project's boss.

JPL had organized Ranger personnel into a hundred subgroups, each focusing on a discrete task. Without any sense of common goal, workers "showed a surprising lack of information or interest" about the impact their item might have on any adjacent circuit or switch, or on the performance of the craft in general.

Project leaders had not the faintest understanding of "systems engineering"—of the need to coordinate individual engineering tasks "into a single complex effort," investigators found. And when machines and procedures did fail in testing, there was no process, beyond water-cooler chatter, to let managers and colleagues know, nor any standard follow-up procedure to ensure that the flaws were corrected (and that the "corrections" did not, in turn, adversely affect other systems). Everything in the tiny craft was connected in one way or another.

JPL's culture was like that of Caltech, its founding institution: it was a place of genius tinkerers who bristled at oversight or any kind of interference with their work. On the Ranger project, it was hard to see where the lines of authority ran, or whether there were any.

The Ranger program was supposed to consist of nine missions. NASA's investigators, however, were convinced that flights six through nine would fare no better than the first five; the space agency threatened to withhold any new projects from JPL until it reformulated its management systems.

The threat of a funding cut worked. As later flights would bear out, the laboratory's leadership did turn things around. New engineering processes and oversight—from the basic (regularly scheduled meetings between team leaders and clear chains of command) to the sophisticated (matrix charts showing the potential interactions of every item on the craft)—were put in place. Such strategies would be employed to near perfection in the later manned space program, observed Stephen B. Johnson, professor of space studies at the University of North Dakota who wrote an insightful 2002 book on the subject. "Systems management," he contended, would turn out to be "the real secret behind Apollo's success."

Just after the moon shot's triumph in 1969, writer Tom Alexander would wonderfully distill the lesson in a piece for *Fortune* magazine:

> The really significant fallout from the strains, traumas, and endless experimentation of Project Apollo has been of a sociological rather than a technological nature; techniques for directing the massed scores of

thousands of minds in a close-knit, mutually enhancive combination of government, university, and private industry.

It took but two and a half years from Neil Armstrong's famous first steps on the moon to forget the lesson. Not long after the passage of the National Cancer Act, it became clear that this second "moon shot" would not have the management it required. There would be no coordinated, multistaged plan for how to target the inner space of the human cell. There would be no "war on cancer." The crusade that began on December 22, 1971, would be one without a strategy, without even basic command and control; in this battle, there would be no corps of engineers building the equivalent of pontoon bridges—the infrastructure necessary to collect and share tumor specimens, or to aggregate data from different gene-chip-readers, or to speed the recruitment of clinical trials. The "war on cancer" would turn out to be a mere slogan, a bumper sticker of an idea.

Which brings us nearer to the end of this inquiry. Nine years ago I began my reporting with a five-word question: How did we get here? The single answer, if there can be one, is that we have lacked the good, smart management to help guide us to our goal.

The argument over whether science can ever be managed is an old one. But often left out of the debate is the fact that scientists, and particularly cancer scientists, are already being managed . . . and middle-managed, and micromanaged. This mismanagement hasn't come from one boss, two, or ten, but rather from a culture that has emerged over the past several decades. As laid out in Part Three of this book, that culture has been constricting science, and hampering the researchers and doctors who work so hard to make headway against cancer. Most worrisome, it is badly failing the young scientists who may offer our best hope for progress.

The challenge, now, is to change that culture. And there are seven areas where we must begin. The first is, simply, to align the funding system with the right goals. The R01 grants framework, and the elaborate study-section review process built around it, as argued in chapters 9 and 10, encourage a cautious incrementalism in cancer science investigations, when what we need, by most accounts, is bold thinking and innovation. The system forces researchers to spend 50 percent of their time applying for a supply of grants that, despite funding increases, go to proportionately fewer applicants each year. The right goal, of course, is to have scientists spend their time doing science. As Stanford University's John Ioannidis contends, we can get closer to both of these goals by switching to a system that funds people, not projects.

The second area where we can make an immediate fix is to pare the multiple layers of decision–makers that preside over nearly every aspect of the cancer research process. David Dilts, a systems engineer and director of "strategy alignment" at Oregon's Knight Cancer Institute, in Portland, has spent much of the past nine years documenting the bureaucracy, inertia, and pointless delay in the NCI's system of cancer clinical trials. Forty percent of NCI-sponsored trials, as noted in chapter 11, take so long to begin that they are never completed. Likewise, the application and review process for research grants is a Rube Goldberg contrivance with more than twenty steps, each of which can consume weeks. Besides the R01, moreover, the NCI has some eighty-plus alphanumeric grant and contract mechanisms, from the "K08" ("Mentored Clinical Scientist Research Career Development Award") to the "U34" ("Clinical Planning Grant Cooperative Agreement"), each with its own program managers, rules, and limitations.

That said, there are straightforward ways to speed the process—many conceived by cancer leaders themselves—that have never been implemented. An obvious reform, for example, involves the patient-protection groups called institutional review boards (IRBs). In the current system, before any clinical trial can begin, the IRB at every medical center where the study is to be conducted (often scores of them) must review and sign off on that study. When one IRB makes an amendment to the protocol, the change must be approved, in turn, by every other IRB, which can entangle the process in a months-long "decision loop," Dilts has shown. Having a single, centralized IRB review and approve the protocol would make the process faster.

On the surface, it might seem that such bureaucratic delays are minor obstacles. But such obstacles pile up, helping to slow the research process to the point where developing and testing a cancer drug now requires an average of thirteen years, nearly twice the time needed in the late 1960s. It does not have to take a revolution to speed the levers, just smart management.

Third, we must build a common language and research infrastructure that can help transform tens of thousands of separate laboratory fiefdoms into a critical mass. For all the NCI's excessive management of cancer research, the agency provides too little management when it comes to bridging far-flung researchers and fostering collaborations. The widely disseminated research effort that emerged from the National Cancer Act in 1971 has created a Tower of Babel of terminology, technical standards, and technological systems. Data produced by one "gene reader" are often not reproducible in another. Specialists in the same types of cancer measure patient status in incompatible ways. Blood tests that measure "routine" cancer-antigen levels in patients are read differently by different test providers. "Bioinformatics platforms"—computer database systems that archive biological information—call individual genes, proteins, and molecular signaling pathways by different names. As oncologist David Agus beseeches, "We need a taskmaster to set standards!"

As chapter 13 makes clear, we can only have a true National Cancer Program, as envisioned in 1971, if we have a common language and networks through which investigators can exchange information. One important step in the right direction would be to turn the fledgling National Biospecimen Network (NBN) into a true and viable system for collecting, storing, and sharing cancer tissue specimens. The NCI, tomorrow, can make participation in the NBN mandatory for those who take taxpayer money. Every day we wait, more valuable information is lost.

The cancer culture's predisposition to inaction, as argued throughout this book, is driven in large part by a mind-set of risk-aversion. That mind-set, which contributes to the delay in clinical trials and discourages scientific investigators from proposing bold ideas in grant applications, will not be easy to change. The "omission bias," in which we reflexively assume that the unfortunate consequences of our actions are worse than those of our inactions, says the University of Pennsylvania's Jonathan Baron, is deeply engrained in most of us. The fourth thing we must do is begin to recognize that we are paying a profound price for our excessive caution. It is costing lives.

Before we can have any hope of changing this mind-set and of charting a new course, however, we must be candid about the rising cancer burden. That is our fifth task. Because, as argued in Part One of this book, we will be able to make the systemic and strategic reforms we need only when we come to terms with the true scope of the cancer crisis, and with our limited success in controlling it so far.

For too long, we have spooned out the truth of our progress in small doses. While some improvements have been made in treating cancer and extending patient survival, the "cancer problem" is, in reality, as formidable a challenge as ever. In the four decades since the modern war on cancer began, the burden of this disease has only grown, as the number of Americans who develop cancer rises inexorably from one year to the next. So, too, the cost of treatment has risen, as breathtakingly expensive new therapies enter the market while offering little improvement in patient survival. So, too, the death count has risen. More Americans, in fact, will die from cancer over the next fifteen months than have died in combat in all the wars the United States has ever fought, combined.

The problem, of course, isn't just an American one. By the year 2020, the number of annual cases worldwide is expected to reach 17 million; by 2030, between 22 million and 27 million—with 70 percent of those projected to occur in the developing world, where even treatments conceived in the 1960s and 1970s remain unaffordable. This is the true face of the cancer burden.

At the same time, we must also be candid about our strategy in attacking the problem. As described in Part Two, the modern cancer enterprise has undertaken what many call a "targeted therapy" approach, developing chemical and biological agents to block the genetic and protein switches that transform cells and enable their deadly spread. The weakness in that strategy, unfortunately, is twofold: it does little to prevent new cancers from developing, and it largely ignores the complexity and evolutionary capacity of the disease.

That complexity was made yet more clear in a March 2012 study by Marco Gerlinger and colleagues in the *New England Journal of Medicine*.

Gerlinger, working in the laboratory of Charles Swanton at the Cancer Research UK London Research Institute, and fellow investigators, mapped out the genomic landscapes within the tumors of four patients with metastatic kidney cancer, showing the mind-boggling variability of mutations within each tumor. The finding, corroborating those of many other studies over the past several years, was yet another blow to the targeted-drug paradigm, as an accompanying editorial in the *Journal* said: "A serious flaw in the imagined future of oncology is its underestimation of tumor heterogeneity—not just heterogeneity between tumors, which is a central feature of the new image of personalized medicine, but heterogeneity within an individual tumor."

Our best hope of success, as argued previously, is to attack a developing cancer much earlier in the process, before the destruction within the cells becomes too rampant. This is our sixth critical task. To be sure, this strategy comes with its own profound scientific obstacles, as laid out in chapter 7. But it offers the only chance we have of reducing both ends of the growing disease burden, the number of people of getting advanced cancers and the number dying from them. Here as well, our collective mind-set of caution has held us back from an aggressive effort to preempt cancer development, even for those at heightened risk for the disease. The strategy of preemption has dramatically reduced deaths from heart disease and stroke, triumphed over a litany of infectious diseases, and even reduced traffic fatalities. Yet, as Dartmouth's Michael Sporn argues, the cautious worldview that reigns in the cancer realm keeps us at arm's length from true prevention efforts in cancer.

Just as important, we must frankly acknowledge that increasing funding for cancer will not, *by itself,* solve the problem. Task number seven is to wean ourselves off the mind-set that "more money for research" will magically reduce the cancer burden. As chapters 8 and 9 make clear, we have tried this "fix," again and again, over the past four decades to no avail. What we need isn't money; it's management.

Management—the *right* management—is, at its heart, story-telling. It conceives of the common enterprise as a great tale, with a beginning, middle and end. Story is what turns any mere aim into a quest, what sketches paths to the impossible, what gets people to reach beyond their own jobs and doorsteps to link arms with another. Story drives and pushes and strives.

The question that must be asked now, forty years after the passage of the National Cancer Act, is, are we ready for another story? Are we ready for another great engineering challenge that we, as a nation—indeed, as a global human community—can pursue together?

I hope and believe we are. The journey to end the cancer threat is no further from the reach of human ability today than was the journey to the moon five decades ago, when President John F. Kennedy promised to land a man there and bring him back.

To accept one opinion survey, most Americans believe the same. Or did. On December 23, 1949. Gallup asked Americans to consider the limits of what they thought achievable by the end of the twentieth century.

Question 14(c) went like this:

Do you think that men in rockets will be able to reach the moon within the next 50 years?

Seventy-seven percent of those asked said, "No."

It was not that the American people did not believe in the power of science and technology. By then, a world war had been won on the strength of an atom, and researchers had descended into the microbial universe, returning with a trove of antibiotics that cured an array of once-fatal infections. Engineers had built jets that flew faster than sound and had sped up time itself, it seemed, with the aid of giant digital computing machines. (IBM had introduced its eight-foot-tall, fifty-one-foot-long Automatic Sequence Controlled Calculator in 1944.)

"American know-how," as the phrase went, could do anything.

But not, it seemed, get man to the moon.

In the same poll, though, was Question 14(a):

Do you think that a cure for cancer will be found within the next 50 years?

This time, 88 percent said, "Yes."

Acknowledgments

This book got its start in the fall of 2003, when I began reporting a story for that extraordinary idea-incubator, *Fortune* magazine. Any writer lucky enough to have written a feature for *Fortune* will no doubt understand my gratitude to this eighty-three-year-old institution. By the time the story ran in March 2004, so many colleagues had improved it—through probing questions, graceful edits, striking graphics, and more—that I feel a little ashamed to have claimed the byline for myself.

As lucky as I was to be working at *Fortune,* I was even luckier to have Joe Nocera edit the story. In a brief conversation at lunch, I mentioned to Joe what I had learned about the war on cancer in some preliminary reporting; thereafter, Joe pressed me (relentlessly) to pursue the story—then served as the consummate cornerman, a seasoned pro who made every paragraph that much stronger. Rik Kirkland, *Fortune's* wonderful managing editor and my long-standing mentor, encouraged me at every turn, and forced me to rethink the end of the magazine story in a way that gave purpose to the beginning and middle.

Fortune also made it possible for me to meet two celebrated corporate chieftains who, in very different ways, helped set this book in motion. In several memorable conversations, Dan Vasella, then chairman and CEO of Novartis, shed light on an important new cancer drug called Gleevec that became the basis for my initial inquiry. Later, in late 2003, Andy Grove, then chairman of Intel, helped, in a few perfect words, to shape the thesis I would pursue for close to a decade.

I am guessing that Dan, for one, won't agree with many of this book's conclusions—or even know how instrumental he was in its germination—but I am grateful both to him and to Andy for their candor and insight. Likewise, I am indebted to John Mendelsohn at the MD Anderson Cancer Center, who saw the critical story in *Fortune,* not as an attack, but as an opportunity to engage me in conversation and to explore the nuances of a subject that was too complex to explain in fifteen or so magazine pages. Our discussions over the years that followed have been some of the most illuminating I've had during the course of this project.

Elaine Jaffe at the National Cancer Institute—and, to my great fortune, my aunt as well—has been an excellent teacher and has been a continual support in this undertaking. I am also thankful that she led me to Michael Sporn, at Dartmouth.

Our first marathon conversation, in his bunker of an office in Hanover, New Hampshire, just after New Year's Day in 2004, lasted from early morning to dusk. Sprawling, expansive, provocative, and ultimately jaw-dropping in its revelations, it would set the mold for the next many years of talks to come. Nobody could have been a better chaperone through the marvelous history of cancer research. And I cannot thank Mike enough for his wisdom, his encyclopedic knowledge, his moral force, his hours of instruction, and his very cherished friendship.

I am also grateful to Dick Rettig, author of the seminal history *Cancer Crusade: The Story of the National Cancer Act of 1971,* who not only shared insights from his own long experience reporting on the war on cancer, but also generously handed me reporting files he had carefully assembled along the way.

Over the past nine years, hundreds of people have led me through the labyrinthine alleys of the cancer realm, translated its language, and explained its intricate customs and rules. In some cases, they challenged my narrow thinking and offered important correctives. At the start of my reporting, Ellen Sigal, the indefatigable force behind Friends of Cancer Research, opened up her Rolodex (yes, there was such a thing back then) and introduced me to dozens of thoughtful experts who, in turn, introduced me to dozens of others. Truly, in all that time, I cannot think of one person who refused to talk, or was anything but generous with his or her time. I wish I could thank each of them by name here—but the list would be too long and not do justice to the contribution of any.

That said, I would be remiss in not acknowledging at least some of the men and women who helped me see things that I would never have seen without their guidance. In a few cases, our conversations were relatively brief and occurred long, long ago; in others, the conversations lasted years. For all the time they spent helping me understand the cancer process—and the cancer research process—I deeply thank John Bailar, Francis Barany, Anna Barker, Mina Bissell, Bruce Chabner, David Dilts, Ray Dorsey, Brian Druker, Josh Fidler, Jay Freireich, Per Hall, John Ioannidis, Genie Kleinerman and Len Zwelling, Kim Lyerly, Peter Nowell, Homer Pearce, Rick Pazdur, Ching-Hon Pui, Kathy Redmond, Raul Ribeiro, Janet Rowley, Victoria Seewaldt, Frank Torti, and Bob Weinberg. In addition, I am particularly grateful to two legendary scientists—Judah Folkman, who died in 2008, and Elwood Jensen, who died at the end of 2012—who were extremely generous with their time with me.

It is important to note that those named above may not agree with all, or even many, of the conclusions of this book. No one should take their inclusion in these pages as a suggestion that any one of these brave souls endorses my message, wholly or partially. For what I've gotten right, they collectively deserve the credit. For what I've gotten wrong, the blame lies solely with me. And in every case, I am entirely grateful for their expertise, memories, arguments, and keen observations.

Over the past many years, there were some who shared so much of their time—and private lives—with me, that a lifetime's worth of thank-yous would not begin to express my gratitude. I am especially indebted to the Quinlan family: Nancy, Pat, Brendan, and most of all, Brian. Their compassion, courage, grace, and humanity are without limit. From the moment I met them at St. Jude Children's Research Hospital in October 2004, the Quinlans have been a profound inspiration to me, and I am beyond grateful for their trust in me and for their friendship.

Deep, heartfelt thanks are also owed to Kathy Giusti, who spent many hours talking with me, enlightening me, and helping me comprehend the inner dimensions of a research culture that she understands better—and has navigated more expertly—than anyone on the planet.

In the course of reporting this book, I have gotten to know many patient advocates who, like Kathy, have worked tirelessly to make cancer's burden lighter for millions of people—who have made preventing and curing cancer, and helping patients and their families, their life's calling. Their heroism is monumental, and yet too often unsung. I have learned so much from them. For inspiration and helpful discussions along the way, I owe special thanks to Diane Balma, Barbara Brenner, Nancy Brinker, LaSalle Leffall, Virgil Simons, Marlo Thomas, and Doug Ulman.

I have been moved and inspired, on a near-daily basis, by the many cancer patients and devoted family members and caregivers I've met over the past nine years. In their eyes, I have seen the hopes and prayers of millions who confront and fight this disease.

And in the lives of four women—Sue Morrow Flanagan, Kate Levin, Anita Roberts, and Laura Ziskin—who died of cancer as I reported this book, I can never forget the stakes.

Sue Flanagan had written me after the publication of the *Fortune* story. I can't recall what it was, in an eloquent letter from a stranger, that clicked—but something did. In the years that followed, we shared an untold number of e-mails, letters, postcards, phone calls, packages, poems, and photographs, and then in July 2010, a funeral. In our six years of friendship, we never met. I am grateful to her for her spirited, nose-bloodying hope—and for everything she taught me about life and death.

So many friends were immeasurably generous in ways that, quite thankfully, have nothing to do with cancer. They cheered me on, rallied me when I slowed, lifted me up when I fell.

Thanks to Lila Cecil and Joy Parisi, for welcoming me into Paragraph, a wonderful writers' workspace—and to the crews at Brownie's and at Vineapple, where I wrote much of the book.

John and Carole Repaci, neighbors who are so gracious as to redefine the term "neighborly," welcomed me into their kitchen at all hours during the past many years—so that John could feed me and, in his words, "keep me strong for the mission." Thank you, both.

For nearly a decade, David Agus has been a valued teacher and friend. I have learned so much from him and am grateful for every nugget.

Edmond Mulaire, my dearest friend from the age of four, offered keen suggestions for tightening and clarifying. His instincts for precision came through each time he reviewed the manuscript—which was too many to count, I'm afraid.

Nick Varchaver, a transcendent reporter, writer, and storyteller, was equally instrumental—and equally generous. Among his serial acts of friendship, Nick spent an entire vacation sequestered in his hotel room, instead of dozing on a warm Florida beach, reading and carefully marking up my manuscript. Indeed, the full truth is that Nick took the time off from work *just* to do that for me. (. . . And the full-full truth is that I begged him to do it.) He has been a constant champion and counselor.

My brother and sister—Marc Leaf and Jenifer Jaeger—offered wisdom, insight, and reassurance in every one of our conversations about the book. I am incredibly lucky to have grown up with them and to call each a friend, in addition to sibling. So, too, my extended family—Slimmers and Viscardis—have offered unlimited love and support. I am grateful for them all.

And it was luck again—a veritable lightning strike of it—that brought this book to Simon & Schuster, a home that could not be more welcoming.

My profound and abiding thanks to Jon Karp for his generosity in letting me pitch a long shot of a book, not once but *twice*—eight years apart, no less—and yet more incredibly, for his willingness to bet on it. I am grateful beyond words for his belief in me.

If mathematically possible, I am doubly thankful for his insight to pair me with Ben Loehnen—an editor, gentleman, and *consigliere* without parallel. There are hawks that can spot a mouse scurrying in the brush a hundred feet below. Ben's eye is at least that keen, and his sense for storytelling sharper still. I am truly indebted to him, not only for improving every single page of the manuscript, but for his unfailing wisdom, unending patience, and, I hope, never-ending friendship. No writer could ask for more.

Sincere and lasting thanks are also due to Brit Hvide for expertly moving these pages through production, and for all the other unseen tasks she has so adroitly fulfilled. Her dedication and kind spirit ought to be celebrated high and low.

I am grateful as well to so many others at Simon & Schuster—especially Richard

Rhorer, Marie Kent, Larry Hughes, Michael Accordino, and Irene Kheradi—for their great efforts in transforming an author's manuscript into a bonafide book.

Thanks also to Steven Boldt for his masterful, incisive copyediting; to Mia Crowley-Hald and Ruth Lee-Mui for overseeing the production editing and design; to John Pelosi and Paula Breen for their legal acumen; and to Wendy Sherman, for her sound counsel and help in making a transition between publishers effortless.

Tracy Brown, my extraordinary agent and friend, has been a rock-steady support throughout. I will be forever grateful for his sage advice, soothing optimism, and perpetual encouragement.

At the start of October 1979, I was eight weeks shy of sixteen years old, entering my junior year of high school a month after my classmates. I had spent September in a subbasement at the NIH's Building 10 getting radiation therapy for Hodgkin's disease. After four weeks of irradiation, I had been exposed to enough gamma rays, I imagined, to power a small city and I was now back at school. The accident at the Three Mile Island nuclear reactor had occurred earlier in the year, and fear of radiation exposure remained pervasive. The fear was palpable.

On my first day at school, though, one classmate welcomed me with "Hey, Cliff, how's it glowing?" and then wrapped his arms around me in a warm bear hug, letting every skittish kid and teacher in sight know that I was safe to approach. Years later, this same friend, Seth Kanor—a truly gifted writer—worked alongside me in one coffee shop and college library after another. He was always willing to read a passage I'd labored over, share a pound cake, walk around the campus at Columbia University, distract me when I needed it, but mostly, to keep me focused on the goal. I am eternally grateful for his thousands of insightful suggestions over the past nine years, his joyful readiness to help at all hours, and most of all, his friendship.

I could not have written this book without the unflagging support of my father, whose confidence in me has been sustaining, and whose guidance has been indispensable. No words can capture how grateful I am—how infinitely grateful I am for him. Were I to try, my dad might only wonder how I could thank him for something that, in his heart and soul, is automatic. No one on the planet is more generous of spirit, wiser, or truer. If ever I embark on another book, it will be to write about him—the man who has taught me more than anyone.

Though my mom died long ago, she, too, has been an ever-present force in my reporting and writing; she has been a voice of hope ringing softly in my ears. When I think of that hope, I cannot help but think first of my daughter, Sofia—in whom I see so much of my mom. To Sofia I sing thanks from hill to valley.

My almost-nine-year-old daughter has given far more to this book, to her grateful father, than she understands. I began the project before she was born. I know that I can never repay the moments I've stolen from us—the missed bedtime songs, weekend games, morning walks to school, days in the park. The book that came out of those stolen moments is in no way a fair trade. I hope, however, that I can make it up to her in the next nine years, and in the nine after that.

And to the person who ultimately filled those moments, my darling wife, Alicia Slimmer, I owe the most thanks of all. There is no part of these pages that did not come from her. There is no observation or argument, no morsel of fact, no character that did not spring out of the generosity of my wife, who surrendered a significant portion of a husband for nearly a decade in order to give them.

If that were all she gave, I would be in debt in this life and the next. But even more than that, my true love read every word of every draft and half-draft, gently alerting me to any note that rang flat or false. Her instinct is and has always been the gut I've relied on. Her heart is and has always been my own. The gift that I can truly never thank my wife enough for is that she chose to make my dream her own.

Notes

Prologue: How Did We Get Here?

1 *The notion had spun:* Originally described in Vasella and Leaf 2002.

2 *Vasella had been surrounded:* Personal interviews with Vasella (February 1 and October 14, 2002, and others); see also Kher and Frey 2007, and Capell 2009.

3 *leukemia drug called Gleevec:* For an extensive discussion on Gleevec, see chapter 5 and related notes.

4 *As for the revolution:* The story of Waksal and ImClone Systems has been covered eloquently by Prud'homme 2004 and in the *Cancer Letter,* where journalist Paul Goldberg broke much of the unfolding news (see Goldberg 2002). The saga has also been well reported in the business press and news dailies: see Pollack 2002, Serwer 2002b, Arnst 2003a and 2003b, Varchaver 2003, and Denby 2004.

4 *Conceived by a well-respected:* Refers to John Mendelsohn, the former president of MD Anderson Cancer Center. Personal interviews with Mendelsohn (November 17, 2003, and November 29, 2005). See also Arnst 2001.

5 *ImClone's antibody:* UBS Warburg 2001, Morgan Stanley Dean Witter 2001 and 2002.

5 *Sam Waksal tried:* See US Attorney 2003, Securities and Exchange Commission 2003a.

5 *The style doyenne:* Securities and Exchange Commission 2003b, US Court of Appeals 2006. See also conviction (March 4, 2004) and final judgments of conviction (July 20, 2004) in the US District Court for the Southern District of New York. For summary of case, see Subcommittee on Oversight and Investigations 2002.

6 *In May 2003:* For a discussion of Iressa (approved May 5, 2003) and Velcade (approved May 13, 2003), see Anon. 2004a, Giaccone and Rodriguez 2005, and Dy and Adjei 2008.

6 *A few weeks later:* ASCO 2003. Avastin presentation was on June 1.

6 *The evidence dangled:* ImClone stock closed at $7.83 on June 12, 2002, and at $36.30 on June 10, 2003. Data from Bloomberg.

7 Fortune's *longtime rival:* Arnst 2003b.

7 *The numbers did not:* Discussed at length in chapters 2 and 3.

7 *Officials used a death rate:* See "Table 108: Age-Adjusted Death Rates by Major Causes: 1960 to 2004," in *HUS 2007.* The annual rate of death due to cancer in 1971 (the year the National Cancer Act became law) was 199.3 per 100,000 people, when deaths are age-adjusted to the Year 2000 Standard Population. In 2003, the rate was 190.1, a percentage drop of just 4.6 percent over the previous three-plus decades. (Using the same measure, the death rate from heart disease over the same period dropped 53 percent.) More extraordinary is that the age-adjusted cancer death rate in 2003 was only 2 percent lower than that in 1950; heart disease rates, by contrast, had fallen by more than 60 percent during this time (see table for Figure 20 in the same publication). For a full discussion of "age-adjusted death rates," see chapter 2.

7   *Every few weeks:* A LexisNexis search on August 27, 2004, of English-language newspapers found 691 articles using the phrase *cancer breakthrough* between 1990 and 2002. See also Brownlee 2003.

7   *The nation was spending:* Martin L. Brown and colleagues at the NCI have done extensive research in the area of cancer costs. See Brown et al. 2001 and Warren et al. 2008.

8   *I wrote a cover:* Leaf 2004.

10 *I served for three:* From April 2006 to March 2009. For more on the experience described here and in the following pages, see Beishon 2008.

11 *What may be surprising:* Among the most critical assessments can be found in the biannual reports of the President's Cancer Panel, a group created by the National Cancer Act of 1971 to assess progress in the US cancer enterprise and report back to the president. See, for example, President's Cancer Panel Reports for 2001, 2005, and 2008. Particularly frank in this regard is the last, as seen in the report's executive summary, which cites "a troubling confluence of trends, including . . . needless inefficiencies in and insufficient collaboration among government, voluntary, industry, and academic components of the cancer research enterprise; growing questions about the focus and principal emphases in cancer research given limited declines in mortality and morbidity and increased incidence and mortality from several cancers [and] an apparent complacency and/or lack of understanding among policymakers, the research and health communities, and the public about the escalating burden of cancer and a lack of urgency to confront the present and looming national cancer crisis."

Chapter 1: Counting

17 *Joe Hin Tjio couldn't believe:* I first read about the discovery by Tjio and Levan in George Klein's elegant memoir, *The Atheist and the Holy City: Encounters and Reflections* (Klein 1990), 3–13. See also Peter Harper (2006), who provides key photographs, including that of the Institute of Genetics at the University of Lund. Additional information on the events, people, and places described here comes from the following sources: Gartler 2006, Levan 1956, Arnason 2006, Hultén 2002, Wright 2001, and McManus 1997.

18 *They were human chromosomes:* Lawler and Reeves 1976.

18 *Thanks to a bit:* Arnason 2006, 203. See also Anon. 1956, 526. An early discussion of the colchicine technique can be found in Hsu and Moorhead 1953. See also Nowell 2007, 2033–35.

19 *Theophilus Shickel Painter:* Painter's earliest "definitive" determination that the normal human chromosome number was forty-eight can be found in Painter 1924, in which he reports, "Recent studies in human spermatogenesis have

cleared up the doubt which has so long existed over the number of chromosomes possessed by mankind. The somatic or diploid number for the female is
48, and this must be taken as the basic number for the race." The recent studies to which he refers, notably, are his own—and in particular Painter 1923.
(In that article, Painter gives an accounting of efforts to count human chromosomes back to 1891.) As late as 1952, the legendary T. C. Hsu "confirmed"
Painter's finding; see Hsu 1952.

19 *The researchers prepared:* Tjio and Levan 1956.

20 *A black-and-white:* Refers to Darlington 1953, cited in Tjio and Levan
1956, 5.

20 *Masuo Kodani:* Kodani 1958.

21 *Why had so many scientists:* George Klein raises the same question in Klein
1990. For more discussion, see Unger and Blystone 1996 and A. Martin 2004.

22 *John C. Bailar III:* Personal interview with Bailar, January 7, 2004, National
Academy of Sciences, Washington, DC; phone interviews (December 19,
2003, and January 20, 2004); and e-mail correspondence.

23 *With Elaine Smith:* Bailar and Smith 1986.

24 *At the time:* See Cohn 1984, which leads: "Top federal health officials yesterday launched an unprecedented program to cut cancer deaths in half." Greenwald and Sondik 1996 offer a description of the plan, which was to reduce
"cancer mortality rates by 50% between 1985 and 2000." Bailar and Smith
directly address the NCI's ambitious goal in their *New England Journal* article,
concluding, "It is clear that the goal will not be attained unless the present upward trend is reversed very soon and there is a precipitous and unprecedented
decline. We do not believe that hopes for such a change are realistic."

24 *Lawmakers in Congress:* See Public Law 99-158 (1985), the Health Research
Extension Act of 1985, which raised funding levels for the next three years.
The fierce funding debate between Congress and President Reagan continued,
however, late into 1986 and was well covered in the journal *Science*: See Norman 1984, Culliton 1985a/b and 1986. The last of these articles ran under a
banner headline and began, "The National Institutes of Health have fared well
in the battle of the budget for fiscal year 1987, thanks to a supportive Congress, which has increased funds by more than $800 million over the amount
available in FY 1986, an increase of 17.3%." To put the funding "victory" in
perspective, the journal also boasted that "NIH will have sufficient resources
to support 6,200 new grants and more than 10,500 trainees—way up from
the Administration's request."

25 *The president of the American:* The quote, attributed to Dr. John Durant,
ASCO's president at the time, is from Haney 1986, which ran the following day in papers around the country, including the *San Francisco Chronicle,*

the *Los Angeles Times,* and the *New York Times.* See also Letters to the Editor 1986.

25 *Perhaps the angriest:* See Cohn 1986 and DeVita 1987. See also later coverage of the continuing debate between the NCI and its critics: Culliton 1987 and Bailar 1987, in which he responds to critics in *Science.* The referenced US General Accounting Office report (GAO 1987b) concluded that biases in the cancer survival data used by the NCI "artificially inflate the amount of 'true' progress." Like Bailar and Smith's *NEJM* article, it created a firestorm within the cancer community. DeVita derided what he called the GAO's "opinion–based analysis," saying it made "the report limited in its accuracy and usefulness." The US Department of Health & Human Services, the NCI's parent agency, joined in rebutting the report, calling the findings from its fellow governmental agency negative in tone, opinion–based, and "counterproductive" (Merz 1987).

25 *Bailar wasn't just offended:* Interviews with Bailar; see also Bailar 1987 and Cohn 1986.

26 *Eleven years later:* Bailar and Gornik 1997.

26 *But as before:* Fellow members of the cancer community laced into Bailar for his "defeatism," "underlying bias," and "cavalier attitude" toward those lives that *had* been saved in the anticancer effort. Others bashed the researcher for being overdramatic and polarizing (see Anon. 1987). "I think Dr. Bailar has gone beyond the data in order to dramatize the issues," the then–chair of the National Cancer Advisory Board told a reporter. "Scientists have, more and more, taken liberties with data to get the attention of the media." For more on the Bailar rebellion, see Groopman 2001.

27 *With a detailed "route map":* Years later, celebrated scientists William C. Hahn and Robert A. Weinberg would indeed publish a route map of such signaling pathways in the journal *Nature Reviews Cancer* (Hahn and Weinberg 2002). Accompanying their article was a now-famous poster, "A Subway Map of Cancer Pathways," designed by artist Claudia Bentley, that hangs on the walls of many laboratories and in the apartments of countless doctoral students.

27 *The argument that somehow:* Bailar and Gornik 1997, 1573. In one example of premature hype, *Fortune* put on its cover a pair of vials of interleukin–2, a protein involved in human immune function. The boldfaced cover line read, "Cancer Breakthrough" (Bylinsky 1985).

27 *A significant number:* See Kolata 1986, who states that "Bailar and Smith's data are not in dispute."

28 *Frederick Ludwig Hoffman:* Sypher 2002, throughout.

29 *None of that quite:* A few writers have acknowledged the importance of Hoffman's speech ("The Menace of Cancer") while stating incorrectly that it was

first delivered at a meeting of the American Gynecological Society in Washington. Hoffman originally presented his remarks to the New Jersey Academy of Medicine on March 26, 1913, at the invitation of Dr. Edward J. Ill, and gave a revised speech in Washington on May 7. See letter from Hoffman to Forrest F. Dryden, president of the Prudential Insurance Company of America, dated May 10, 1915, in Hoffman 1915. For a transcript of speech, see Hoffman 1913.

29 *Hoffman had, by then:* Sypher 2002, bibliography.

30 *Hoffman, the in–house:* Sypher 2000.

30 *He had caused a stir:* Hoffman's most offensive and troubling error may understandably lead many to question his insight into the cancer problem and his judgment overall. In "Race Traits and Tendencies of the American Negro" (Hoffman 1896), he attributes the higher rate of death in African–Americans to what he calls a "constitutional weakness" (66), then regurgitates a litany of data and other "evidence" to support his insidious theory of racial inferiority. Beatrix R. Hoffman (no relation to Frederick) points out that Hoffman's treatise established him as "a foremost practitioner of scientific racism" and elevated him to prominence in academic circles (B. Hoffman 2003). The book, she writes, citing a fellow historian, became "the most influential discussion of the race question to appear in the late 19th Century." For more on the disturbing acceptance of such theories in early-twentieth-century academic circles, see DiKötter 1998, Krieger 2001, and Wolff 2006.

30 *W. E. B. Du Bois had been:* See Du Bois 1906. But in fact Du Bois did not wait long to challenge Hoffman's assertion and underlying data. That first salvo came in a scholarly book review (Du Bois 1897), which is amply worth reading for both its graceful evisceration of Hoffman's argument and its dismissive humor. As Du Bois writes in his concluding paragraph: "As a piece of book-making [Hoffman's] work invites criticism for its absence of page headings or rubrics, and its unnecessary use of italics. Moreover, Mr. Hoffman has committed the unpardonable sin of publishing a book of 329 pages without an index."

30 *years later, Hoffman:* See Sypher 2000, Anon. 1926, and Sypher 2002, 80ff. In a meeting of the National Urban League, the *Times* notes, Hoffman "virtually reversed the statement" he had made some thirty years earlier. The occasion was marked by a satisfying "quirk of history," says Sypher (2002, 81): W. E. B. Du Bois was present at that 1926 meeting and got to hear Hoffman recant firsthand.

30 *Recorded by physicians:* Several writers have done an "archaeological" study of the disease, of which L. J. Rather's classic (1978) stands out. A pathologist at Stanford, Rather traced the "idea" of the tumor as it morphed (and

occasionally evolved) through history, from the ancient Greeks to the close of the nineteenth century. Also notable is the short history by the late Swiss medical historian Erwin H. Ackerknecht (1958). More recent studies include Weiss 2000a, Weiss 2000b, Donegan 2006, and David and Zimmerman 2010.

30   *"It must be admitted":* Hoffman 1913, 400.

31   *The disease was feared:* For a lively exploration of this deep-running "cancer phobia," see Patterson 1987, 12–35 and 36–55. See also Jasen 2002. The depth of fear can readily be seen in newspaper headlines of that era, of which the following from the *New York Times* are representative: "Alfred Tate Kills Himself, Noted English Rose Grower Had Cancer and Feared Impending Doom" (February 1, 1913); "Tuttle Ends Life as Nurses Sleep, Brooklyn Man, Suffering from Cancer, a Suicide by Gas . . ." (May 4, 1915).

31   *During the first decade:* Hoffman 1915, 13: "In the Ordinary [whole life insurance] experience of The Prudential Insurance Company of America, 1880–1913, the proportionate mortality from cancer at ages 45 and over was 8.5 percent for males and 17.8 percent for females."

31   *Hoffman told his:* Hoffman 1913, 402ff.

31   *By his calculation:* Ibid., 449.

32   *As terrifying:* The crude rate from tuberculosis (TB) fell from 194.4 per 100,000 people in the United States in 1900 to 143.5 in 1913. See NCHS, *Leading Causes of Death, 1900–1998* (undated report). TB's share of all death fell by a much smaller margin, dropping from 11.3 percent in 1900 to 10.4 percent in 1913. The precise reasons for the decline, which began earlier in the nineteenth century, have been the subject of an enduring argument, with credit variously going to nutritional factors, improvements in social condition, the segregation of TB patients, public health campaigns, natural selection, and other factors. See McKeown and Record 1962, 94–122, and McKeown's seminal book, *The Role of Medicine: Dream, Mirage or Nemesis?* (1979). For more recent discussion, see Fairchild and Oppenheimer 1998.

32   *even if his dire warnings:* Anon. 1921, cited in Patterson 1987, 75.

33   *There were now more than eighty thousand:* Hoffman 1915, preface, vii.

34   *Combining the returns:* Ibid., 38. The combined death rate had climbed from 44.8 per 100,000 individuals in 1881, to 59.6 in 1891, to 76.3 in 1901, to 90.4 in 1911.

34   *He also found:* Ibid., 185. Hoffman 1931, which concluded, "Smoking habits unquestionably increase the liability to cancer of the mouth, the throat, the esophagus, the larynx and the lungs." As for the US health officials' arrival to the same conclusion, see Office of the Surgeon General 1964.

34   *"It is for this reason":* Hoffman 1915, 103.

34   *In 1913:* NCHS, *Leading Causes of Death,* 58–63.

35   *It took just weeks:* Strickland 1971.

35   *"The people":* Parran 1939, 428.

35   *America's first assault:* Anon. 1937, 278. See section 7(a) of Public Law 75-244. President Franklin D. Roosevelt signed this three-page bill (the National Cancer Institute Act) into law on August 5, 1937, the aim of which was "to provide for, foster, and aid in coordinating research relating to cancer; to establish the National Cancer Institute; and for other purposes."

35   *Ninety-six senators:* Parran 1939, 428, citing speech by Senator Homer T. Bone at the laying of the cornerstone of the new NCI building on June 24, 1939. For a full accounting of this period, see Strickland 1972, 1–14.

35   *The following year:* NCHS, *Leading Causes of Death,* 54–58. From 1933 through 1935, cancer briefly surpassed pneumonia and influenza (a combined cause of death) to claim the number two spot, but returned to the number three killer in 1936 and 1937. The following year, and for thereafter, cancer became the second-leading cause of death in the United States.

36   *Until 1971:* The National Cancer Act of 1971 (Public Law 92-218). The law is discussed in depth later in this book (see chapter 8, "The Wrong Bill"). Richard Rettig has written a masterful legislative history of this law in *Cancer Crusade: The Story of the National Cancer Act of 1971* (1977). See also Strickland 1972, 158–291.

36   *Consider the progress:* The crude death rate fell from 362.0 deaths per 100,000 people in 1970 to 193.6 in 2010, a drop of 46.5 percent. Data for 1970 can be found in *HUS 2010,* Table 30, and in *MVSR* 22 (11), Table 2. Note: Based on some population estimates for 1970, including that cited in the note below, the crude death rate for heart disease would have been 359 per 100,000. For consistency, I have used the official estimates published in *HUS* throughout. For 2010 data, see *NVSR* 61 (6), Table 2, and *NVSR* 61 (4), "Selected Tables," Table 9.

37   *From 1970 to 2010:* US Census Bureau. Population estimate for July 1, 1970, is 205,052,174 (Census: Historical, revised June 28, 2000). The estimate for July 1, 2010 is 309,330,219 (Census: NST-EST2011-01). Using this estimate, crude rate of death from heart disease in 2010 would have been 193.2 per 100,000, so it is likely that NCHS is using a different population estimate for the year.

37   *Yet there were 138,000:* There were 597,689 deaths from heart disease in 2010 compared with 735,542 in 1970. For 2010, see *NVSR* 61 (6), Table 2, and 61 (4), Table 10; for 1970, see *MVSR,* Final Mortality 1970, Table 4.

37   *The crude rate of death:* There were 207,166 deaths from cerebrovascular diseases (strokes) in 1970, which equals a crude rate of 101.9 deaths per every

100,000 individuals: *MVSR* 22 (11), Table 1. By 2010, the number had been cut to 129,476 deaths, for a crude rate of 41.9—which dropped stroke to fourth place on the list of leading causes of death in the United States: *NVSR* 61 (6), Table 2. Respective deaths and crude death rates for influenza and pneumonia, grouped as the fifth leading cause of death in 1970, were 62,739, or 30.9 per 100,000 residents: *MVSR,* Final Mortality 1970, Table 4; by 2010, there were 50,097 deaths, or 16.2 per 100,000. For liver disease, deaths went from 31,399 in 1970 to 31,903 four decades later, a gain of about 500 deaths. But given the gain in population, the crude death rate fell by more than a third, from 15.5 per 100,000 Americans to 10.0.

38 *The pattern holds:* For comparative statistics on fire-related fatalities, accidental drownings, and lightning-strike fatalities between the years 1970 and 2010, see NCHS 1975, Table 1-23, "Deaths and Death Rates for Each Cause," and *NVSR* 61 (6), Table 10.

38 *America's highways:* US Department of Transportation 2012a, Table 1-11: "Number of US Aircraft, Vehicles, Vessels, and Other Conveyances." In 1970, there were 111 million registered vehicles on US highways, a figure that would more than double by 2010, to 250 million. Yet traffic-related fatalities would drop considerably between these years, from 54,633 in 1970 to 35,332 in 2010. See NCHS 1975, 1–154, and *NVSR* 61 (6), Table 2. Per data from the National Highway Transportation Safety Administration (*Traffic Safety Facts for 2010*), fatalities fell significantly whether one compares deaths per passenger-car occupant, per registered vehicle, or per miles traveled. Also, notably, deaths have primarily been avoided by preventing traffic accidents, as seen in the drop in the number of passenger-car occupants injured each year. In 1988, the first year for which such statistics are available, there were 2,585,000 traffic-related injuries. By 2010 that number had fallen by more than half, to 1,253,000 (Table 4). For one view of how this came to be, and for some striking data on the lives saved through the use of seat belts, see Longthorne et al. 2010 and NHTSA 2010 (DOT HS 811 153). For insights into how vehicle improvements have reduced death and injury on the road, see NHTSA 2012 and Al-Marshad et al. 2013. (Note, NHTSA and NCHS offer differing fatality figures for certain years.)

38 *The tale can be:* For crude rates of death from all causes for years 1970 and 2009, see *HUS 2010,* Tables 29 and 32, and *NVSR* 61 (6), Table 2. While the crude cancer death rate climbed 14.4 percent from 1970 through 2010, the death rate for all causes except cancer dropped 24.2 percent.

38 *Some 580,000:* ACS 2013, 3. Estimate for 2013 is 580,350. The actual number of cancer fatalities in 2010, according to death certificates, was 574,743. The American Cancer Society estimates the global number of deaths from

cancer at 7.6 million, or roughly 21,000 deaths each day (ACS 2008, 1). The World Health Organization previously estimated the number as high as 7.9 million, but has since put the figure at 7.6 million.

Chapter 2: The Truth in Small Doses

39 *The method is:* The actual number of US deaths from cancer in 2010, the latest year for which final data were available in January 2013 from the National Center for Health Statistics (NCHS), is 574,743.

39 *Here, a group:* Espey et al. 2007, 2120.

39 *The study prompted:* ACS 2007b, 17. The charity repeated the claim in its *2009 Strategic Plan Progress Report,* 16 ("Death rates continue to decline in measurable, inspiring numbers"); and again, in the same report for 2010, 16.

39 *The NCI, meanwhile:* NCI 2007b.

40 *"Cancer Death Rates Dropping Fast":* Neergaard 2007. Other media outlets, from Fox News ("Cancer Death Rates Falling Faster Than Ever in America") to the *Seattle Times* ran the same story.

40 *"The news has never":* On–air report, *CBS Evening News,* October 15, 2007. The *NewsHour,* on PBS, broadcast the same news: "Overall death rates have been dropping for the past fifteen years," said the PBS correspondent. "Essentially what's happened here is that that steam has really picked up."

40 *Over the next few years:* See, among many reports, Edwards et al. 2010.

40 *Andrew von Eschenbach:* As the NCI director wrote, "I believe that the progress has been so great that today it is within our grasp to eliminate suffering and death due to cancer by the year 2015" (von Eschenbach 2005). Von Eschenbach reportedly first announced this "challenge goal," later known as the Year 2015 Goal, at a February 2003 meeting of the National Cancer Advisory Board (Simone 2004, 3), and he spoke and wrote about it often. See also von Eschenbach 2004. The American Cancer Society and other groups were hardly shy about using this radical "stretch target" in their lobbying efforts on Capitol Hill and even succeeded in getting 92 US senators and 280 members of the House to sign a letter promising to support the 2015 goal. See Eastman 2004, 4.

40 *The numbers arriving:* Siegel et al. 2013. For all cancers (and both genders) combined, the age-adjusted death rate fell 20 percent during the period cited, from 215.1 per 100,000 individuals at the peak in 1991 to 173.1 in 2009. Wrote the authors, "The reduction in overall cancer death rates since 1990 in men and 1991 in women translates to the avoidance of approximately 1.18 million deaths from cancer, with 152,900 of these deaths averted in 2009 alone." The report is largely an echo of earlier upbeat assessments. In 2009, the ACS issued a press release to accompany that year's cancer statistics, saying,

"New American Cancer Society Report Says 650,000 Cancer Deaths Avoided between 1990 and 2005" (ACS 2009c).

41 *How was it possible:* According to the NCHS, 505,322 Americans died of cancer in 1990 and 567,628 died in 2009, a difference of 62,306. By comparison, 58,193 US soldiers died in the entire Vietnam War, of whom 38,502 were killed in action. See CACCF 2013. Apart from the number of dead, more than 150,000 US servicemen were wounded. As of November 2001, the most current report from the Library of Congress's Vietnam-Era Prisoner-of-War/Missing-in–Action Database, an additional 1,910 US servicemen and 38 civilians are still unaccounted for.

41 *Cancer accounting:* Much has been written on the subject of malleability of financial accounting. Particularly insightful are Henry 2004, Collingwood 2001, Mandel 2002, Serwer 2002a, Morgenson, 2002, and Norris 1999, the last of whom provides a notably prescient analysis. See also Glassman 2003, Byrnes et al. 2002, Browning and Zuckerman 2002, Macdonald with Kruger 2002, and Rosato 2002. For a thorough survey of these issues in academic journals, see Stolowy and Breton 2004.

41 *The annual death toll:* For a straightforward explanation of the terms to follow, see Buescher 2010. See also "Glossary of Statistical Terms," *SEER*, NCI, http://www.seer.cancer.gov/cgi-bin/glossary/glossary.pl.

41 *There is nothing:* Elandt-Johnson 1975, 267–71. "Epidemiologists," she explains, "calculate the *proportion of fetal deaths* = (No. of fetal deaths)/(No. of conceptions) and call it (incorrectly) the 'fetal death rate.' It is a *relative frequency* of fetal deaths among all conceptions and can be used as an estimate of the *probability* of this event. . . . Ratios and proportions are useful summary measures of phenomena which have occurred under certain conditions. In particular, in studies of populations, the conditions are often determined by factors such as race, sex, space, and often in a definite period of time (for example, in a year)."

42 *Go back to the start:* The crude cancer death rate rose from 162.8 in 1970 to 184.9 in 2009, a 13.6 percent increase. By the measure health officials prefer, which adjusts for changes in the age of the population being studied (more on that in a bit), the death rate fell from 198.6 in 1970 to 173.2 in 2009—a decline of 12.8 percent. See *HUS 2011,* Table 32 (updated data files that include 2009 are available online) and *NVSR* 60 (3), Table B.

43 *In 2009, the Sunshine:* In Florida in 2009, there were 40,817 deaths from cancer, fewer than the number estimated by the ACS (41,270). Based on a population of 18,819,000 that year, the crude death rate from cancer was about 217 per 100,000 residents. In Texas, the same year, there were 35,531 cancer deaths (below the ACS estimate of 36,030) in a population of 24,782,302,

resulting in a crude death rate of 143. See State of Florida Department of Health 2010, Charts P-3 and D-6; Texas Department of State Health Services, Vital Statistics Annual Report 2010, Table 16. For estimate of Texas population in 2009, see Nazrul Hoque and Population Estimates and Projections Program, Texas State Data Center, Office of the State Demographer, "Estimates of the Total Populations of Counties and Places in Texas for July 1, 2009 and January 1, 2010," posted November 2010, 10. For state population estimates, see also US Census Bureau 2010a. In 2009, cancer was the leading cause of death in Florida for individuals aged 45 to 84, accounting for 45.4 percent of deaths in this age group.

44 *Such an exercise:* Neison 1844, 40–68. See also Curtin 1992, 11–16.

45 *Thanks to Neison's:* For all cancer sites, African–American males had an age-adjusted death rate of 304 in the period 2002–6, compared with 227 for white males. In some cancer sites, including the stomach and prostate, the age-adjusted death rate for blacks is more than twice that for whites. See Jemal et al. 2010, Table 11. The academic literature on outcome disparities by race is extensive. See, for examples, Dignam 2000 and Brawley 2002. Such differences were apparent, notably, even in the earliest years of the cancer war. See Schmeck 1975, 25.

45 *Or that, since:* CDC, United States Cancer Statistics (USCS) 2005 State vs. National Comparisons; and "Cancer Incidence Rates by Site and State, US, 2002–2006" in ACS 2010a, 7.

45 *Or that women:* ACS 2006, 34; Parkin 1998, 227–34.

46 *Table 1:* To complicate matters, the comparable death count in NCHS, *MSVR* 41 (7s), 1993, is 50,194; I use the lower number to be conservative. Prior to 2003, age-adjusted rates were calculated using standard million proportions based on rounded population numbers. *SEER CSR, 1975–2005* (Ries et al. 2008) is based on nineteen age groups in the US Census Bureau's *Current Population Reports,* document p25-1130.

47 *Warns one of the:* Anderson and Rosenberg 1998, 3.

47 *Cautions another:* Curtin and Klein 1995, 3. The quote begins, "Because of the method of computation, the age-adjusted rate is often interpreted as the hypothetical death rate that would have occurred if the observed age-specific rates were present in a population whose age distribution is that of the standard population."

48 *The country's population:* July 1 estimates for each year. US Census Bureau 2010a.

48 *The nation's median:* The median age went from 32.9 in 1990 to 36.7 in 2009. US Census Bureau 2000; US Census Bureau 2010a, Table 1, "Population by Age and Sex: 2009."

48 *Over this brief:* US Census Bureau 2002; US Census Bureau 2010a.

48 *America in 2009:* NCI's SEER website.

48 *For here, in this:* See National Center for Health Statistics, *HUS 2011,* Tables 26 and 27 (updated tables online include data for 2009). For share of annual cancer cases, see Howlader et al. 2012, Table 1.10, "Age Distribution (%) of Incidence Cases by Site, 2005–2009."

49 *So if for no:* There were 22,703 more cancer deaths in this age group in 2009 than in 1990. *MVSR* 41 (7s), Table 7, and *HUS 2011,* Table 27. The group's share of total cancer mortality (all age groups) rose one-tenth of a percentage point, to 27.8 percent.

49 *By the NCI's: HUS 2011,* Table 32. The standardized death rate for the 45–54-year-old cohort fell 28.6 percent; that for 55–64-year-olds dropped 31.7 percent. Calculating both segments together, using the Year 2000 standard population, the age-adjusted death rate fell just under 31 percent.

49 *As high as: HUS 2011,* Table 32.

49 *Already, according:* US Census Bureau 2011c, Table 1. For 2025 estimate, see US Census Bureau 2008a, Table 9. For a more comprehensive look at the implications of this age boom, see the Federal Interagency Forum on Aging-related Statistics 2011. Particularly telling is Table 15a. From 1981 to 2006, the age-specific death rate from cancer for Americans sixty-five and older fell less than 3 percent, even as the same rate for heart disease dropped by 49 percent. For more discussion on the cancer burden and aging, see Yancik and Holmes 2001 and Smith et al. 2009.

50 *After all:* NCI SEER 2013. SEER data sets.

50 *America's aging population:* It's important to note that, while official NCI assessments of progress in the cancer war are still generally rosy, a number of prominent researchers have sounded the alarm on the effect that America's demographic changes are likely to have on the cancer burden. See, for examples, Smith et al. 2009 and Theisen 2003. As Martin L. Brown is quoted in the latter: "We all know that the US population is aging, and even if nothing else were to change, or if things do change, the aging of the population will have a major effect on the number of cancer cases." Brown, who since 1999 has been chief of the Health Services and Economics Branch in the NCI's Division of Cancer Control and Population Sciences, is the man charged with estimating the annual cost of America's cancer burden.

50 *According to the:* Howlader et al. 2012 *(NCI SEER CSR, 1975–2009),* Table 2.9, "SEER Relative Survival (Percent) by Year of Diagnosis." In Table 1.4, which averages outcomes for patients diagnosed between 2002 and 2008, the five-year relative survival rate is 65.4 percent. For a more comprehensive discussion on the survival measure, see Dickman and Adami 2006.

51 *The overall survival:* Howlader et al. 2012, Tables 4.15, 11.9, and 13.17.

51 *The National Center for Health Statistics: HUS 2010,* Appendix II, Definitions and Methods, 529.

52 *Fewer than a fifth:* Data here and in Figure 4 derives from Howlader et al. 2012 and reflects outcomes for patients diagnosed between 2002 and 2008.

53 *"We're making":* Interview with Gwen Fyfe, January 2004.

53 *In 2013 alone:* Annually, nearly four hundred thousand Americans are diagnosed with a cancer of the pancreas, liver, lung, esophagus, stomach, brain, ovary, or with multiple myeloma, each of which has a five-year relative survival rate of less than 50 percent (see Figure 4). Tens of thousands more will be diagnosed with an advanced stage of breast, colorectal, prostate, or other cancer, in which the survival rate is similarly low (see Figure 5).

53 *That is far:* In 1971, the overall five-year relative survival rate for the roughly 635,000 patients diagnosed with cancer that year was projected to be 49 percent. An analysis of cases by specific disease and stage at diagnosis suggests the number of patients facing a survival rate of 50 percent or less, however, was well more than half of those new patients, and perhaps as high as 380,000. See Silverberg and Holleb 1971. Smith et al. 2009 point out that among the cancers with the fastest-growing rates of incidence are several of the lethal cancers shown in Figure 4.

55 *At first glance:* Johnson, Williams, and Pazdur 2003.

55 *The JCO is:* In May 2012, ASCO said it has "nearly 30,000 members worldwide"; see ASCO 2012. In 2010, *JCO* was ranked fourth among 184 oncology journals in terms of its "impact factor," a well-cited measure of academic importance, published in the Thomson Reuters *Journal Citation Reports.* By another measure, *JCO* then ranked seventeenth out of 8,005 active scientific, technical, and medical journals in terms of its "total influence on the research community" (ASCO Connection website, July 1, 2011).

55 *The authors concluded:* Silvestri et al. 2003.

57 *In some cases:* The immense cost of many newer cancer drugs has been well covered in the press. See, for examples, Berenson 2005; Goodman 2006, A. Johnson 2009; and Anon. 2011b. In an op-ed for the *New York Times* in March 2013, Ezekiel Emanuel and twenty-one leading oncologists reported another dismal statistic in cancer drug efficacy. "Of the 13 anticancer drugs the Food and Drug Administration approved in 2012," they wrote, "only one may extend life by more than a median of six months. Two extended life for only four to six weeks. All cost more than $5,900 per month of treatment."

57 *"The overwhelming":* Interview with Richard Pazdur, January 2004.

57 *The definition:* Johnson, Williams, and Pazdur 2003, 1405. See also Miller, Hoogstraten, Staquet, and Winkler 1981, 211.

58 *The problem is:* As Joan Massagué, a leading cancer biologist at Memorial Sloan–Kettering and the Howard Hughes Medical Institute, said in a 2006 interview: "Metastasis is responsible for ninety percent of deaths from solid tumors and yet we know very little about its cellular and molecular underpinnings. There's a vast literature suggesting that this or that gene may be involved, but that still hasn't given us much knowledge about how the metastasis process really works and about how it could be therapeutically attacked. So metastasis is one of the last big frontiers in tumor biology. We have to understand it, because it really is, quite literally, killing us" (Massagué 2006). For a more thorough explanation, see Naora and Montell 2005 and Naumov et al. 2002.

59 *Nonetheless, during:* In May 2012, a Google search of *cancer breakthrough* (in quotes) yields 309,000 hits.

60 *The cover of:* ACS 1959.

Chapter 3: A War of Attrition

62 *On a Sunday:* Interviews with the Quinlan family. I first met the Quinlans at St. Jude Children's Research Hospital in Memphis on October 18, 2004. The story in this chapter unfolded during several interviews in 2006 (July 28, August 15, September 16, September 29), in October 2007, and by e-mail.

67 *Much of what:* Tortora and Anagnostakos 1987, 440–57; Alberts et al. 1994, 1160–75; de Duve 1984, 34–36; Tsiaris and Werth 2004, 130–63. The estimate of "tens of trillions" includes red blood cells; without mature red blood cells (which contain no nucleus), the overall number of blood cells would be significantly smaller.

68 *Fundamentally:* Robert Weinberg writes elegantly about how cancer cells subvert normal cell function and interaction in *One Renegade Cell* (1998). Many other scientists have also discussed aspects of this subversion in detail: Emmanuelle Passegué, citing work by Andrei V. Krivtsov and others, theorizes that certain cancer genes subvert key progenitor cells called stem cells, which then produce cancer cells rather than normal cells (Passegué 2006, 754–55). Mark P. de Caestecker and colleagues describe how tumor cells subvert important growth-signaling mechanisms (de Caestecker et al. 2000, 1388–1402). Noël Bouck and colleagues discuss how, in developing cancers, a blood vessel-generating process known as angiogenesis is altered, subverting the normal physiological system for wound healing (Bouck et al. 1996, 141). Garth R. Anderson and colleagues relate how the cohesive "society of cells" in a human being can quickly erode (Anderson et al. 2001). And Glenn Dranoff delineates

how tumor cells can subvert normal immune responses and cell migration (Dranoff 2004).

68   *Laid end to end:* Hixson 1967, 546–47; National Institute on Aging 2012, 1161–75.

68   *The challenge is:* Estimates vary widely as to the total number of erythrocytes and other human cells; the most commonly cited estimate for red blood cells appears to be 30 trillion, which is thought to be between a quarter and third of the total cell count in an adult human body. See, for example, Föller 2008; Muzykantov 2010; and Finch et al. 1977.

69   *The result is:* Ogawa 1993 and Hodges et al. 2007, 140.

69   *Reinforcing and replacing:* For more on stem cell renewal in the blood, see Orkin and Zon 2008 and Dick 2003, 231–33. For hematopoiesis generally, see Weinberg 2007, 468–70.

69   *Information about which:* Weinberg provides an accessible explanation in Weinberg 1996a, 62–70. Note he cites a much-smaller figure for total cell count.

70   *Once in a rare:* For a discussion of this breakdown in cancer, see Reya et al. 2001; Wicha et al. 2006; and Huntly and Gilliland 2005.

70   *In the case of:* le Viseur et al. 2008. See also Yale Medical School 2012.

70   *Additional mutations:* As early as the 1950s scientists debated how many mutations, or "hits," are necessary to transform a healthy cell into a malignant one and eventually to produce a viable metastatic tumor. By 1957, British medical statisticians Peter Armitage and Richard Doll developed what they called a "two-hit" model for carcinogenesis, which then seemed to explain the connection between cancer risk and advancing age. According to that theory, the first mutation increased a cell's rate of division, and the second, often coming much later, released it from normal cellular controls (Armitage and Doll 1957), a theory later explored by D. J. B. Ashley in 1969. In 1971, Alfred G. Knudson Jr. demonstrated how two genetic mutations could transform a normal type of eye cell into a malignant one, even in young children (Knudson 1971). Since then, a number of scientists have shown that additional mutations are typically needed to create most cancers. See Fearon and Vogelstein 1990; Balmain et al. 1993; Tomlinson, Sasieni, and Bodmer 2002; and Loeb 2011.

70   *With each cell:* Douglas Hanahan and Robert A. Weinberg have described the traits and abilities that any cancer cell must acquire in their seminal paper, "The Hallmarks of Cancer" (2000), which the authors updated in 2011.

70   *Fail-safes fail:* The remarkable extent of the systems failure is reflected in the multiple ways human cells have to identify DNA damage and repair it. For a clear explanation, see Gibbs 2003. See also Sancar et al. 2004 and Lombard et al. 2005.

70   *Even in this:* Rubnitz and Pui 1997; Gaynon, Trigg, and Uckun 2000, 2140–50 and Escalon 1999, 83–89. The NCI's PDQ website has a helpful fact sheet on childhood ALL: http://www.cancer.gov/cancertopics/pdq/treatment/childALL/Patient.

71   *Every human cell:* Spivak 2005; Hodges et al. 2007.

71   *Along with anemia:* Pui 2003, 9, 87.

71   *The biological breakdown:* Bodey et al. 1966, 328–40; Frei et al. 1965a, 1511–15.

71   *And as recently:* The NCI's SEER program records five-year relative survival rates for leukemia for patients diagnosed in 1960–63 as 14 percent (Ries et al. 2008, Section 13, Table XIII-11). But prominent oncologists Joseph H. Burchenal and M. Lois Murphy surmised, in 1965, that some of the patients with reported "long-term remissions" and "so-called 'cures'" may have had diseases that were "different from the majority of cases of acute leukemia which, even in spite of excellent drug-induced temporary remissions, do not survive more than 2 years from the onset of the disease." Clinical trial reports from the late 1950s and early 1960s also suggest the percentage of ALL survivors was lower. Surveying forty-three leukemia specialists around the country, Burchenal and Murphy received reports of only fifty-three children and eighteen adults who were still alive five years or more after diagnosis. In most chemotherapy clinical trials undertaken through the year 1963, the share of leukemia survivors approached 10 percent or less by two years of follow-up. See patient survival graphs in Frei et al. 1958, 1130. See also Frei et al. 1961, 445; and Frei et al. 1965b, 649. For a thorough, but accessible discussion, see Löwy 1996, 57ff.

71   *In 2003:* ACS 2003, 4, 10–11.

72   *As best he could:* Ibid., 11; Jemal et al. 2003, Table 13. For children diagnosed from 1992 through 1998, five-year relative survival was 46 percent. Such rates, by necessity, reflect the outlook of patients diagnosed several years earlier, so they sometimes underestimate treatment advances that may have occurred in the interim. At the same time, as many epidemiologists have pointed out, the rates may be also be inflated if, thanks to improvements in screening and diagnosis, a greater share of patients are diagnosed earlier in their disease (a phenomenon known as lead-time bias). The two effects may or may not balance out.

75   *In 1963:* See Ries, et al. 2008, Table XIII-11.

75   *At St. Jude:* Ching-Hon Pui, in–person discussion, October 18, 2004. In 2006, Pui and William E. Evans wrote in the *New England Journal of Medicine*, "Emerging results suggest that a cure rate of nearly 90 percent will be attained in the near future," citing results from the "Total Therapy Study XV," conducted at St. Jude.

75 *Indeed, as with ALL:* See Laszlo 1995; Nathan 2007, 38–67; and Chabner and Roberts 2005, 65–72. For a detailed analysis of the statistics, see M. Smith et al. 1999. Jemal et al. 2003, 25, show comparative survival data for other childhood cancers going back to 1974. As will be discussed in chapter 13, however, the most dramatic paradigm shifts in treatment occurred not during the age of the modern cancer war, but in the roughly two decades prior to 1971. For some perspective, see Frei 1972; Frei and Sallan 1978; and Lacher 1985, 35, 88.

75 *To be sure:* Howlader et al. 2012, Table 28.8. Five-year relative survival for children under fifteen diagnosed with any form of cancer in the years 2002–8 was 82.8 percent.

75 *Cancer remains:* Miniño et al. 2011, Table 10.

75 *But had death:* M. Smith et al. 2010, 2625–34.

76 *The reason can:* ACS 2012, 11.

76 *The annual count:* See the ACS's annual *Cancer Facts & Figures* going back to 2000. In 2000, there were an estimated eighty-six hundred new cases of cancer in children aged zero through fourteen (*CAFF 2000*, 9). For population comparisons in the age group, see US Census Bureau 2012b, Table 7. The population of children aged zero to fourteen grew by a mere 1.6 percent between 2000 and 2010.

76 *Correcting for differences:* M. Smith et al. 2010, 2626.

76 *No one quite:* Ibid., 2631–32. The authors attribute the overall rise in incidence mostly to the increase in ALL cases. Ries et al. chart the rise of childhood cancer incidence from 1975 to 1995 in the introduction to the NCI's *SEER Pediatric Monograph* 1999, 5.

76 *But remarkably:* NCI, *2010 Fact Book*, B-2, "Program Structure Fiscal Year 2010." The NCI spent $364 million, or 7.1 percent of its budget, on "Cancer Prevention and Control," down from 10.7 percent in 2006 (v). In fiscal year 2009, the NCI eliminated "Cancer Prevention and Control" as a separate budget mechanism, making some line-item comparisons more difficult. The prevention issue is discussed in detail in chapter 7. For another important perspective, see Davis 2007a, who explores our lack of cancer prevention efforts, particularly our failure to control and protect against known environmental carcinogens. For a summary, see Davis 2007b.

76 *"I'm not saying":* Interviews with Bailar. Carl Nathan, a leading researcher of infectious diseases and cancer at Weill Cornell Medical College, has argued the broad point strenuously (Nathan 2007). See also Kanavos 2006.

77 *They also had a telltale:* Pui and Evans 2006, 167.

77 *He had responded:* Ibid., 170.

77 *And still:* The late effects of treatment in childhood cancers are, unfortunately, dramatic. See Oeffinger et al. 2006; Geenen et al. 2007; Alvarez et al. 2007; Allan and Travis 2005; Li et al. 1983; Inskip and Curtis 2007; Brouwer 2007; Adams et al. 2004; Dores et al. 2005; and Greenfield et al. 2006.

77 *Pediatric cancer survivors:* Studying the outcomes of 16,541 three-year survivors of childhood cancer treated in Britain through the end of 1987, Helen C. Jenkinson and colleagues found an approximately sixfold greater risk of developing a secondary cancer than for untreated children (Jenkinson et al. 2004). Bhatia and Roberts (2005) report similar numbers: "Excluding retinoblastoma as the first primary tumor (as there is increased risk of SMN [secondary cancers] following inherited retinoblastoma), 201 SMNs occurred in 15,452 cases, for a mean follow-up of 9 years and 6 months, corresponding to 147,163 person–years of observation. As 34.7 SMNs were expected, [the standardized incidence ratio—a measure of comparative risk] was 5.8 (95% CI 5.0–6.7)." The comparative risk of getting a later cancer was highest for those who had had a childhood cancer of the bone; the next-highest risk group was those who had soft-tissue cancers (sarcomas) as children, followed by those who had survived endocrine tumors or brain cancer. Bhatia and colleagues note that several big studies have found between a threefold and sixfold increased risk in such populations (Bhatia et al. 2006, 1794). As they and others have reported, childhood survivors of Hodgkin's disease, in particular, have much higher excess risk (18.5-fold) than the general population of developing (a new) cancer (Bhatia 2003). The NCI is continuing to study the topic through the Childhood Cancer Survivor Study; see the NCI website http://www.cancer.gov/cancertopics/coping/ccss.

77 *That number has soared:* The ACS estimated the number of new cancer cases diagnosed in 1971 at 635,000 (Silverberg and Holleb 1971). In 2012, the annual estimate was 1,638,910 (ACS 2012, 4), an increase of 158 percent over 1971's caseload. Over this same period the US population grew 53 percent, from 205 million to 314 million.

77 *Nor do the:* ACS 2012, 9. Graves and Bland 2009, 1509–21, provide an overview. See also Burstein et al. 2004, 1430–41. Li and colleagues report that incidence rates of such preinvasive cancers occurring in the breast duct (called DCIS, for "ductal carcinoma in situ") jumped more than sevenfold from 1980 to 2001, driven largely by increased screening by mammography (Li et al. 2005,1008–11). The impact that in situ disease has on the national cancer burden is significant, as many have explored: See Kumar 2005; Jones 2006, 204–8; Ernster et al. 200; Leonard and Swain 2004; and Baxter et al. 2004.

78 *There is heated:* See Silverstein 1998; Leonard and Swain 2004.

78 *Americans spent:* The NIH estimated the overall costs of cancer in 2010 at
$263.8 billion, of which $102.8 billion was spent on medical outlays; the
rest were "indirect costs," such as that from lost productivity due to illness
and premature death (ACS 2010, 3). In 2002, direct medical costs related to
cancer were estimated to be $56.4 billion (ACS 2002, 3). Population changes
come from the US Census Bureau; inflation adjustments from the US Department of Labor, Bureau of Labor Statistics, CPI Inflation Calculator. In
2011, the NIH began calculating these costs based on data from the Agency
for Healthcare Research and Quality's Medical Expenditure Panel Survey
(MEPS), making direct comparisons with previous years' estimates impossible.
The MEPS data suggest that direct medical costs for cancer are actually higher
than previous estimates, with direct medical expenditures on cancer calculated
at $103.8 billion in 2007 (ACS 2012, 3). Based merely on population projec-
tions, and assuming that rates of cancer incidence, survival, and medical and
drug costs remain constant through 2020, Angela B. Mariotto and colleagues
projected that the United States will spend between $125 billion and $158
billion (in 2010 dollars) on cancer care in the year 2020 (Mariotto et al.
2011). See also Yabroff, Lund, Kepka, et al. 2011. The global cost of cancer is
so great—and so quickly growing—that health officials around the world are
now concluding the obvious: this burden is unsustainable. See, for example,
Kelland 2011.

78 *Cancer patients spend:* Agency for Healthcare Research and Quality 2002. See
also Tsimicalis et al. 2011 for an enlightening review of the cost of childhood
cancer from the family's perspective.

78 *Even for those:* For a comprehensive public survey, see *USA Today*/Kaiser Family Foundation/Harvard School of Public Health 2006. See also Meropol et
al. 2009. See also Himmelstein et al. 2009, presenting the results of a national
study on medical bankruptcy, which found that, of some twenty-three hundred US bankruptcy filers in 2007, more than 62 percent attributed the cause
to medical debts. See also Pisu et al. 2010; and Thorpe and Howard 2003.
In an abstract submitted to ASCO's 2009 annual meeting, Oatis and colleagues (2009) showed how such out-of-pocket expenditures—and, particularly, copayments for medical care—disproportionately affect lower-income
cancer patients. For a look at how trends in cancer care expenditures have
changed over time, see Warren et al. 2008. The exorbitant cost of the new
breed of "targeted" cancer drugs has been widely discussed in both the popular
media and academic literature. On October 14, 2012, for example, Peter B.
Bach, Leonard B. Saltz and Robert E. Wittes, three physicians at Memorial
Sloan–Kettering Cancer Center, authored an op-ed for the *New York Times,*

decrying the high cost of cancer drugs that offer little benefit to patients. They announced that Memorial Sloan–Kettering would refuse to include one new agent, Zaltrap, on the hospital's formulary. (Full disclosure: I edited that opinion essay for the *Times*.) As Bach and his colleagues pointed out, "The typical new cancer drug coming on the market a decade ago cost about $4,500 per month (in 2012 dollars); since 2010 the median price has been around $10,000." In a letter to the *Times* (October 19, 2012), Sandra M. Swain, president of the American Society of Clinical Oncology, called such stratospheric cancer prices "the elephant in the room."

79   *Some of the 1.6 million:* The topic has been well studied in the case of breast cancer, where the issues of both overdiagnosis and overtreatment have been heatedly debated. For a collection of discussions, see Gilbert and Black 2010; Day, Duffy, and Paci 2005; and Bangma et al. 2007.

Chapter 4: The Soldier

82   *When my father:* Interview with Martin Leaf, February 14, 2008, and follow-ups.

82   *It was likely:* My mother, Louise Leaf, had several carcinoid tumors in her liver and intestines, which gave rise to a constellation of pathological effects grouped under the name carcinoid syndrome. Though, typically, such cancers are considered indolent (or slow-growing), her cancer had already spread at the time of diagnosis and seemed to be aggressive.

84   *Some ten months:* The remarkable combination therapy that saved my life and the lives of so many others—called MOPP for its component drugs: nitrogen mustard (the *M* in the acronym), vincristine sulfate (often called by its original trade name, Oncovin), procarbazine hydrochloride, and prednisone—was developed in 1964 by Vincent T. DeVita Jr. and colleagues at the National Cancer Institute. Forty-three patients were treated from 1964 to 1967; thirty-five of them went into complete remission, though just over half of them had relapsed by the time DeVita and two colleagues submitted their report to the *Annals of Internal Medicine* (DeVita, Serpick, and Carbone 1970). The treatment quadrupled the number of patients who went into complete remission, according to one early assessment (Maugh 1974, 974), with Stage III patients (who had an advanced form of the disease) remaining in remission for roughly three years on average (Young, DeVita, and Johnson 1973, 170n5). This was an extraordinary development in the early 1970s, and refinements to the treatment would boost remission—and genuine cure—rates even more (see DeVita et al. 1980 and DeVita and Hubbard 1993). For elegant histories of the challenge of treating Hodgkin's disease and the breakthrough with MOPP, see Bonadonna and Santoro 1982 and Aisenberg 2000.

85 *The combination therapy:* As effective as the drug and radiation therapy was in destroying any residual cancer cells, the combination—like so many other childhood cancer therapies—had powerful short- and long-term effects on the body. Since the early 2000s, oncologists have tried to scale back on therapy, especially with regard to combining drug and radiation therapies. "The long-term carcinogenic effect of combining chemotherapy with radiotherapy has turned out to be far too severe, however, to warrant continuing with this approach" (DeVita 2003).

Chapter 5: The Little Orange Pill

89 *Unlike acute:* Weinberg 2007, 517ff; Sawyers 1999; Moloney 1978. A summary can be found on the NCI PDQ website: http://www.cancer.gov/cancer topics/pdq/treatment/CML/Patient/page1.

89 *In 2000:* ACS 2000, 4; 2006, 4; 2009a, 4.

90 *Gleevec, according:* Deininger, Buchdunger, and Druker 2005, 2650.

90 *The drug represents:* Ibid.

90 *Nobel laureate:* Varmus 2006, 1162.

90 *Another veteran scientist:* Sausville 2003, 1400.

90 *A third told:* Altman 2001.

90 *A fourth put:* Society for Medicines Research Committee 2004, 217.

90 *Andrew von Eschenbach:* von Eschenbach 2002, 792.

91 *The excitement was:* Lemonick and Park 2001.

91 *The drug had been:* FDA 2001.

91 *Tested on fewer:* A single Phase I study with 83 patients was followed by three Phase 2 studies (with a combined 1,027 patients). See Druker et al. 2001a; Talpaz et al. 2002; Sawyers et al. 2002; and Kantarjian et al. 2002. Investigators also conducted a fourth Phase II study with 56 patients, but it is not clear whether these results were considered in the FDA approval process (Ottmann et al. 2002). For an excellent history, see Deininger, Buchdunger, and Druker 2005.

91 *But even in:* Lemonick and Park 2001.

92 *One writer:* Leaf 2003.

92 *For as lifesaving:* The Gleevec story has been told by many scientists. The tale in these pages draws in part from interviews with Peter C. Nowell, Janet Rowley, Brian J. Druker, and Daniel Vasella as well as from the following published accounts: Druker and Lydon 2000; Heisterkamp and Groffen 2002; Hunter 2007; Nathan 2001; Nowell 2002, 2007; Patlak 2001; Rowley 2008, 1990a, 1990b; Vasella with Slater 2003; Waalen 2001, 10–15; Weinberg 2007, 757–65; Wong and Witte 2004; and Ziegler 2003.

92 *In the spring:* Interview with Peter C. Nowell, September 5, 2007.

93 *After staining:* Ibid.; Nowell 2002, 2.

93 *Without knowing it:* Brinkley 2003; Pathak 2004; German 2004, 1.

94 *Hsu went on:* Hsu 1952. Hsu describes the "mistake" in the addendum on page 72.

94 *The stunning:* See discussion of Joe Hin Tjio and Albert Levan in chapter 1, pages 17–22.

94 *This wide open:* Osgood and Krippaehne 1955; Nowell 1960, 462–66; Moorhead 1960.

96 *in one of the tiniest:* Caspersson et al. 1970, 238–40.

96 *Of the seven:* Nowell and Hungerford 1960, 1497; Nowell 1985, 19; Nowell and Hungerford 1961; Lynch 2009, 1–2.

96 *The findings:* Nowell and Hungerford 1960.

96 *A decade earlier:* Interview with Janet Rowley, November 16, 2009; Rowley 2008, 2189; Beutler 2000, 511–12.

97 *The so-called:* Rowley 1980, 3818.

97 *But in contrast:* Rowley interview 2009; US National Library of Medicine.

97 *Using a new:* Rowley 1973a, 1973b; Rowley and Ultmann 1983, 57–60.

98 *Researchers gave:* Groffen 1984.

98 *A group of:* de Klein et al. 1982; Heisterkamp and Groffen 2002.

98 *In 1986:* Davis, Konopka, and Witte 1985; Ben–Neriah et al. 1986; Daley et al. 1987; Daley and Baltimore 1988; Daley et al. 1990; and Lugo et al. 1990. See also Patlak 2001, 10; and Goff 1980.

99 *The monster BCR/ABL:* Witte, Dasgupta, and Baltimore 1980; Konopka, Watanabe, and Witte 1984; Davis, Konopka, and Witte 1985; Ben–Neriah et al. 1986; Lugo et al. 1990.

99 *That was due to the critical:* Hunter 1998. For a summary of key events in the understanding of this process, see Table 1, "A Brief History of Tyrosine Phosphorylation," ibid., 584. See also Schlessinger 2000; Blume-Jensen and Hunter 2001; Lemmon and Schlessinger 2010.

100 *Medicinal chemists:* Silverman 2004 gives a wonderful primer on drug discovery and development (lead modification) from the chemist's eye view; see pages 8–86; for a more summarized explanation, see Ng 2004, 15–41.

101 *Jürg Zimmermann:* Ziegler 2003; Vasella with Slater 2003, 44–56; Zimmermann et al. 1997.

101 *Lydon, a biologist:* Ziegler 2003, 21.

101 *But phosphorylation isn't:* Goodsell 1998, 28–45; Khakh and Burnstock 2009, 84–92. For some historical perspective, see Lipmann 1941, 100–162. For a discussion of the challenges of ATP inhibition, see Bogoyevitch and Fairlie 2007.

102 *In an average:* Garrett and Grisham 2012, 69; Kornberg 1991, 65. Note: Kornberg estimates that ATP is synthesized and broken down some four

thousand times a day. See also Buono and Kolkhorst 2001, 70–71; and Kush-merick 1995, 178. For an early and compelling discussion of this balancing act, see Lehninger 1960, 105–6 in particular.

102 *"We almost cannot":* Ziegler 2003. Vasella confirms the account in his memoir, saying, "There was little enthusiasm from the senior management at Ciba-Geigy. No one would have been surprised to learn on any given day that the project had been scrubbed and resources put into other projects." Vasella with Slater 2003, 57.

103 *"Because of that"* (and following): Interview with Brian Druker, February 1, 2012.

104 *As is nearly:* The high failure rates in drug development will be discussed in chapter 11. See also GAO 2006b, 1–5, 25–28; Owens 2007; DiMasi and Grabowski 2007; and David, Tramontin, and Zemmel 2009. For some insight into drug binding with receptors, efficacy, and metabolism, see Silverman 2004, 138, 415–16, et passim.

105 *When given low:* Druker interview, 2012; Druker and Lydon 2000, 4.

105 *Even if the drug:* Vasella with Slater 2003, 62.

106 *As the company's:* Interview with Vasella; in his own telling of the Gleevec story, the former Novartis CEO recalls that Druker made the case that STI571 would be an ideal "proof of concept" test for targeted cancer therapy to Nick Lydon. Vasella with Slater 2003, 46–47, 63–72.

106 *The first three:* Vasella with Slater 2003, 77.

106 *Of the fifty-four:* Druker et al. 2001a, 1031, 1034–35.

107 *The second phase:* Talpaz et al. 2002 reported on 235 patients enrolled at eighteen centers in France, Germany, Italy, Switzerland, the United Kingdom, and the United States between mid-1999 and mid-2000; Sawyers et al. 2002 studied 260 patients; and Kantarjian et al. 2002 reported on 532 patients.

107 *The company got:* FDA 2001. NDA was filed February 27, 2001. Cohen 2002, 941, calls the seventy-two-day review for Gleevec "the fastest approval ever for an antineoplastic drug." Redmond 2004 offers some perspective on the speed of the drug approval in United States compared with Europe.

108 *Rick Klausner:* Quoted in Ackerman 2001, A1.

108 *The secretary:* Ibid.

109 *Some top cancer:* Weinstein 2002, 63–64; Jain et al. 2002; Weinstein and Joe 2008; and response by Felsher, 3080. See also Garber 2007.

109 *These still-mysterious:* Regarding the genetic instability that is a hallmark of cancer, see Lengauer, Kinzler, and Vogelstein 1997; Stoler 1999; Radisky and Bissell 2006; Lingle 1998; Sieber, Heinimann, and Tomlinson 2003; El-Deiry 2005; and Beckman and Loeb 2005. For some helpful historical perspective, see also Bignold 2006, 1–24. Regarding the evolution of drug resistance, see

Shojaei and Ferrara 2008, 219–30; McCarthy 2004, 924–25; Fletcher 2010; and Hedley 1993, who gives a fascinating and early cell's-eye-view account of the problem. Regarding the role of cancer stem cells in this vexing complexity, see Reya, Morrison, Clarke, and Weissman 2001; Wicha, Liu, and Dontu 2006; Dean, Fojo, and Bates 2005; and Ward and Dirks 2007. And in a marvelous 2012 paper for *Nature Reviews Cancer,* Robert Gillies, Daniel Verduzco, and Robert Gatenby at the Moffett Center, illustrate why targeted therapy is no match for the "dynamically evolving clades of cells" in a malignant tumor—each of them living in "distinct microhabitats that almost certainly ensure the emergence of therapy-resistant populations."

109 *For a glimpse:* Rowley 1975a, 1975b, 1977, 1980.

109 *In 1973:* Interview with Janet Rowley, November 16, 2009. The paper in question was Rowley 1973. Further discussion can be found in Rowley 1980, 2184; Rowley and Testa 1982, 118; and Nucifora, Larson, and Rowley 1993.

110 *In those cancers:* Nowell, Dalla-Favera, Finan, Erikson, and Croce 1983, 165–82; Yunis 1983.

110 *When it comes to:* Worth noting is how long researchers have recognized this enormous variability of cancer subtypes and understood how the disease's ever-changing nature would make the notion of successful treatment by a single targeted agent, on any large scale, profoundly unlikely. See, for example, Heppner 1984, 2259–65. For further (and more recent) discussion on the mind-boggling heterogeneity of both genetic mutation and nongenetic change in cancer, see Gerlinger et al. 2012; Shibata et al. 1993; Lonn et al. 1994; Shah et al. 2009; Heng et al. 2009; Welch and Wei 1998; Flintoft 2009 (who cites work by B. C. Christensen in *PLOS Genetics, Nature Reviews Genetics*); Rak and Yu 2004; Klein et al. 2002; Clark et al. 2010; Suzuki et al. 1998; Joyce and Pollard 2009; and Dueñas-González et al. 2005. In the last of these papers, the authors reveal a surprising degree of variability in methylation status—which genes are silenced or expressed—within different tissue samples of the same patient.

110 *the damage keeps piling on:* William C. Hahn, of Dana-Farber Cancer Institute, sums up the heterogeneity issue in Gibbs 2003: "If you look at most solid tumors in adults, it looks like someone set off a bomb in the nucleus."

110 *Details of this:* Sjöblom et al. 2006. A year after the Sjöblom paper, Vogelstein and a yet-bigger team (Wood et al. 2007) reexplored the genomic landscape of breast and colorectal cancers, examining more than 18,000 human genes in twenty-two tumors. This time, they found, the number of mutated candidate cancer genes per tumor averaged fifteen in colorectal tumors and fourteen in breast tumors. In this topology, wrote the study authors, "There are a few 'mountains' representing individual [candidate cancer-causing] genes mutated

at high frequency. However, the landscapes contain a much larger number of 'hills' representing the [candidate] genes that are mutated at relatively low frequency. It is notable that this general genomic landscape (few gene mountains and many gene hills) is a common feature of both breast and colorectal tumors" (1112).

110 *For in addition:* Sjöblom et al. 2006, Table 1, 270. The team found 673 mutated genes in their breast cancer samples, of which 122 were thought to be "driver" genes in cancer development, and the rest "passengers."

111 *But more challenging:* Gerlinger et al. 2012. See also Salk, Fox, and Loeb 2010. As the authors explain (59): "From a clinical perspective, a chronologically ordered series of mutations driving malignancy is particularly attractive, as it implies that the evolutionary process must bottleneck through a defined set of genes that could be therapeutically targeted. Unfortunately, even in the most-studied model, early investigations indicated that fewer than 10% of advanced colon cancers simultaneously bear mutations in the three most frequently mutated genes."

111 *"The heterogeneous nature":* Interview with Isaiah "Josh" Fidler, January 29, 2004.

111 *The same holds:* This was well known several decades ago. See Mitelman 1974, 315; and Erikson 1986.

111 *When, in early testing:* Druker et al. 2001a; Deininger, Buchdunger, and Druker 2005, 2649; and Shah et al. 2002.

112 *A second barrier:* The issue has been well studied (and of concern to cancer researchers and physicians) since before even Gleevec's approval. See, in chronological order: le Coutre et al. 2000; Gorre et al. 2001; Barthe et al. 2001, 2163a; Hochhaus et al. 2002; Azam et al. 2003; Branford et al. 2003; Al-Ali et al. 2004; Shah et al. 2004; McCarthy 2004, 924; Branford and Hughes 2005; Deininger, Buchdunger, and Druker 2005; Weisberg et al. 2007; Hutchinson 2007; Savona and Talpaz 2008; and Garg et al. 2009.

112 *But once a patient:* Garg et al. 2009, 4361, 4367.

112 *What the laboratory:* Merlo et al. 2006; Greaves 2007; Otto 2007; Loeb, Bielas, and Beckman 2008; Loeb, Loeb, and Anderson, 2003. For a fascinating and broader discussion about evolution and "the cell-individual," see Gould 2002, 694–701.

Chapter 6: Missing the Target

113 Epigraph: Rhoads 1954, 77.

113 *Among the major:* Breast cancer offers a good test case of the targeted therapy paradigm, in part because the cancer community has tried harder to make it work here than in any other disease. One measure of that public commitment,

of course, is money. By the NCI's own estimates, it devotes far more money ($631 million in 2010) to studying breast cancer than any other cancer. For the past decade, breast cancer's share of NCI research dollars has been greater than that of colorectal, lung, stomach, and uterine cancers and multiple myeloma combined, though these five diseases typically kill six times as many Americans each year as breast cancer does (NCI, *2010 Fact Book*; ACS 2012). Just as the academic research and philanthropic communities have focused on breast cancer, so, too, has the pharmaceutical industry. In 2006, according to one research report, forty-two drugs were currently approved in the United States for breast cancer, which was twice the number approved for any other cancer indication with the exception of leukemia (see Bionest Partners and Exane BNP Paribas 2006, 21, Table 3). Most of the cancer drugs approved between 1990 and 2002, for example, were for an indication of breast cancer, according to the FDA's Richard Pazdur and colleagues (Johnson et al. 2003, 1406–7, Table 2). See also DiMasi and Grabowski 2007, 211, Table 1. The pharmaceutical industry's trade group (PhRMA) also compiles lists showing medicines in development for cancer. For many years, drugs aimed at breast cancer outnumbered those for other cancers, though today medicines targeting lung cancer, leukemia, and lymphoma lead the tally by small margins.

114 *Estrogen, of course, is the female:* Jensen and de Sombre 1972; Jensen, Jacobson, Walf, and Frye 2010; Katzenellenbogen 1996; Mendelsohn and Karas 1999 (cardiovascular system); Magness and Rosenfeld 1989 (vasodilation); Mirand and Gordon 1966 (the making of red blood cells); Hewitt, Harrell, and Korach 2005; and Toran–Allerand, Singh, and Sétáló 1999 (brain function).

114 *It helps maintain:* Frasor et al. 2003, 4562 in particular.

114 *That one hormone:* Jensen and Jordan 2003; Ekena, Katzenellenbogen, and Katzenellenbogen 1998.

114 *And a few of those chains:* Yager and Davidson 2006; Tyson et al. 2011.

114 *Estrogen in some:* Russo, Hu, Yang, and Russo 2000. The NCI provides a straightforward explanation of estrogen's effects on breast tissue on its website; see "Understanding Cancer Series: Estrogen Receptors/SERMs," http://www .cancer.gov/cancertopics/understandingcancer/estrogenreceptors/.

115 *It typically takes:* See the discussion on page 70 (chapter 3) and related end notes (under "Additional Mutations") on the number of mutations believed necessary to create a cancer cell capable of spreading and producing a viable tumor.

116 *External factors:* There may be no greater debate in cancer research circles today than over what role elements in the environment play in carcinogenesis. For a general overview, see Luch 2005; Farber 1984; Carbone and Pass 2004; OTA 1993b; Thilly 2003; and Weinberg and Komaroff 2008. For thoughtful

discussions from very different perspectives, see Davis 2007a (throughout) and Ames and Gold 1998. For more on the potential mechanisms of this process, see Milo et al. 1996; Barrett 1993; and Lewtas 2007. The International Agency for Research on Cancer (IARC) has also been an active participant in the debate. For more, see Grosse et al. 2009 and Bouvard et al. 2009.

116 *Here, in the cellular:* For an overview, see Jackson et al. 2002. The journal *Cancer Letters* devoted its July 2008 issue to this complex subject; see in particular Panayiotidis 2008, 6–11; Nishikawa 2008, 53–59; and Goetz and Luch 2008, 73–83. See also Yu and Anderson 1997 and Genestra 2007. For a discussion of how ultraviolet light can cause DNA damage, see the seminal Stubbe and van der Donk 1998.

116 *The hormone raises:* Henderson, Ross, and Bernstein 1988, 246 in particular; and Nandi, Guzman, and Yang 1995. The precise ways in which this happens, however, are still not fully known; see, for example, Russo, Hu, Yang, and Russo 2000, 19.

117 *The risk adds up:* Howlader et al. 2012, "Table 1.10, Age Distribution (%) of Incidence Cases by Site, 2005–2009."

117 *Some 70 to 80:* Keen and Davidson 2003. Younger, premenopausal women are less likely than older women to be diagnosed with estrogen–receptor-positive breast cancer. Harrell, Dye, and Allred et al. 2006 write that 70 to 80 percent of all breast cancers are sensitive to either estrogen or progesterone. Estimates in the medical literature of estrogen–positive breast cancer vary widely, however. For two different ranges, see Neubauer et al. 2008 and Roodi et al. 1995. Furthermore, although many women test positive for the estrogen receptor, Jensen et al. 2010 point out that as few as one third of those diagnosed with breast cancer will be rich in functional receptors and therefore be likely to respond to therapy.

117 *It was the understanding:* In 1896, George Thomas Beatson, surgeon to the Glasgow Cancer Hospital in Scotland, reported that advanced, inoperable breast tumors in some younger patients got smaller and less vascular once the women's ovaries were surgically removed. The phenomenon, as well as anecdotal evidence from Australian farmers, led him to suggest that the female ovaries (as with testicles in men) "send out influences more subtle and more mysterious than those emanating from the nervous system." These substances were capable, surmised Beatson, of controlling the proliferation of epithelial cells (those that comprise the lining of organs) in the breast. The notion that the ovaries might be "the seat of the exciting cause of carcinoma, certainly of the mamma" was then radical; it flew in the face of what was then the dominant theory of cancer's beginnings—that the disease was caused by some sort of local parasite in the affected organ. His now-famous *Lancet* paper (Beatson

1896) also introduced an entirely new physiological concept: that one organ could hold "control over the secretion of another and separate organ." More than a half century later, Charles Huggins of the University of Chicago's Ben May Laboratory for Cancer Research, who was then primarily studying the endocrine control of prostate cancer, removed the adrenal glands (a source of estrogen in women postmenopause) in several older patients with advanced breast cancer and saw striking remissions. (In 1966 Huggins would win a Nobel Prize for his discoveries leading to advances in the hormonal treatment of prostate cancer.)

117   *led to the first:* For more on this history, and the unusual story of tamoxifen's discovery, see Jensen and Jordan 2003; and Jordan 2003 and 2008. Jordan calls tamoxifen the first targeted therapy for breast cancer.

117   Footnote: The role of the progesterone receptor is perhaps less well understood than even that of the estrogen receptor, though the consensus view is that progesterone modulates the growth-stimulating effects of estrogen.

118   *Other drugs:* Osborne and Tripathy 2005; Johnston and Dowsett 2003.

118   *Critical to the:* Salomon et al. 1995; Yarden 2001; and Citri and Yarden 2006.

118   *Technically speaking:* Coussens et al. 1985; Slamon 1987; Slamon et al. 2001; and Hudis 2007.

119   *What makes:* Harari and Yarden 2000, 6102 in particular; Ross et al. 2003; and Ross et al. 2004. Ross et al. state that the HER2 gene is amplified, and/or the HER2 protein overexpressed, in 10 to 34 percent of invasive breast cancers.

119   *Less understood:* Hynes and Lane 2005; Moasser 2007, 6579 in particular.

119   *In women who test:* Vogel et al. 2002, 719; Green 2004, 2191; Harries and Smith 2002.

119   *In each of the:* "The ErbB2 antagonist Herceptin is unquestionably an example speaking for the new generation of targeted cancer drugs," write Thomas Holbro and Nancy Hynes (2004, 207). "Instead of indiscriminately targeting cells with a high proliferative potential using standard chemotherapeutics, this antibody selectively targets a deregulated pathway, which is directly involved in tumor progression."

119   *Even the more:* As the opening epigraph of this chapter makes clear, cancer doctors and researchers in the 1950s and 1960s also viewed their cytotoxic approaches to cancer as both rational and focused on specific biological mechanisms in the disease. See also Fildes 1940; Elion 1988; Stock et al. 1950; Bertino et al. 1971; Rall 1968, 576–78 in particular; Rhoads 1957, 141; Galton et al. 1961; and, from a surgical standpoint, Devitt and Beattie 1964. That these older approaches were both rationally designed and targeted has been acknowledged by many researchers in recent years; see, for example, Kamb, Wee, and Lengauer 2007, 115; and Atalay et al. 2003, 1346.

120 *During the 1990s:* Johnson, Williams, and Pazdur 2003, 1406–7 in particular.

120 *An additional six:* FDA, "NME Drug and New Biologic Approvals," retrieved from FDA website for each year. http://www.fda.gov/Drugs/Development ApprovalProcess/HowDrugsareDevelopedandApproved/DrugandBiologic ApprovalReports/ucm121136.htm.

120 *The last of these:* IMS Health, annual data on cancer drug sales from 2006 to 2011, provided by the company in February 2012. In 2011, nearly $2.7 billion worth of Avastin was prescribed to US patients. Prior to its purchase by Roche, Genentech broke out US sales data for Avastin on its corporate website, http://www.gene.com/gene/about/ir/historical/product-sales/avastin .html. Avastin's $3.09 billion in 2010 sales represents nearly 14 percent of total US oncology drug sales ($22.3 billion) that year, according to IMS Institute for Healthcare Informatics (IMS Health 2012, spreadsheet; and IMS Institute for Healthcare Informatics 2011, 23–24).

121 *After continuing to:* Berry et al. 2005. The CISNET authors report that in 1990 "the rate of death from breast cancer among women 30 to 79 years of age, adjusted for age to the 2000 population," was 49.7 deaths per 100,000 women. A decade later the rate was 38.0 per 100,000, a decline of 24 percent from 1990 (1785).

121 *To its credit:* Ibid. Detailed findings of the study can be found in CISNET 2006.

121 *drug treatment:* Berry et al. 2005 summarize the findings in Table 3, 1790. Averaging the estimates of the seven groups, the CISNET team found that all forms of adjuvant drug (chemotherapy) and hormonal treatment were responsible for just over half (54.6 percent) of the reduction in the age-adjusted death rate from breast cancer over the period. The range of estimates was relatively wide, however, with the group from Dana-Farber Cancer Institute estimating that drug treatment was responsible for little more than a third (35 percent) of the decline and the University of Rochester pegging the contribution at 72 percent. Eliminating the high and low estimates, the average contribution of all therapy to the decline in death rate was 55 percent.

121 *But the full:* Ibid. The University of Rochester's model did not offer separate estimates for the contributions of the hormonal treatment tamoxifen and other forms of adjuvant drug treatment (chemotherapy). And the remaining six teams assumed a slight synergistic effect from combining both forms of therapy. But when separated out, each of the models, save for Dana-Farber's, attributed more than half of the benefit of breast cancer treatment overall to the single estrogen blocker tamoxifen; Dana-Farber assumed tamoxifen's contribution was equal to that of other therapy.

121 *Tellingly, tamoxifen:* Jordan 2003a–b, 2009, and 2006. In the last of these,
V. Craig Jordan gives a wonderful and detailed account of the discovery of
the compound ICI46,474 (tamoxifen) by Arthur L. Walpole, who led a team
of reproductive endocrinologists at Imperial Clinical Industries (ICI) Pharmaceuticals Division, which has since been absorbed into the pharmaceutical
giant AstraZeneca. "Walpole never saw the tremendous success of this discovery," writes Jordan, "as he died suddenly on July 2, 1977." The ICI's group first
published a study on the compound in 1966 (Harper and Walpole 1966). A
year later, the team published a report on the molecule's effect of preventing
the implantation of fertilized eggs in the uteruses of female rats, suggesting
that it might have useful antifertility applications in humans. By the spring
of 1971, researchers at the Christie Hospital and Holt Radium Institute in
Manchester, England, had published the results of the first clinical trial of the
molecule in breast cancer, showing a response in ten of forty-six patients (see
Cole, Jones, and Todd 1971). That was months before the National Cancer
Act would be enacted into law in the United States.

121 *Nine years later:* Tamoxifen (trade name Nolvadex) was originally approved
in the United States on December 30, 1977, for the treatment of postmenopausal women with advanced breast cancer; then in 1986, to delay breast cancer recurrence in women who had had both breasts removed; then in 1989, for
premenopausal women with metastatic breast cancer who chose not to have
their ovaries (the primary source of estrogen in younger women) removed or
irradiated; then in 1990, for women whose breast cancer had yet to spread to
nearby lymph nodes; then in 1993, to fight metastatic breast cancer in men;
then in 1998, to prevent breast cancer in women at high risk for the disease;
then in 2000, for women diagnosed with DCIS, a preinvasive form of breast
cancer, to reduce the risk of getting invasive cancer later on. For more, see
FDA, "List of Approved Oncology Drugs with Approved Indications" on the
FDA website, http://www.accessdata.fda.gov/scripts/cder/onctools/druglist.cfm.

122 *Yet what is perhaps most compelling:* While the data in the CISNET study show
little benefit from traditional mitosis-targeting regimens, they are less informative about the impact of Herceptin (for which human clinical trials began in
1992 and US marketing approval was granted in 1998) or any of the drugs that
came afterward. In the case of Herceptin, however, the results of various clinical trials demonstrate that to the extent that the antibody delays progression
of breast cancer or keeps patients alive longer, it is likely to be only for a few
months in the vast majority of cases. In the so-called pivotal Phase III trial of
Herceptin begun in June 1995, which compared the results of patients treated
with both Herceptin and traditional chemotherapy versus chemotherapy alone,

women in the combination group lived roughly five (4.8) months longer. For a significant number of patients, however, this benefit came with a side effect of "potentially severe, and in some cases, life-threatening" heart problems. In a second trial, investigating more than two hundred HER2-positive patients whose cancers were still progressing despite other chemotherapy regimens, 16 percent showed a response to Herceptin, with treatment failing in these patients after eleven months on average. See Slamon et al. 2001, 783–92; and Cobleigh 1999. For an overview, see Harries and Smith 2002.

122 *So what accounts:* The seven research groups in Berry et al. 2005 estimate that between 28 percent (University of Rochester) and 65 percent (Dana-Farber) of the total benefit was derived from breast cancer screening—mammography, essentially; the mean estimate is 45.4 percent, although the research teams do acknowledge synergistic effects between screening and therapy that make singling out any one factor difficult.

122 *The answer is:* The relationship between the advent of breast cancer screening and smaller and early-stage tumors has been well documented. See Elkin et al. 2005; and Cardoso et al. 2002. The trend has been tracked in many cancers beside breast cancer. See Etzioni et al. 2003; Battat et al. 2004; and Galper et al. 2006. In some cases, paradoxically, earlier detection—and particularly the ability to catch disseminated (metastasized) disease earlier—has led to stage inflation (or what some call stage migration). This can make it hard to compare stage-specific survival in various cancers over time. See Feinstein et al. 1985: "By demonstrating metastases that had formerly been silent and unidentified . . . many patients who previously would have been classified in a 'good' stage were assigned to a 'bad' stage. Because the prognosis of those who migrated, although worse than that for other members of the good-stage group, was better than that for other members of the bad-stage group, survival rates rose in each group without any change in individual outcomes." Giordano et al. 2004 explore this issue as well in breast cancer.

123 *"I saw breast":* Interview with John Mendelsohn, November 2005.

123 *It appears likely that:* Welch and Black 2010; Barry 2009, 8; and Welch, Schwartz, and Woloshin 2000. The problem of overdiagnosis is most notorious in the case of prostate cancer. See, for example, Welch and Albertsen 2009 and Parker-Pope 2011.

124 *Such "overdiagnosis":* For an excellent discussion, see Brownlee 2007. See also Woloshin, Schwartz, and Welch 2005 and Parker-Pope 2010.

124 *(Such questioning):* See, for example, Stein 2009 and Lerner 1998.

124 *Even when authentic:* Jackman et al. 1999.

125 *for it suggests that:* Yie 2008, 157–58 in particular; Lumachi, Basso, and Basso 2008, 109–15; and Temple et al. 1999.

125   *In one 2008:* Brewster et al. 2008.

126   *In the previous:* In 2009, 8,230 Americans between the ages of thirty-five and fifty-four died of breast cancer, up from 8,110 in 2008. See NCHS 2011b, "Table 10: Number of Deaths from 113 Selected Causes," as well as the previous year's report, NCHS 2011a. For crude death rates in Table 3, see NCHS, *HUS 2011,* "Table 34: Death rates for malignant neoplasm of breast among females, by race, Hispanic origin, and age: United States, selected years 1950–2008," 146; as well as the same in *HUS, 2008, HUS, 2009,* and *HUS, 2010.*

126   *The Pap test:* Carmichael 1973, 73ff. George Papanicolaou published a mono-graph on the technique, *Diagnosis of Uterine Cancer by the Vaginal Smear,* in 1943, but he had described it as early as 1928. Carmichael (59) reprints a January 5, 1928, newspaper story from the *New York World* that emphasizes the benefit of detecting early lesions: "Although Dr. Papanicolaou is not will-ing to predict how useful the new diagnostic method will be in the actual treatment of malignancy itself, it seems probable that it will prove valuable in determining cancer in the early stages of its growth when it can be most easily fought and treated. There is even hope that pre-cancerous conditions may be detected and checked by the cytological method." See also Casper and Clarke 1998, 257: the authors cite a 70 percent reduction in age-adjusted mortality from 1947 to 1984.

127   *The colonoscopy:* Wolff and Shinya 1971, 1973, and 1974. For a recent study on colonoscopy's impact on cancer mortality, see Zauber et al. 2012. For a good, clear discussion of the importance of colorectal cancer screening, see American Cancer Society 2005b, 39–44.

128   *By the time:* Interview with Isaiah "Josh" Fidler, January 29, 2004.

128   *This population:* Talmadge and Fidler 2010, particularly 5652. See also Black and Welch 1997, 4 in particular.

128   *By then, at:* Talmadge and Fidler 2010, 5652.

Chapter 7: Preemption

130   Epigraph: Quoted in Zhivotovsky and Orrenius 2009, 3 and notes.

130   *When I first met:* Interview with Michael Sporn, Hanover, NH, January 2004. Direct quotes from Sporn throughout this chapter come from this and twelve additional interviews conducted from May 2005 through March 2012, as well as from written correspondence with the scientist.

131   *He had sent:* Sporn 1996, 1377.

131   *The NCI director:* DeVita 1997, 867.

131   *In his innumerable:* Interviews and correspondence with Sporn. See also Sporn 1996, 1379. In his original, unpublished draft for "Dichotomies" (Sporn 2006), he compares a mosaic in Venice's Basilica di San Marco with a diagram

of cellular networks proposed by the pioneering British cancer researcher Leslie Foulds (see also Foulds 1969, 266–72).

131   *Elegant as the imagery:* Carl Nathan, a leading immunologist at Weill Cornell Medical College and a friend of Sporn's, captures this blunt edge wonderfully: "At one point," Nathan recalled during a 2006 interview, "the establishment tried to cover its tracks with Mike and gave him the Bristol-Myers Squibb Award for Distinguished Achievement in cancer research. I went to the dinner. And he just hammered them. He doesn't care that he's got a tuxedo on and he's standing under a glass chandelier and all the executives are sitting around. He just let them have it. And I was so proud of him."

132   *Sporn is the sort of:* Thomson Reuters 2010; Google Scholar search.

132   *Following the citation:* Sporn et al. 1976.

132   *Inspired by:* Wolbach and Howe 1933.

133   *Just as famously:* For discussion of the discovery, see Moses and Roberts 2008 and Sporn 1999. For the early scientific papers, see Moses et al. 1981 and Roberts et al. 1981. And for a particularly influential paper, see Roberts and Sporn et al. 1986.

133   *With another accomplished:* Sporn and Todaro 1980.

133   *In 2004: NCI* 2004, 7.

133   *For all his:* Sporn et al. 1976; Sporn 1976, 1978, 1980, and 2011.

134   *Lee Wattenberg:* Wattenberg 1966.

134   *To distinguish:* Sporn et al. 1976.

134   *Such a view:* Interviews with Sporn. The issue is also discussed in Leaf 2004.

134   *Cancer is not:* Sporn 2006 and 1991. For a detailed discussion of the multistep process, see also Hanahan and Weinberg 2000 and 2011.

135   *But most:* Kelloff et al. 2006, see figure on 3669.

135   *Long before:* O'Shaughnessy et al. 2002; Farber and Cameron 1980.

136   *The boundary between:* See, for example, Fleskens and Slootweg 2009, 11; Warnakulasuriya et al. 2008; and Iatropoulos 1983.

136   *When it comes to:* Kambic 1997, 9 in particular; Hellquist et al. 1999, 227 in particular.

137   *Biologists and geneticists:* Hahn and Weinberg 2002.

137   *This is the long-enshrined:* Michor et al. 2005; Beerenwinkel et al. 2007, e225; and Speer et al. 1984. For an early classic paper on the subject, see Whittemore 1978.

137   *Over time:* The NCI has calculated that 41 percent of Americans will be diagnosed with cancer during their lifetimes, a percentage that rises slightly higher (to nearly 44 percent) if in situ cancers are included. The share of males expected to be diagnosed with an invasive cancer is 45 percent, while the "lifetime risk" for females (percent likely to be diagnosed) is 38 percent.

Figures are based on data from patients diagnosed in 2007 through 2009. See Howlader et al. 2012, Table 1.14.

137 *While half:* Ibid., Table 1.11.

138 *That, after all:* Topol 2004; Cannon et al. 2004; Nissen et al. 2005; Stossel 2008; Glassberg and Rader 2008; and Mosca et al. 2004.

139 *What if we had treated:* As with the case of reducing the burden of cardiovascular disease, one way cancer chemoprevention may be effective is in delaying, if not ultimately preventing, cancer development. Scott M. Lippman and Waun Ki Hong, of Houston's MD Anderson Cancer Center, have argued this approach compellingly in Lippman and Hong 2002.

139 *A cadre of:* Hong, Lippman et al. 1990; Talalay et al. 1988; Prochaska et al. 1985; Weinstein 1988.

139 *This was also the change:* Bailar and Smith 1986. Even Sidney Farber, the Boston doctor who, with his use of antifolates on childhood leukemia patients, opened the door to the first genuine pharmacological "cures" of an advanced cancer, thought it misguided to focus the national cancer effort almost exclusively on finding cures. "I notice that the term 'cancer cure program' has been introduced in the last few months," Farber told the Senate in 1971. "We are very much interested in the over 900,000 people who have cancer and the more than 300,000 who will die this year, so the word 'cure' is terribly important. But of great importance also is prevention. We wouldn't want to have this identified as simply a program for 'cure' without prevention, too." Senate Hearings 1971, 406. For more on Farber, see chapter 12.

139 *In 1976:* The journal *Cancer Research* compiled the nearly forty papers delivered at the conference in its July 1976 issue.

139 *A quarter-century:* In November 2006, AACR held a four-day international conference, "Frontiers in Cancer Prevention Research," in Boston, which was particularly well attended. The strategy of pursuing (very) early detection of cancer gained more prominence in the early 2000s as a number of leading scientists began to argue for it. Nobel Prize–winning scientist Leland Hartwell coauthored one such article (Etzioni et al. 2003); see page 2 for emphasis on precursor lesions.

139 *Shortly after:* Grady 2003.

140 *When he and:* Interview with Michael Sporn.

140 *When I later:* Interview with Elias Zerhouni, January 9, 2004.

141 *Even with the aid:* Siegel et al. 2012, 27, Figure 8, "Stage Distribution of Selected Cancers by Race, United States, 2001 to 2007." In the case of cancer of the uterine cervix, 48 percent of women diagnosed in the years 2001 through 2007 were diagnosed while the cancer was still thought to be localized; in 35 percent, the cancer had already spread within the ovarian region but had

not metastasized further; in 13 percent, the cancer had spread distantly, affecting other organ systems in the body. In the case of colorectal cancer, 39 percent of patients were diagnosed with localized cancers, 37 percent with regional disease, and 20 percent with advanced disease in which tumor cells had already spread through the blood or lymph system and colonized elsewhere in the body. (Data is drawn from the NCI SEER program.)

141   *Macromolecules:* Much of the focus has been on finding the telltale proteins of a cancer-in–development. But researchers have also scoured the human body for biomarkers in the form of carbohydrates, lipids, glycoproteins, nucleic acids (DNA, RNA, microRNA, mitochondrial DNA), gene expression, immune cells and factors (cytokines), and much more. See, for examples, Sell 1990; Xu et al. 2005; Galli-Stampino et al. 1997; Ugorski and Laskowska 2002; Nigam and Canter 1973; Calin and Croce 2006; Danovi 2008; Fliss et al. 2000; Gal-Yam et al. 2008, 273–74 in particular; Verma and Manne 2006; Seruga et al. 2008; Petricoin et al. 2006; and Lilja et al. 2007.

141   *So little:* Srivastava et al. 2008. "Recent reductions in cancer mortality are due in part to risk reduction behaviors like smoking cessation and more strongly to early detection of cancer coupled with appropriate therapy," say the authors in the report's "Executive Summary" (8). "Yet, there are no validated molecular biomarker tests for the early detection of any cancer (see Table I). Among the list of FDA-approved biomarkers, none have been approved for cancer early detection and screening."

142   *The US company:* Throughout the late 2000s, the company, Myriad Genetics, charged approximately $3,000 for its full analysis of the "breast cancer genes" BRCA1 and BRCA 2; since 2010, however, the price for a complete sequencing plus a supplemental genomic rearrangement test has approached $4,000; see Leaf 2005, 266 in particular. In a high-profile civil case (*Association for Molecular Pathology v. Myriad Genetics,* No. 11-725), plaintiffs have challenged the validity of Myriad's initial BRCA gene patents as well as the company's right to bar other firms from offering tests to detect mutations in them, an exclusivity that has helped keep the testing price high. For discussion, see Stempel 2012; Pollack 2012a; Conley and Vorhaus 2010.

142   *A separate crop:* In the United States, three prognostic tests have been approved for breast cancer: Oncotype DX, MammaPrint, and the Breast Cancer Gene Expression Ratio, each of which looks at a different subset of genes. See Benson et al. 2009; van de Vijver et al. 2002; and Jansen et al. 2007.

142   *Biomarkers are now:* Cheok and Evans 2006; and Christensen 2002.

142   *Best known of all:* Ludwig and Weinstein (2005) provide a comprehensive review in "Biomarkers in Cancer Staging, Prognosis and Treatment Selection."

142 *Perhaps no marker* (and following paragraphs): Bast 1981; Bast and Knapp 1998; Bast et al. 2005; Cragun 2011; and Greenwood 2007.

143 *Such false:* Robert Bast and colleagues point out that an early-detection method must have not only a high sensitivity for early-stage disease (catch more than 75 percent of cases), but also an extremely high specificity (the positive cases that are identified by the test must be accurate 99.6 percent of the time) in order to "attain a positive predictive value of at least 10 percent." And even that relatively high predictive value would mean that ten women would have to undergo surgical intervention (laparoscopy or laparotomy) to detect just one case of ovarian cancer. See Bast, Hennessy, and Mills 2009, 416 in particular. Ian Jacobs and Usha Menon (2004) also emphasize that "the consequence of a positive screening test for ovarian cancer is surgical intervention of some kind."

143 *In a study:* Einhorn et al. 1992.

144 *A single ovarian:* Gortzak-Uzan et al. 2008.

144 *Out of this swarm:* Faça and Hanash 2009; and Faça et al. 2008. While relatively few academic studies have assessed the number of proteins and protein fragments released in this process, two classic papers have examined the shedding of cancer cells from tumors. See Liotta, Kleinerman, and Saidel 1974 and Butler and Gullino 1975. In addition, Paul H. Black has written about the process in depth in Black 1980.

144 *But perhaps a fraction:* Interview with Lance Liotta at NIH, January 8, 2004; and Petricoin and Liotta 2004. As Petricoin and Liotta point out, there are conceivably tens of thousands of proteins (or parts of proteins) in human blood, which makes isolating an individual protein marker that's wholly specific to a single disease akin to searching for a needle in a haystack. And given the great variability between ovarian cancer patients, finding a single protein tumor marker is all the more difficult. Their approach has been to look for a "signature" based on a large number of proteins, a strategy that has also met with controversy. For more on this general approach, see Anon. 2002; van der Merwe et al. 2006; and Diamandis 2004.

144 *That is why:* In Lutz et al. 2008, Amelie M. Lutz and colleagues calculated what size an ovarian tumor would have to be in order to be detected by way of screening the blood for CA-125 antigen. Even assuming that only malignant ovarian cells secreted the antigen, it is likely that a tumor smaller than one-tenth of a millimeter cubed would be undetectable, the authors conclude. But the "minimally detectable tumor size" might be hundreds of times larger than that. In other words, tumors would already be well advanced, in most cases, before a CA-125 test would detect them.

144 *Rather, the failed:* "Despite the increasing rates of publications on biomarkers," Joseph A. Ludwig and John N. Weinstein (2005) note, "the number of US Food and Drug Administration (FDA)-approved plasma-protein tests is decreasing," and few of those that are approved are used in standard clinical practice. One additional challenge, as Jacobs and Menon (2004) point out, is that to the extent that existing biomarkers have been validated, the evidence has come retrospectively. As the scientists write, "It is important to note that most of these studies use samples from women with clinically diagnosed ovarian cancer as opposed to asymptomatic women with preclinical disease."

144 *There has never been:* Veteran cancer researcher George Poste wrote a scathing commentary on this for the journal *Nature* (Poste 2011). "The dismal patchwork of fragmented research on disease-associated biomarkers," he argues, "should be replaced by a coordinated 'big science' approach."

144 *In the fall:* NCI 2000, 38–39. The directors of the NCI-designated cancer centers came to a similar conclusion in Cancer Center Directors Working Group 2006: "In spite of the great interest in identifying markers in blood or cells that can identify the presence of cancers at the earliest possible time," the author concludes, "progress in research has been slow." See also Dalton and Friend 2006, in which the authors argue that political and cultural barriers to biomarker research and implementation are just as formidable as the technical hurdles.

145 *What was actually:* The study compared circulating levels of two proteins already used in the diagnosis of hepatocellular carcinoma (primary liver cancer)—alpha-fetoprotein (AFP) and des-gamma-carboxy prothrombin (DCP)—to determine if either could be predictive of early disease; team members also looked at a subset of AFP (AFP-L3%), which has a different molecular structure. Notably, AFP was identified as a potential marker for liver disease by a Russian tumor immunologist named Garry Abelev in 1963, a discovery that predates even the start of the modern cancer war; see Abelev et al. 1963, and Abelev 1968. Moreover, researchers were comparing the predictive value of AFP and DCP as early as the late 1980s. See, for example, Buffet et al. 1989.

145 *Sporn and others:* See, for example, Rapkiewicz et al. 2004; Gormally et al. 2007; Mills, Bast, and Srivastava 2001; Irish, Kotecha, and Nolan 2006; Ludwig and Weinstein 2005; and Brennan et al. 2010. See also Goetz 2009, 80ff.

145 *Years ago:* Interview with Eric Lander, January 23, 2004.

146 *To take one:* Tuttle et al. 2009. For broader context, see Baxter et al. 2004 and Eisen and Weber 1999.

147 *Many, if not most:* Berman et al. 2006, 391–92 in particular. The regression rate (or more accurately, in some cases, the nonprogression rate) differs from

one cancer type/site to the next. "For unknown reasons," Berman and colleagues report, "most in situ neuroblastomas do not evolve into clinically apparent tumors." Similarly, in a 2005 study of patients with precancerous lesions of the bronchi, Roderick H. Breuer and colleagues report that slightly over half (54 percent) of the lesions regressed. More remarkable—and certainly far more rare—are cases in which established "clinical cancers" or high-grade dysplasias have regressed. For discussion, see Challis and Stam 1990; Cole 1981; Trimble et al. 2005; Krikorian et al. 1980; Del Giudice et al. 2009; Halliday et al. 1995; Iihara et al. 2004; and Papac 1996.

147 *The damaged tissue:* Interview with Michael Sporn. For more, see Novak 2005; Dvorak et al. 1995; Coussens and Werb 2002; Schäfer and Werner 2008; and Martins-Green, Boudreau, and Bissell 1994. In the case of precancerous lesions specifically, several research groups have studied this healing process. See, for instance, Mera et al. 2005.

147 *The notion:* Haddow 1973 and 1974; and Dvorak 1986. Other cancer scientists have since taken up the notion as well. See, for example, Bouck et al. 1996; O'Byrne and Dalgleish 2001; and Schäfer and Werner 2008.

148 *One of the more:* Mintz and Illmensee 1975.

148 *But it was the work:* Interviews with Mina Bissell, December 9, 2006, and February 8, 2007; Bissell, Hall, and Parry 1982; Dolberg and Bissell 1984; Dolberg et al. 1985; Sieweke, Thompson, Sporn, and Bissell 1990; Weaver et al. 1997; Bissell and Radisky 2001; Nelson and Bissell 2005; and Bissell 2007.

149 *The implications of:* An early, and often overlooked, pioneer of the conception of cancer as a "disease of organization" was Sir David W. Smithers, a professor of radiotherapy at the University of London and a prominent radiologist at the Royal Marsden Hospital and Institute of Cancer Research in London. "Cancer is no more a disease of cells than a traffic jam is a disease of cars," Smithers wrote in a 1962 essay for the *Lancet*. "A lifetime of study of the internal-combustion engine would not help anyone to understand our traffic problems. The causes of congestion can be many. A traffic jam is due to a failure of the normal relationship between driven cars and their environment and can occur whether they themselves are running normally or not." Smithers 1962, 497.

149 *Such interventions:* It's important to note that the strategy of preemption should not preclude traditional cancer *prevention* efforts. Many leading scientists, in fact, argue that the path to reducing the cancer burden is rather simple: commonsense lifestyle and behavioral changes and screening. In a January 2004 interview, the Nobel laureate and current NCI director, Harold Varmus, made the point stridently: "We have the knowledge [to prevent cancer]. We

don't know how to *apply* it. What's the big knowledge? It's that tobacco causes cancer. And still a quarter of the population smokes. . . . Genetic risk assessment: We've made a lot of progress there in understanding what ought to be looked for. But are we really ready to offer that kind of information? Do people want it? How would they use it? Colonoscopy—there's a huge, huge advance in preventing colon cancer by detecting polyps. And yet we have the issue of cost-benefit analysis. Is society willing to pay for a colonoscopy for everybody every ten years? And motivation: A lot of people would seem that they'd rather take risks on cancer than tolerate an enema—or purging. Which I find pretty absurd. That's one thing I'm happy to subject myself to. This is one of most undervalued ways to control cancer. Colon cancer is the second-biggest killer of cancer. And we could come close to eliminating it." Regarding, tobacco's effect on cancer rates, see also Rodu and Cole 2001. In "The Fifty-Year Decline of Cancer in America," the authors state that if lung cancer mortality were to be stripped out of the picture, age-adjusted death rates for the remaining cancers would have declined from 1950 to 1990.

150 *Aspirin and nonsteroidal:* Agus 2012. (Disclosure: I assigned and edited this editorial.) See also Agus 2011, 44–45, 62ff; Rothwell et al. 2011.

150 *An alternative plan:* Sporn and Roberts 1992; Siegel and Massagué 2003; and Sporn 2005. Rakesh K. Jain, a Harvard scientist, proposed in Jain 2008 that restoring the normal vasculature (blood vessels) around developing cancers may be one way to "tip the balance toward normalcy."

150 *Indeed, some researchers:* Prestera et al. 1993; Surh 2003; and Issa et al. 2006.

150 *The longer the destructive:* Slaughter, Southwick, and Smejkal 1953; and Braakhuis et al. 2003.

151 *Statin drugs, while:* Wilson 2010; Wolfe 2005; US GAO 2006a, 43ff; Blood Pressure Lowering Treatment Trialists' Collaboration 2003; Kelly et al. 1996; FDA 2007; and Larson et al. 2005. Risks and side effects for various ACE inhibitors, beta-blockers, and other classes of medicine can be found at the US National Library of Medicine's MedlinePlus service, http://www.nlm.nih.gov/medlineplus/druginformation.html, and at the FDA's Drugs@FDA website, http://www.accessdata.fda.gov/scripts/cder/drugsatfda/index.cfm.

151 *Health care researchers:* McWhinney 2000, 6.

151 *So whereas the idea:* Grabowski and Moe 2008. For a broader discussion on the effects of such fear on drug development, clinical trials, and, ultimately, adoption of a chemopreventive strategy for cancer, see chapter 11 of this book and also Kelloff, Lippman, Dannenberg et al. 2006, 3689 in particular.

151 *"The issue here":* Interview with Richard Pazdur, January 21, 2004.

152 *But he has been:* Faust and Menzel 2006 offer a thorough discussion of this mind-set and the challenges it raises. See also Leaf 2006.

153 *Anita Roberts:* Interviews with Anita Roberts, Bob Roberts, and Michael Sporn.

153 *On* ScienceWatch's *list: ScienceWatch* 2003.

153 *According to one:* Based on a June 30, 2004, survey by Eli Lilly of all molecules in active Phase II development or higher, according to the PJB (now Informa) Pharmaprojects database. Includes new chemical entities (NCEs) and previously marketed ("launched") drugs with new indications. Interestingly, in oncology, the share was slightly higher, at 3.1 percent. Meeting of Eli Lilly Prevention Task Force, Indianapolis, January 10–11, 2005.

153 *Theirs will continue:* See, for example, Kelloff et al. 2006; Herberman et al. 2006.

153 *The more important:* Dan Troy, a former chief counsel of the FDA, framed the trade-off as "risk versus risk" in a panel discussion; see Milken Institute Global Conference 2005.

Chapter 8: The Wrong Bill

157 *The ever-popular:* Ann Landers, "Ask Ann Landers," syndicated newspaper columns for April 1, April 3, April 8, and April 14, 1971, in the *Hartford Courant,* and elsewhere. Stephen P. Strickland (1972, 271) notes that Landers's column was then syndicated in some 750 newspapers with a estimated circulation of 54 million people.

157 *The offering:* Ann Landers, "Ask Ann Landers," *Washington Post,* April 20, 1971, B5, and elsewhere.

158 *One senator from New Jersey* (and following): Rettig 1977, 176ff.

158 *The cascade of:* Ibid., 176. Landers herself writes about the IMPEACH ANN LANDERS signs in her May 18, 1971, column.

158 *They knew:* Rettig 1977, 177.

158 *Members of the House:* US House of Representatives 1971b, 142–51.

159 *The former all-star:* Ibid., 740. On Kemp, see Otten 1971, 22.

159 *Dick Shoup: Congressional Record* 1971, 41147. On Shoup, see *Biographical Directory of the United States Congress.*

159 *According to death:* For the official cancer death count in 1971, see NCHS 1974b, 2, 8. For the tally of US servicemen deaths in Vietnam the same year, see CACCF 2013. During 1971, 2,357 US servicemen were killed in Vietnam, compared with 337,398 Americans killed by cancer.

159 *Over the previous:* CACCF 2013. Of the reported 58,193 servicemen who died in Vietnam, more than 56,000 died in the ten–year period 1962–71. In the same period, 67,637 Americans age fifteen through thirty-four died of cancer. See NCHS 1974b, 3; NCHS 1977 (unpublished tables), 40, Table 290A; and NCHS 1982 (unpublished tables), 72, Table 290A.

160   *But Cornelius: Congressional Record* 1971, 41158–59.

160   *That notion of:* It would be difficult to overstate how bitterly divided the country was in 1971—an era that offers striking parallels to the present one. The unpopular war in Vietnam seemed without end; indeed, the year before, President Nixon had announced the invasion of Cambodia, a move that escalated the conflict and split America even more profoundly. The US economy was mired in the worst stagflation it had experienced in twenty years, and in months a presidential campaign was set to begin anew. The two men who many believed would be facing each other, Nixon and Ted Kennedy, had already squabbled on virtually every issue prior to the cancer bill—all of which made their cooperation here more remarkable. For background, see Anon. 1970a, 1970b, and 1971a.

161   *That day: Public Papers of the Presidents of the United States* 1972, No. 408.

161   *The special implements:* Semple 1965.

161   *Schmidt had chaired:* Rettig 1977, 86–89; Oppel 1999; Gupta 2000, 95–100.

162   *The cancer legislation:* National Panel of Consultants on the Conquest of Cancer 1970; Bazell 1970.

163   *While the bill had:* Rettig 1977 gives a masterful account of the legislative wrangling that produced these similar-looking, yet drastically different, bills.

163   *The citizens' committee* (and following): Senate Hearings 1971, Benno Schmidt testimony, June 10, 1971, 396–406; and letter from Benno Schmidt to Senator Edward M. Kennedy, dated March 22, 1971, 277–85. See also testimony of R. Lee Clark, president of MD Anderson Cancer Center, March 10, 1971, 194–95; and testimony of Anna Rosenberg Hoffman, former undersecretary of defense, March 10, 1971, 200–202.

163   *The committee had:* See Rettig 1977, 93ff.

164   *"We would have":* Senate Hearings 1971, Benno Schmidt testimony, March 10, 1971, 196.

165   *On July 7:* Rettig 1977, 196.

165   *On September 16:* US House of Representatives 1971b, 197ff.; Rettig 1977, 197–247.

165   *The congressman:* Rettig 1977, 199; Davis 1996, particularly 2587; Bazell 1971a.

166   *The Wisconsin senator:* Estimates of letters received range from six thousand to eight thousand; see Rettig 1977, 176, 212.

166   *The letters warned:* US House of Representatives 1971b. Dozens of witnesses called to testify during Rogers's eleven days of subcommittee hearings voiced their concerns about removing the cancer mission from the folds of the NIH. For a summary, see 12–17. Many of the same scientists and academic

administrators testified or submitted letters of concern to Senator Kennedy's subcommittee as well.

166 *One professor:* Senate Hearings 1971, statement by Philip R. Lee, chancellor, University of California, San Francisco, before the Health Subcommittee, March 9, 1971, 130–68. Attached to Dr. Lee's lengthy statement was a twenty-four-page letter detailing myriad achievements of the NIH during the previous three and a half decades.

166 *Dr. Sol Spiegelman:* US House of Representatives 1971a, 204.

167 *One by one:* The mobilization started with the Senate bill (Rettig 1977, 143–47, 171–74, 351–52nn24–27). When that passed overwhelmingly, the medical and scientific guilds took their fight to the House subcommittee (Rettig 1977, 233–41). Many of these same groups sent letters to members of both chambers, as well as to newspapers. See also Schmeck 1971a.

167 *Dr. John Hogness:* US House of Representatives 1971a, 584.

167 *Thirteen scientists:* Nobel Prize winners Arthur Kornberg, Severo Ochoa, Edward Tatum, Julius Axelrod, and Marshall Nirenberg, for example, were among thirteen scientists who wrote a letter to the editor of the *Times* on August 9, 1971 (Martin et al. 1971), which was harshly critical of the Senate plan; the last two of these men had, notably, conducted some of their research in the intramural program of the NIH. See also Strickland 1971, 1098. A similar letter was published in the *Washington Post,* September 5, 1971.

168 *The barrage:* Rettig 1977, 164–65, 191, 221; Bazell 1971b.

168 *"Much of the great":* US House of Representatives 1971a, 191.

168 *The program:* Ibid., 791.

168 *The director of:* Ibid., 794.

168 *As with nearly:* Rettig 1977, 248–77.

168 *This committee was the proverbial:* Anon. 1971b, 20–21. See also Schmeck 1971b, 1971c, and 1971d.

169 *The cancer legislation:* Rettig 1977, 272–77.

169 *There were orders:* "The National Cancer Act of 1971," Public Law 92-218. The complete text of the law can be found at http://legislative.cancer.gov/history/phsa/1971.

169 *Cancer researchers in 1972:* Note that 1970's appropriation is reported slightly differently in various sources. It is also important to emphasize how remarkable this doubling of funds was in those tough economic times. The rate of inflation had been rising so rapidly for so long that only a few months before, President Nixon had imposed mandatory wage and price controls across the land. Budgets for popular programs were in the midst of being slashed, even as an unpopular war continued to drain the nation's coffers; the dollar was in

a swirl of devaluation, and the United States was suffering its first annual trade deficit since 1893.

169   *By 1976:* In 1976, the federal government changed the dates for its fiscal year and thus dispensed additional funds to the agency to cover the "transitional quarter" (between the end of the old fiscal year and the beginning of the new one). Such funds are not included in the 1976 figures stated here. The NCI provides a timeline for its congressional allocations in its annual *Fact Book*. For a breakdown of all years from 1938 through 2011, see *Fact Book* for 1973 (24), 1990 (77), 2006 (H-1), and 2011 (H-1). The NIH also lists allocations to each of its agencies (in rounded numbers) in one online source; see National Institutes of Health, NIH Almanac, Appropriations (Section 1), http://www.nih.gov/about/almanac/appropriations/index.htm.

169   *It would have:* See chapter 9 for more discussion.

Chapter 9: The "Door" Question

171   *Mr. Sam Donaldson:* Senate Hearings 1997, 32.

171   *the spring ritual:* Typically, spring is the markup season for Appropriations subcommittees; the full-committee markups are held in the summer and fall.

172   *But if Arlen Specter:* The subcommittee was formally known as the Subcommittee on Labor, Heath and Human Services, and Education, and Related Agencies. Senator Specter, at that time, was the senior Republican senator from Pennsylvania. He later became a Democrat.

172   *The extra money:* Senate Hearings 1997, 30.

173   *Tom Harkin:* Ibid., 25.

173   *The man was Sam:* Ibid., 32.

174   *Participants in the PCP's:* President's Cancer Panel 2008, 3.

175   *That was the message:* Casey et al. 2007.

175   *A year later:* Casey et al. 2008.

175   *So, too, Congressman:* Higgins 2010.

175   *That is the message:* As Andrew Thorburn (2010), professor and chair of Pharmacology at the University of Colorado School of Medicine, has explained, "We need more research into cancer biology, because without really understanding what is going on, our efforts to apply that research will be doomed to failure. Understanding cancer biology isn't just the best way forward; it is the only way forward, if we really want to solve the cancer problem." Just as often, however, the message has been conveyed through stark warnings about the failure to properly fund biomedical research. See, for example, the written congressional testimony of Margaret Foti (2011), the chief executive officer of the American Association for Cancer Research, the world's largest guild of cancer researchers: "Since 2003, appropriations for the NIH have fallen well

below the biomedical research inflation rate, resulting in shrinking, rather than expanding, the nation's biomedical research capacity. Flat funding means thousands of lost scientific opportunities. Worse, it means the loss of promising young researchers to the field of cancer research and delays—unforgivable delays—in the delivery of new therapies, and new hope, for thousands of cancer patients." See also Mitka 2007. Mitka quotes Joan S. Brugge, chair of the department of cell biology at Harvard Medical School, as saying that the recent flat funding of the NIH was having "a devastating impact on the trajectory of cancer research," that it was continuing to damage "the research infrastructure," and that it would, if not reversed, "delay relief from the cancer burden." Despite the high drama of the rhetoric, such views are standard fare in biomedical-research circles today.

176 *From the founding* (and data in following two paragraphs): NCI *Fact Book, 2006*, H-1. Worth noting is how, even in these early decades of the NCI's history, many scientists regarded the funding as bountiful. "American cancer research grew dramatically in the 1940s," writes the historian of science R. F. Bud (1978, 425). "Its funding rose twenty-fold in the fourteen years after 1937, reaching more than 14 million dollars annually by 1951. The scale made possible by such large funds was new to medical enquiry, but a precedent did exist in American industrial research." Donald S. Fredrickson, a former director of the NIH and, later, the Howard Hughes Medical Institute, captures this feeling of largesse in "Biomedical Science and the Culture Warp" (1993, 33): "The ascent of the annual NIH obligations for extramural research was swift. The approximately $4 million in fiscal year 1947 rose to $15.6 million in fiscal year 1950, to $36.6 million in 1955, and by 1960 was $203 million. This last figure represented two-thirds of all NIH obligations in 1960 ($338 million)."

176 *Total appropriations:* Just as Sam Donaldson and other well-known figures would do a decade later, the industrialist Armand Hammer (with help from celebrities such as Bill Cosby) began a high-profile push for more cancer funding in the spring of 1988. Hammer, who was then chairman of the President's Cancer Panel, announced a campaign to raise an additional $1 billion in public and private cancer funding, "convinced that the cure to cancer lies in more money for research," as *Science* reported (Culliton 1988).

176 *Congress would:* For some perspective, funding for the NCI over the past ten years (2002 through 2011) has totaled $48 billion. That's roughly equal to what Congress allocated to the NCI in the previous sixty-four years. (NCI funding from 1938 through 2001 totaled $48.8 billion, in nominal dollars.)

176 *After adjusting:* Inflation adjustment is from Bureau of Labor Statistics, CPI inflation calculator. For comparison, the entire federal budget, using the same

inflation measure, grew by between three and three and a half times over the same time. If calculated with GDP-based inflation adjustments, the 2010 NCI budget is roughly 6.5 times larger than the one in 1970. It is important to note, however, that the NIH itself prefers to use an inflator based on the Biomedical Research and Development Price Index (BRDPI), which assumes much larger cost increases from year to year than do other standard measures of inflation. Recently, the BRDPI's estimate of inflation, for example, has averaged some 2 percentage points higher per year than the CPI's. For more discussion on the possible distorting effects of BRDPI, see below.

177   *While the NCI:* The federal government allocated $6.036 billion "to continue to expand research related to cancer" in fiscal year 2011, according to Office of Management and Budget 2010, 21. The roughly $1 billion not spent by the NCI was allocated through other agencies within the NIH (such as the National Institute of Environmental Health Sciences and the National Heart, Lung, and Blood Institute); the NIH's parent, the US Department of Health and Human Services (such as the Centers for Disease Control and Prevention); and even by departments seemingly remote from the mission of cancer science. In 2011, the Department of Veterans Affairs spent $252 million on "biomedical laboratory science," and the Department of Defense devoted more than $500 million to its Congressionally Directed Medical Research Programs (CDMRP), most of which focus on cancer research. Since CDMRP began, the Pentagon has spent $2.8 billion on breast cancer research alone. See American Association for the Advancement of Science 2012; Department of Veterans Affairs, http://www.aaas.org/spp/rd/fy2013/; and the CDMRP's website, http://wwwcdmrp.army.mil/about/fundinghistory.shtml. For more, see Heath 2012, 83; and US GAO 2012, 96–101.

177   *The pharmaceutical:* This estimate is almost surely conservative. PhRMA, the pharmaceutical industry's main trade group, estimates that its member companies spent close to $39 billion on domestic research and development in 2011, which accounts for some 78 percent of its global R&D spending. In addition, scores of smaller biopharmaceutical firms not included in the PhRMA figures spend roughly $15 billion a year on drug R&D, according to PhRMA and Burrill & Company, a San Francisco firm that studies the biotech industry. The share likely spent on cancer drug development is based on conversations with industry analysts and other published estimates. See PhRMA 2012, 51ff, and profiles for previous years.

177   *The American Cancer Society:* American Cancer Society 2010b, 3–4. The cancer charity raised $903 million in "total support from the public" in 2010; that same year, it spent $681 million on "total program services"—of which $149 million went to support academic research.

177 *Several other nonprofit:* See IRS Form 990 (Return of Organization Exempt from Income Tax) for the 2010 calendar year, for the following: Susan G. Komen Breast Cancer Foundation, Inc. (which raised $175 million through contributions and grants); the Leukemia & Lymphoma Society, Inc. ($270 million in contributions and grants); American Institute for Cancer Research ($21 million). Leading cancer research centers also raise hundreds of millions of dollars each year. Dana-Farber Cancer Institute received $441 million in contributions and grants in 2010—apart from the $540 million the hospital received that year from "net patient service revenue." At Memorial Sloan–Kettering Cancer Center in New York, "total contributions and pledges raised through fund raising efforts were $301,374,000 and $237,666,000 for 2011 and 2010, respectively" (Memorial Sloan–Kettering Cancer Center 2011, 7). MD Anderson in Houston received $107,364,150 for its operations from gift contributions (MD Anderson Cancer Center 2010).

177 *As of the end:* Author's calculation, based on charity search of Internal Revenue Service's "Online Version of Publication 78" (now called "Exempt Organizations Select Check"), IRS.gov website, October 1, 2010. Note: Includes charities with any of the words *cancer, leukemia, lymphoma, melanoma, sarcoma, carcinoma, blastoma,* or *carcinoid* in their names. Charities with multiple keywords in their name were counted only once, as were individual charities listed in multiple locations.

177 *All told:* Author's calculation. For more discussion, see Leaf 2004, 82. For two historical examinations, see Ruzek et al. 1996; and McGeary and Burstein 1999. "In 1974, after the initial buildup of federal funding in the War on Cancer," write McGeary and Burstein, "NCI accounted for nearly two-thirds of all funding of cancer research in the United States. By 1997, NCI was the source of less than half of all funding (46 percent). Industry's share increased from 2 percent in 1974 to 31 percent in 1997" (17).

178 *However, America's:* Author's calculation. Again, this is likely to be a conservative estimate. In nominal dollars, congressional appropriations to the NCI from 1938 through 2011 total nearly $97 billion (NCI *Fact Book, 2011,* H-1), a figure that would be dramatically higher if calculated in current (inflation–adjusted) dollars.

178 *Though the overall:* NIH Office of Extramural Research, Office of Research Information Systems, "NIH R01 Equivalent and RPG Success Rates FY 1970–2009"; NIH, Research Portfolio Online Reporting Tools (RePORT), Research Project Success Rates by NIH Institute for 2011. See also Kalberer 1975.

179 *Current grant:* In 2011 NCI grant applications had a success rate of 13.8 percent compared with 27.6 percent in 2002.

179   *The dreary success:* Interview with John P. A. Ioannidis, April 10, 2012. See also Ioannidis 2011.

179   *In 1980:* Matthews et al. 2011; Cech et al. 2008, 10; and NIH Office of Extramural Research, Office of Research Information Systems, "NIH Research Project Grant Principal Investigators and Medical School Faculty Age Distributions, 1980–2006."

180   *Four decades ago:* Matthews et al. 2011, 4. A critical issue is that young investigators typically need to win an R01 grant to secure a tenure-track position at most leading research institutions. See, for example, Franko and Ionescu-Pioggia 2006, 38–39, 41–45, 153–74.

180   *"Exceptionally bright":* Anon. 2011a; and Collins 2010b, 635. See also Couzin and Miller 2007, 359, quoting the chairman of one university neurobiology department: "It's just about inconceivable for a brand new investigator to get an NIH grant funded on their first submission these days. . . . I see it as this dark shadow hanging over people who are just starting out their labs. They're having to spend so much time being anxious over funding, to the detriment of having time to think creatively about their research."

180   *Collins, for his:* See Cech et al. 2008; Tilghman et al. 1998; Cech et al. 2005; and Monastersky 2007.

180   *If the current:* Kaiser 2008. The average age of NIH principal investigators rose from 39.1 in 1980 to 50.8 in 2006. Cech et al. 2008, 11.

180   *Making it harder:* Zerhouni 2006, 1088 in particular.

180   *Senior investigators:* Brainard 2004 provides a thorough explanation. For additional perspective on why the touted NIH doubling did not increase grant success rates, see Mandel and Vesell 2001 and Malakoff 2001.

180   *In 1975:* NCI *Fact Book, 1977,* 47; and *2010,* E-2. In 2010, the NCI awarded 1,041 new competing grants for investigator-initiated research projects compared with 581 in 1975.

181   *This grant-size:* The NIH measures such inflation with the Biomedical Research and Development Price Index (BRDPI). Like the better-known consumer price index (CPI), the BRDPI is a weighted average of a basket of components (including, in the latter case, such things as investigator and technician salaries, equipment, and supplies). The actual weighting of the forty-five BRDPI components was provided on February 15, 2011, by the NIH's Division of Program Coordination, Planning, and Strategic Initiatives—though only after a formal request under the Freedom of Information Act. Together, expenditures for compensation and benefits (for NIH personnel, academic and nonacademic workers, and consultants) accounted for 66 percent of the total index weighting in 2010. By contrast, scientific instrumentation, equipment, laboratory supplies, and research animals, in sum, accounted for 9.8 percent

of the index. It is not just the relative weightings that are telling, however; so is the annual growth rate in the cost of these components. In the case of "instruments and apparatus," for example, the average annual growth rate from 1993 through 2009 was 0.79 percent. During this same period, academic "salary and wages" grew by 3.83 percent per year, on average. "Fringe benefits" for academic personnel, meanwhile, grew at an astounding rate of 5.15 percent a year. Since 1980, the rate of inflation for biomedical research, according to the BRDPI, has outpaced ordinary inflation (as measured by the gross domestic product index) by about 1.5 percentage points annually—a dramatic difference. But it is important to understand that this has been driven largely by personnel wages and benefits, not by some imagined higher premium for "doing science."

182 *Academic salaries:* American Association of University Professors 2010, 4–32. See also Rapoport 1998; Zemlo et al. 2000, 229 in particular; and Patton 2012.

182 *Three of every:* The issues surrounding "indirect" research costs have been fiercely debated since the early 1980s. See, for example, Comptroller General of the United States 1984; Sundro 1991; Goldman et al. 2000; and Friendly 1996.

182 *At Johns Hopkins:* Rate agreement, dated May 5, 2010, between Johns Hopkins University and the Department of Heath and Human Services. The 64 percent rate applies to federally sponsored research conducted on campus between July 1, 2009, and June 30, 2010.

182 *in 2010 alone:* Johns Hopkins received some $610 million in medical-research funding from the federal government in 2010, which works out to nearly $238 million in facilities and administrative costs, if its standard rate is applied to all the funding.

182 *The money adds:* Bascetta 2007. The United States paid research institutions $3,945,506,253 in 2003, $4,203,165,147 in 2004, and $4,304,951,026 in 2005 for overhead related to NIH-funded biomedical-research grants (8).

182 *As made clear:* Cech et al. 2008, 42.

183 *The current system:* Interview with E. Ray Dorsey, March 15, 2012.

183 *One obvious cost:* This was a resounding theme in conversations with dozens of veteran and younger scientists. In particular, I am grateful to Michael Sporn (various interviews, see notes to chapter 7) and Francis Barany, Weill Cornell Medical College, July 10, 2007, for their candor. At a meeting of organizers for "Stand Up to Cancer" (November 26, 2007, Century City, CA), the late Judah Folkman was passionate about the problem. "They think it's their fault," Folkman said of young cancer investigators. "Among those who are leaving are superstars. I'm worried it's all going to stop. We are losing so many young people."

183 *"For the first":* Robert Weinberg, comments at the end of his Kirk A. Landon Prize lecture at the 2006 AACR annual meeting, transcribed in the *Cancer Letter* 32 (April 7, 2006): 5–6. Kirsten Boyd Goldberg reports in the same issue of the *Cancer Letter* (2), that "Weinberg's statement triggered a 25-second burst of applause—an unusually long interruption for a scientific lecture."

183 *The profound danger:* Vastag 2006.

184 *Between 1980 and:* Matthews et al. 2011.

184 *in short, we keep:* Hand with Wadman 2008. Examining grants given by the NIH in 2007, the authors found "a whopping 200 scientists received six or more grants each." In addition, "one principal investigator was awarded 32 grants, the data reveal, and many others got eight or nine."

184 *More striking* (footnote): Dietrich and Srinivasan 2007.

185 *NIH leaders:* Collins 2010a; Blackburn et al. 2011, 13; Sargent 2012, 25; NIH 2009, statement from the NIH director, February 25, archived at http:// www.nih.gov/about/director/02252009statement_arra.htm.

185 *In 2011:* Data for 2006 through 2011 are drawn from the Blue Ridge Institute for Medical Research, "Ranking Tables of National Institutes of Health (NIH) Award Data," available at http://www.brimr.org/NIH_Awards/. (In these calculations, I have used data tables for "all institutions.") BRIMR obtains the annual figures from the NIH's Research Portfolio Online Reporting Tool (RePORT), at http://report.nih.gov/award/trends/AggregateData.cfm, and orders the institutional recipients of funding in ranking tables, as the NIH itself did prior to 2006. The NIH stopped publishing its own lists, it said, in part because of "responses received from the grantee community suggesting that ranking tables were not necessary." (Data for years prior to 2006 are drawn from the NIH's own published rankings.)

185 *And so it has gone:* GAO 1987, throughout. See also OTA 1991, 8–13, 90, 198, 263–65, and Appendix B.

185 *As the CEO:* Miller 2005. Retrieved at http://www.hopkinsmedicine.org/ webnotes/newsletter_draft/editorials/0507.cfm, accessed January 14, 2011.

187 *Brian Druker:* Interview with Brian Druker, February 7, 2012.

189 *In 1963:* Hoeschele 2009 and Christie and Tansey 2007, 20. Rosenberg and colleagues published their findings in a seminal *Nature* paper (Rosenberg, Van Camp, and Krigas 1965).

Chapter 10: Publish and Perish

190 *Among them:* Nowell and Hungerford 1960, discussed in chapter 5.

191 *The study of:* Tjio and Levan 1956, discussed in chapter 1.

191 *They had no theory:* Interview with Peter C. Nowell, September 5, 2007; Nowell 1985, 19. See also chapter 5, 106–11.

191 *Their research:* Nowell 1977, 53.

191 *When I asked:* Interview with Nowell.

191 *Gracious and:* The allusion is to lines Horace Walpole had written in a 1754 letter to a friend: "I once read a silly fairy tale, called 'The Three Princes of Serendip'; as their Highnesses traveled, they were always making discoveries, by accidents and sagacity, of things which they were not in quest of." Nowell told me amiably that this was the same route he had taken (Merton and Barber 2004, 1–2).

192 *Their discovery was yet more proof:* Pasteur said the now famous line—which Vallery-Radot (79) translates as "In the fields of observation, chance only favours the mind which is prepared"—in a speech to the Faculté des Sciences in Lille, France, on December 7, 1854.

192 *In the same:* Rosenberg, Van Camp, and Krigas 1965, discussed in chapter 9.

192 *Francis Peyton Rous:* Rous was thirty-one years old, the same age as Peter Nowell, when he reported, in a January 1911 paper for *JAMA,* a discovery that would leave a lasting mark on cancer science. Researchers, by then, had shown that transplanting aggressive tumor cells into a healthy animal could cause cancers to develop. But Rous wanted to investigate what within those transplanted cells was responsible for transmitting the cancer. So he took cells from an aggressive chicken tumor, ground them in sterilized sand, and spun the mulch in a centrifuge to make sure there were no viable cells left. Then he pressed the mixture through a fine porcelain apparatus known as a Berkefeld filter, which strained out organisms as infinitesimal as bacteria. He injected a few drops of this faint yellow soup into the breast muscle of a healthy fowl and waited. Weeks later a malignant tumor formed at the spot of injection. The only things known to pass through the Berkefeld filters were viruses. But Rous was cautious enough not to reach that conclusion openly; in fact, in his one-page *JAMA* paper, he avoided mention of the word *virus* altogether. And for good reason: everyone, in 1911, *knew* that viruses didn't cause cancer. Rudolph Virchow, the nineteenth-century German whom many acclaimed as the father of pathology, had shown that the cause of cancer was to be found *inside* the cell, not outside of it. His famed dictum, *Omnia cellula e cellula*—all cells arise from cells—implied that cancer could not be imported, so to speak. Rous's finding was heresy. (*JAMA* editors thought so little of it that they didn't bother to list it in the issue's table of contents.) Despite Rous's avoidance of the word *virus,* his discovery was roundly rejected as an impossibility. "Among oncologists of the day," recalled Richard Shope, who took up the hunt for the cancer-virus connection some twenty years later, "the immediate reactions to Rous's finding and its interpretation were violent and critical." Not until many decades later did others show precisely how Rous's sarcoma virus could

transform a normal cell and explain what this process revealed about the genetic basis of cancer. (For more, see footnote on page 271.)

192 *Temin's heresy:* The prominent cancer scientist Robert A. Weinberg gives a thorough account of Temin's ostracism in Weinberg 1996b, 52–65. See also Milt 1969, 220; and Beeman 2005, 284, who point out that Ludwik Gross received much the same treatment as Temin and Rous did when, in 1953, Gross suggested that an oncogenic virus could cause leukemia in mice. A Polish refugee who'd fled the Nazis in 1940, Gross was then working for the US Army in a VA hospital in the Bronx—a place unknown to the mandarins of cancer research. Indeed, his main job wasn't research at all—it was tending to patients. One day a week, however, his military supervisors allowed him to pursue his own biological studies in a makeshift lab in the building's basement. Gross had laid out the experimental protocols in masterful detail so that anyone might repeat them. But despite his precision and the provocative nature of his findings, his paper was initially cast aside by those *better informed.* Later, when Gross's experiments were finally reproduced, the payoff was yet another surprise. It seems a few of the mouse cells that Gross had painstakingly transformed with his leukemia virus had been harboring a stowaway: a second virus. And that virus, as Sarah Stewart and Bernice Eddy at the National Institute of Health later revealed, led to the formation of *solid* tumors, not leukemia. Not only that, it caused many types of tumor—and in a large number of species, too. Hence, it earned the name *polyoma virus.* For more, see Gross 1974a and 1974b and Stewart 1960.

193 *As David Baltimore:* Baltimore 1997. Retrieved from http://www.ncbi.nlm.nih .gov/books/NBK19376/.

193 *A similar treatment:* Interview with Judah Folkman, November 12, 2006, and conversations with several other scientists, including Bruce A. Chabner at Boston's Massachusetts General Hospital and Michael Sporn at Dartmouth. Robert Cooke 2001 provides a compelling account of Folkman's work and the "almost unending ridicule" he endured at the hands of fellow cancer researchers. See also Linde 2001.

193 *Science, without question:* This has always been the case. When Galileo endorsed the Copernican notion that the earth revolved around the sun, for example, he was summoned by the Holy See in Rome, tried and convicted by the Inquisition, and sentenced to house arrest for the rest of his life.

193 *A 2008 report:* Cech et al. 2008, 28.

193 *Young investigators, the risk-takers of yore:* For a thoughtful discussion on the need for such risk-taking by young scientists, see Maxmen 2009.

194 *The NIH defines:* NIH Office of Extramural Research, "NIH Research Project Grant Program (R01)," http://www.grants.nih.gov/grants/funding/r01.htm, retrieved on September 12, 2012.

195 *The cash, as much:* Though the dollar awards in R01, as a rule, are not limited, few are above $600,000.

195 *The point of:* See, for example, Casey et al. 2008, 5. "The Research Project (R01) grant," say the authors, "is the gold standard in science—it launches careers. A scientist is not considered established and independent until he or she is awarded an R01, which provides multi-year funds that enable scientists to hire staff and buy equipment and materials necessary to conduct experiments." See also *Science* Careers Online 2001–7: The GrantDoctor, July 25, 2003, November 10, 2006; Nextwave from the journal *Science,* "Getting an NIH R01," September 28, 2001; and updated version of the guide, "The NIH R01 Toolkit," July 27, 2007.

195 *The changes have:* Resistance to new ideas is hardly new, as many scholars of the history of science have pointed out. The phenomenon is captured in an adage that has gone through various permutations since the early nineteenth century: "First, a new theory is attacked as absurd; then it is admitted to be true, but obvious and insignificant; finally it is seen to be so important that its adversaries claim that they themselves discovered it." The saying (in a different phrasing) is often credited to the English biologist Thomas Henry Huxley, but Jeffrey Shallit (2005, 2) traces it back to the German philosopher Arthur Schopenhauer. For a different history, see Gould and Eldredge 1986, 143. For a more comprehensive discussion, see Kuhn 1970.

195 *and now, it:* Cech et al. 2005, 18–19, 56–57, and throughout; Ioannidis 2011; President's Cancer Panel 2008, 8; and Bonetta 2008.

195 *"There is no":* Quoted in Kolata 2009.

195 *Or as Leonard:* Interview with Leonard Zwelling, January 30, 2004.

196 *In 1980:* National Institutes of Health, NIH Office of Extramural Research, Office of Research Information Systems, "NIH Research Project Grant Principal Investigators and Medical School Faculty Age Distributions, 1980–2006." In 2006, just 4.7 percent of NIH principal investigators were thirty-six or younger, compared with 26.4 percent in 1980; the share of investigators thirty-two or younger dropped from 7 percent to 0.8 percent over the same time. Such numbers have raised alarms, as Cech et al. 2005 point out. Typical are the remarks the authors cite from Bruce Alberts, president of the National Academy of Sciences, in his 2003 President's Address: "[In the early 1970s] many of my colleagues and I were awarded our first independent funding when we were under thirty years old. We did not have preliminary results because we were trying something completely new. [Now] almost no one finds it possible to start an independent scientific career under the age of thirty-five."

197 *Like other proteins:* Search of scientific papers on NIH's PubMed, http://www.ncbi.nlm.nih.gov/pubmed, on April 15, 2012.

197 *The higher the:* Yaffe 2009. For some background, see Garfield 2005; and Moed and Van Leeuwen 1995.

197 *A middling position:* Search of scientific papers on NIH's PubMed, http://www.ncbi.nlm.nih.gov/pubmed, on April 15, 2012.

199 *The SF424(R&R):* SF424(R&R) 2011.

199 *Arriving first:* Buscher 2002. This 126-page volume goes through the entire process. The NIH's Center for Scientific Review has posted a video of the process, "NIH Peer Review Process Revealed," at http://public.csr.nih.gov/Pages/default.aspx.

199 *Meanwhile, it:* In previous years, there were 220 scientific review groups. Today, besides the 182 standing study sections, an additional 22 groups review fellowships, with 34 for small-business applications, along with 157 "special emphasis panels," for a total of 395 different study sections. See http://public.csr.nih.gov/StudySections/Standing/Pages/default.aspx. Regarding the NIH scoring system, see "Enhancing Peer Review: The NIH Announces New Scoring Procedures for Evaluation of Research Applications Received for Potential FY2010 Funding," NIH Notice Number NOT-OD-09-024, released December 2, 2008. Until recently, the scoring was based on a scale of 1 to 5. For a history of study sections, see Fredrickson 1993, 32.

199 *In some funding institutes:* Martin, Kopstein, and Janice 2010.

200 *The NCI's central:* Rockey 2011. For more, see K. Goldberg 2009, 1–2; and Harvard School of Public Health 2011.

200 *The check goes:* See earlier discussion of indirect costs in chapter 9, 182.

201 *"It's not that":* Interview with John Iaonnidis, April 10, 2012.

202 *Stanford University biochemist:* Quoted in Lee 2007.

202 *Veteran cancer:* Interview with Michael Sporn, February 21, 2005, and e-mail exchange, January 29, 2011; interview with Genie Kleinerman, January 30, 2004. See also Cech et al. 2005, 10–19; Cech et al. 2008, 20–22; Vastag 2006, 1436–38; Kolata 2009.

203 *Inside the study:* I served as a "peer reviewer" for the Congressionally Directed Medical Research Program's (CDMRP) Breast Cancer Research Program in 2006.

203 *That even goes:* Interview with Isaiah "Josh" Fidler, January 29, 2004.

204 *It was Fidler and colleagues:* Paget 1889. For background, see Fidler, Gersten, and Hart 1978, 167ff in particular; Fidler 1990 and 2003; and Talmadge and Fidler, 2010.

204 *"It's all about":* Interview with Robert Weinberg, January 23, 2004.

204 *At the venerable:* Lane 2005, 489; and search of PubMed, April 15, 2012. See also Real 2007.

205 Footnote: *The term may:* Kuipers 1974.

206 *In actual practice:* See, for example, Beveridge 1960, who describes the roles of not just experimentation, but also of chance, intuition, and imagination in scientific inquiry. Citing the words of W. H. George, Beveridge sums up what many scientists know to be true: "Scientific research is not itself a science; it is still an art of craft." For more perspective, see Ayala 2009; Kell and Oliver 2004; and, for a particularly provocative point of view, Feyerabend 2010, 1ff.

206 *Good science:* Sulston and Ferry 2002, 44. For a thoughtful commentary on the subject, see also McKnight 2009.

206 *"My first studies":* Ibid.

206 *So one straightforward:* Ioannidis 2011. For more discussion, see O'Malley et al. 2009.

207 *Somehow, Silicon Valley:* Interview with Andy Grove, January 20, 2004; March 20, 2006; and follow-up conversations.

207 *All of the funding:* Ioannidis 2011, 531.

208 *In a 2005:* Interview with Judah Folkman, April 25, 2005.

208 *As a young:* For more, see Cooke 2001.

209 *"Your hands feel":* Interview with Judah Folkman, November 12, 2006.

Chapter 11: Deadly Caution

210 Epigraph: Ackoff 2006.

210 *Somewhere in the:* Lind 1772, 149–50.

211 *"The consequence":* Ibid., 150.

211 *This was the first:* Thomas 1969, 932–33; Hughes 1975, 342–51; Chalmers 1981. See also the many academic articles on the subject gathered at the James Lind Library, http://www.jameslindlibrary.org/, a web resource curated by Iain Chalmers, James Lind Initiative, Oxford, UK.

211 *The "plague of the sea":* Krehl 1953, 4 in particular. Krehl cites Louis Roddis (1950, 48), a biographer of Lind's, for the claim that "although no exact statistics are available, it is certain that during that period [1500–1800], scurvy killed as many seamen as were lost by deaths in naval battle, shipwreck, other nautical hazards, and all other diseases affecting the sailor." Roddis may, in turn, have been relying on a 1940 report in the *Military Surgeon* (see Gilchrist 1940, 448). There it was reported that "in the 300 years between 1500 and 1800 scurvy killed as many seamen as all other nautical hazards combined. This includes not only deaths from battle and shipwreck but from all other diseases as well."

211 *"Some 250 years":* Anon. 2004b, 5.

212 *And yet, of all:* It's important to stress that this view in no way reflects the views of the James Lind Alliance or, perhaps, most authorities on clinical trials. The speed of studies is rarely, if ever, discussed as an important component of the clinical trials process—though I argue that it should be.

212 *Today, testing:* DiMasi and Grabowski (2007, particularly 212) calculate the mean clinical development time for new oncology drugs approved by the FDA from 1990 to 2005 at 7.8 years, with an additional 1.3 years required on average for regulatory approval. The respective times for new drugs in other therapeutic categories are 6.3 years for the "clinical phase" and 1.8 years for approval (see Figure 1 in ibid., 212). These times are significantly shorter than what DiMasi reported in his widely cited 2001 paper. Then, DiMasi calculated that, for new chemical entities approved by the FDA from 1990 to 1999, the clinical phase for cancer (antineoplastic) drugs lasted 10.4 years on average, compared with 8.6 years for therapies in all classes. In this paper, DiMasi also estimates that the "prehuman testing phase" for cancer drugs approved during the period was 4.4 years on average, compared with 3.8 years for drugs overall. Prehuman testing is the period between the first synthesis of the agent and its first testing in humans. While the clinical-phase time reported by DiMasi and Grabowski for the period 1990–2005 is notably shorter than that for 1990–99, it is higher than that for the period 1970–79 (7.1 years) and dramatically higher than in the previous decade, 1963–69 (3.1 years); see DiMasi 2001, Figures 5 and 6, 212.

212 *What makes this problem:* For more discussion, see Leaf 2006. The public interest group Public Citizen, for example, has argued vocally (and generally quite credibly) that the huge marketing muscle of global drug companies, a willing "take a pill for it" American culture, and a lax regulatory apparatus have combined to allow many unsafe drugs on the market. For more, see Public Citizen's website http://www.worstpills.org/ or http://www.citizen.org/Page.aspx?pid=4374.

213 *From that reasonable:* Many, if not most, of those who have commented on the issue find the FDA's caution and the pace of regulatory approval of new drugs to be appropriate—or if anything, not cautious enough. See, for example, Hilts 1995. Others find the delay less reasonable. See Huber 1998; Miller 2008; and Philipson et al. 2006.

213 *Drug developers worry:* Leibfarth 2008, 1286–89 in particular, provides a thorough appraisal, as well as criticism, of the FDA's "gold standard" drug-approval process.

213 *And because this lengthy:* DiMasi, Hansen, and Grabowski 2003; and English, Lebovitz, and Griffin 2010, 3. For some historical perspective, see Le Fanu 2012, 282–87. Some have sharply questioned the pharmaceutical industry's own assessment of drug-development costs, saying the costs are much lower. See, for instance, Light and Warburton 2011.

213 *Which pushes them:* As discussed in chapter 7, this dynamic discourages investments in chemopreventive agents for cancer, therapies that could help reduce

the burden of cancer. See Grabowski and Moe 2008; and Kelloff et al. 2006, 3689.

213 *They fear anything* (and following): Milken Institute Global Conference 2005: discussions with panel participants in "Starting Over with the FDA." See also Friends of Cancer Research 2004. The perspective described is also drawn from interviews with Alex Tabarrok and Henry Miller in November 2004, and from multiple discussions with pharmaceutical-industry executives, industry analysts, and US drug regulators over the past nine years. For more, see Kola and Landis 2004; Holzman and Hebert 2005, 62; Office of Technology Assessment, US Congress 1993a, 1–37 and passages throughout; GAO 2006a, 27–33 and passages throughout; comments on marketing exclusivity by McKinnell (Pfizer) 2004; and Zemmel and Sheikh 2010.

213 *Firms fear rivals'*: The process is known in the industry as "free-riding." See Roin 2009, 537 in particular. See also Slavin 2006; and Fisk and Atun 2008.

213 *Sponsors are so guarded:* A big part of this game is, quite simply, to exclude older patients from clinical drug studies. See Lewis et al. 2003. Analyzing data for 495 NCI-sponsored cooperative-group trials active from 1997 through 2000, the authors found that just 32 percent of participants in phase II and III studies were sixty-five years old or older—though this age group represents nearly twice the share (61 percent) of cancer cases in the United States. The authors also found that exclusion criteria are largely responsible for this dramatic underrepresentation. See also Hutchins et al. 1999; Littlewood, Schenkel, and Liss 2005; Benson 1991; and Aapro et al. 2005. More broadly, Freemantle and Strack (2010) argue that the modern techniques of clinical trials (randomization, standardization, and rigid control) give "internal validity" to trial data, but also reduce "external validity, that is, generalizability of results and conclusions" to the real world.

214 *Medicare, hoping:* US House of Representatives 2006, 6. The need to "get on the list" is critical; see, for example, Cohen, Stolk, and Niezen 2007, 727–34.

214 *"That element of risk"*: Interview with Richard Pazdur, January 21, 2004.

214 *As the Government:* GAO 2006b, 29.

214 *(A tweak):* Tabarrok 2000, in particular 32n14. See also Booth and Zemmel 2003.

214 *"With all of the hype"*: Pazdur interview, January 21, 2004.

215 *The once-unstoppable:* E-mail correspondence with Dr. John P. Swann, FDA historian, US Food & Drug Administration, March 12–13, 2012. For more on pre-1983 drug approvals, see de Haen 1976 and de Haen 1983. The pioneering oncologist Irv Krakoff provides a wonderful timeline for the approval of key cancer drugs from the 1940s through the 1980s, in the unpublished

manuscript for his Karnofsky lecture at ASCO's annual meeting in 1993. For the published lecture, see Krakoff 1994. See also Krakoff 1977.

215 *The decline in new-drug:* Scannell et al. 2012, particularly 191. The original Moore's Law, coined by Intel cofounder Gordon Moore in 1965, was: "The number of transistors incorporated in a chip will approximately double every twenty-four months." For more background on this principle, see Jorgenson 2001, 3–15. "Between 1974 and 1996," writes Jorgenson, "prices of memory chips decreased by a factor of 27,270 times or at 40.9 percent per year, while the implicit deflator for the gross domestic product *increased* by 1.3 times or 2.6 percent a year!" See also Schaller 1977, 53–59; and Rutten et al. 2001.

215 *"It is no exaggeration":* Woodcock 2011.

215 *Drug companies argue:* PhRMA 2002.

215 *Many blame the FDA:* Walker 2005; Anon. 2011c; Flook 2012. Among the more strident critics of this caution (and the sclerotic process it engenders) are the members of the editorial board of the *Wall Street Journal.* See, for example, Editors 2004, 2005a, and 2005b.

216 *Woodcock says the FDA:* Woodcock 2011.

216 *Medical researchers:* Cutler, Rosen, and Vijan 2006, 924 in particular; Peters 2004, 9–10 in particular; and Bennani 2011. Scannell and colleagues (2012) say the "low-hanging fruit" factor is not as significant as other reasons for the declining efficiency in drug development.

216 *Jonathan Baron:* Interview with Jonathan Baron, December 22, 2005; Leaf 2006. Spranca, Minsk, and Baron (1991) provide a thorough description and experimental evidence for the concept. See also Ritov and Baron 1990; and Baron and Ritov 1994.

216 *In what he calls:* Interview with David Dilts, February 2, 2012.

217 *In the 1990s:* For some background, see Clark, Chew, and Fujimoto 1987, 731–36 in particular; and Dilts, Boyd, and Whorms 1991.

217 *Trial recruitment is:* The 3–5 percent figure is well cited. See, for example, Comis and Crowley 2006, 3. See also Cassileth 2003.

218 *Nearly as many:* For more on this process, see National Cancer Institute, "NCI's Clinical Trials Cooperative Group Program." A search of www.clinical trials.gov, the official NCI registry of clinical trials, on April 28, 2011, found 703 US Phase III trials sponsored by the NIH compared with 740 sponsored by industry.

218 *Dilts and Sandler began:* Dilts, Sandler et al. 2006. For more on CALGB, see Schilsky et al. 2006. See also the web site for Cancer and Leukemia Group B, http://www.calgb.org/.

219 *The actual protocol:* Dilts and colleagues repeated the analysis for other prominent cooperative groups and for the NCI's Cancer Therapy Evaluation

Program. As with the CALGB study, these are essential reading: Dilts, Sandler et al. 2008 and 2009; and Dilts et al. 2010.

219   *Before an "investigational":* Office for Human Research Protections, US Department of Health and Human Services, IRB Guidebook. "The biggest risk aversion occurs in our own IRBs," said John Mendelsohn, the former president of MD Anderson Cancer Center in Houston and one of the nation's most respected clinical scientists. "They are the ones slowing things down more than anything. We must work with them to teach them that if the patient wants to accept the risk, it's okay" (quoted in Patlak, Balogh, and Nass 2012, 44). Lee A. Green et al. 2006 provide some striking data to back up that assessment. Examining data from forty-three IRBs overseeing primary-care clinics operated by the Department of Veterans Affairs, the researchers found it took a median 286 days to get IRB approval for studies. In addition, over a twenty-nine-month period (from May 2001 to December 2003), the IRB process consumed 4,680 hours of staff time. See also Wagner et al. 2003; and Humphries, Trafton, and Wagner 2003. In 2001, the NCI set up a centralized IRB (CIRB) for its cooperative-group Phase III oncology trials, but participation is voluntary—and even here, under current rules, individual study sites still conduct their own review, albeit a "facilitated one," in addition to that of the CIRB (Murray et al. 2010). See also Nass, Moses, and Mendelsohn 2010, 131–36.

220   *The number of procedures:* Getz 2012 reports that the median number of procedures done per study protocol rose from about 106 in 2000–3 to 158 in 2004–7 to 167 in 2008–11. The cost of so-called noncore procedures—those not directly related to the trial end points agreed upon at the start of the study—is estimated to be between $3 billion and $5 billion (Mansell 2012). See also Tufts Center for the Study of Drug Development 2010. Similar data are reported in Getz, Campo, and Kaitin 2011. See also Getz et al. 2008. It's worth noting that the pharmaceutical industry has complained of this procedural burden since 1981, when the Pharmaceutical Manufacturers Association and nine member drug companies commissioned three studies on the issue (OTA, US Congress 1993a, 137).

220   *An astounding 40 percent:* Cheng et al. 2009 examined data from more than five hundred NCI-sponsored trials (Phases I through III) run through its Cancer Therapy Evaluation Program (CTEP). They found that four in ten failed to recruit the minimum number of patients required to conduct the study. Among the Phase III trials examined, 64 percent failed to recruit enough volunteers, with nearly 50 percent of the total closing with enrollments of less than a quarter of what was required. For more perspective on the dimensions of this failing, see Nass, Moses, and Mendelsohn 2010, 143. Said the authors

of this Institute of Medicine report, "The ultimate inefficiency is a clinical trial that is never completed because of insufficient patient accrual, and this happens far too often."

220   *It is "a terrible":* Nass, Moses, and Mendelsohn 2010, x.

220   *"I do think":* Interview and follow-up correspondence with Irv Krakoff, March 20, 2005.

221   *Even in the latest:* Kola and Landis 2004, 712 in particular. Examining a different time period and database of drugs, DiMasi and Grabowski (2007, 212) found that half of cancer drugs "that entered the expensive phase III clinical testing phase never make it to US regulatory approval." For more discussion, see Govindan 2007; Gordian, Singh, and Zemmel 2006, 1–3; and David, Tramontin, and Zemmel 2009. See also Schein and Scheffler (2006), who provide an insightful analysis of the barriers to cancer drug development.

221   *This inability:* FDA 2004b, 9.

221   *Attrition rates:* Ibid., 8; Scannell et al. 2012.

221   *According to one analysis:* Kola and Landis 2004, 712.

221   *Such late-stage losses:* FDA 2004b, ii.

221   *The big pharma companies:* Desdouits et al. 2006, 43.

222   *Or make that:* Search of www.clinicaltrials.gov, February 1, 2011. At the time, the government's database listed an additional 185 studies with Avastin for indications other than cancer. A search on November 16, 2010, listed 1,177 clinical studies. Roche, the maker of Avastin, hints at this strategy in a 159-page presentation on the company's fiscal year 2010 results, delivered by group chief executive officer, Severin Schwan (2011, 71) in London and New York.

222   *Avastin—researchers:* Hurwitz et al. 2004; Ferrara et al. 2004; Miller et al. 2005.

222   *It earned:* Hurwitz et al. 2004; FDA 2004a.

222   *As for metastatic:* See the National Cancer Institute's web page on bevacizumab, http://www.cancer.gov/cancertopics/druginfo/fda-bevacizumab, updated November 18, 2011; FDA commissioner statement and news release, "FDA Commissioner Removes Breast Cancer Indication from Avastin Label," November 18, 2011, http://www.fda.gov/NewsEvents/Newsroom/ucm279485.htm, and related "Questions and Answers: Removing Metastatic Breast Cancer as an Indication from Avastin's Product Labeling," http://www.fda.gov/NewsEvents/Newsroom/ucm280533.htm. See also Pollack 2010 and Stein 2011.

222   *The antibody:* Stein 2011. He cites a cost of $88,000 a year; the drugmaker capped the cost of the drop at $57,000 for women with income of less than $100,000 per year. Mundy 2011 and Berenson 2006.

223   *though unlikely to change:* Mijuk 2011.

223   *Of this money, roughly:* See Schwan 2011, 7, 15. For a glimpse of the dramatic effect approval in an indication such as breast cancer can have on sales, see Jinks and Sargent 2008. The writers report that shares of Genentech, the US maker of Avastin, jumped nearly 9 percent, its biggest rise in almost three years, after the FDA approved the drug to treat breast cancer. Its previous biggest one-day gain was an 18 percent surge on April 15, 2005, after Genentech released results from a study suggesting that Avastin slowed the progression of breast cancer. Until 2008, Genentech broke out the US sales of its various cancer drugs on its corporate website. In 2005, the first full year after Avastin's FDA approval, Genentech sold $1.1 billion worth of the drug to American patients; by 2008, US sales of the drug had reached $2.7 billion.

223   *Ironically, the sizes:* Parazzini 2005.

223   *The purported benefits:* Friedman and Goldberg 1996.

223   *Yet, such an analysis:* Berman and Parker 2002, 10.

223   *To cite one striking:* Bennett et al. 2008. The twenty-one authors of the meta-analysis concluded that "erythropoiesis-stimulating agent administration to patients with cancer is associated with increased risk" of venous thrombo-embolism (blood clots) and a modest increase (1.10-fold) in mortality risk, but stopped short of suggesting any course of action other than "concern." See also Bohlius et al. 2006a, who aggregate the data from thirty trials published between 1993 and 2002 (Figure 2); and Bohlius et al. 2006b. In a more recent analysis, involving sixty studies and 15,323 patients, Glaspy et al. 2010 found "no significant effect of ESAs on survival or disease progression" and had arrived at the same conclusion in a prominent review the year before (2009). In that review, the authors concluded, "Although the preponderance of the data suggests that ESAs do not alter survival when used to treat chemotherapy-induced anemia, large well-controlled trials addressing this issue are needed." See also Rizzo et al. 2007. For a good discussion of anemia in cancer patients, see Spivak 2005.

224   *Dozens upon dozens:* Ioannidis 2005 reveals how strikingly common it is for a clinical study demonstrating the effectiveness of a given medical intervention to be contradicted by a later study—and the more high profile the original finding is, the more likely a later study will dispute it. See also LeLorier et al. 1997. Such debates can be found in every area of clinical medicine, not just the treatment of cancer. Typical is the question of whether flu vaccine makes sense for children under two. In "Vaccines for Preventing Influenza in Healthy Children," the *Cochrane Database of Systematic Reviews* investigators attempted to answer this question by culling data from fifty-one studies involving 263,987 children. While they could not find enough evidence to answer the

question, they were able to conclude that "large-scale studies . . . are urgently required." See also Higgins 2003.

224 *Two meta-analyses:* Harrington 1999 and Mamounas et al. 1999. The question here was whether a standard regimen of chemotherapy (5-fluorouracil plus leucovorin) improved patient survival over doing nothing at all for those with Stage II colon cancer (a stage sometimes referred to as Dukes' B or Modified Astler-Coller B2 and B3). See IMPACT B2 1999; and Midgley and Kerr 2005. Yet another investigation, known as the QUASAR study, also struggled to come up with any definitive answer that would be meaningful to patients— which prompted a debate in the *Lancet.*

224 *So they set up:* English, Lebovitz, and Giffin 2010, 51. These IOM investigators report that some women who tried to enter a cancer clinical trial were "disqualified because of: past treatment regimens (i.e., 'extensively pretreated' or too much chemotherapy); stage of disease (i.e., not recently diagnosed) or the presence of brain metastases; or the presence of advanced disease when many drug trials test first-, second-, or third-line treatments."

224 *The extent to which:* Petryna 2007, 27.

225 *After all:* ACS 2012. See also chapter 3, Figure 6, for new cancer cases and chapter 2, Figure 4, for some perspective on patient survival. Nearly four hundred thousand Americans will be diagnosed this year with one of seven cancers (ovary, myeloma, brain, esophagus, lung, liver, and pancreas) in which the overall five-year survival rate is under 50 percent.

225 *Drug companies have:* DeRenzo 2000; Eichenwald and Kolata 1999; Ferris and Naylor 2004. Some institutions prohibit their clinical investigators from receiving finder's fees or other incentive payments for recruitment. For a discussion, see Conference on Human Subject Protection and Financial Conflicts of Interest 2000.

225 *Sponsors have begun:* Glickman et al. 2009; Thiers, Sinskey, and Berndt 2008, 13–14; Getz and Vogel 2009.

225 *(A recent study):* Glickman et al. 2009, 816.

226 *Some in the cancer:* See Cheng 2009. For a thorough discussion of this and other problems with the clinical-trials enterprise, see English, Lebovitz, and Giffin 2010, 27–28, 49–51 in particular. In the spring of 2010, the NCI and the American Society of Clinical Oncology jointly held a Cancer Trial Accrual Symposium on this issue. Congress has also held several hearings as well: US House of Representatives 2004. For more discussion, see Young 2010, 306–9; Rettig 2000; C-Change 2005, 24; and Comis et al. 2000.

226 *"When you talk":* Interview with Richard Pazdur, January 21, 2004.

226 *Before the first:* Ibid. Daniel Vasella, the former CEO of Novartis confirmed this as well in a 2002 conversation. See also Johnson, Williams, and Pazdur 2003.

227 *But somehow, the modern:* It's worth emphasizing that leaders of the national cancer enterprise have repeatedly concluded that the clinical-trials system is broken. In 1997, an NCI review known as the Armitage Report (NCI 1997) found the trials process so complex and inefficient that it "eroded the ability of the system to generate new ideas to reduce the cancer burden." In 1998, a blue-ribbon "implementation committee" promised to make the clinical-trials system—what it called an "intricate and large research laboratory without walls"—more efficient, streamlined, and relevant (NCI 1998). A 2003 assessment published in *JAMA* called the process "increasingly encumbered by high costs, slow results, lack of funding, regulatory burdens, fragmented infrastructure, incompatible databases, and a shortage of qualified investigators and willing participants" (Sung et al. 2003). A 2003 NIH Roadmap, laid out by its then director, Elias A. Zerhouni, concluded that the United States had no choice but to "recast its entire system of clinical research," and that such a reengineering must be the health agency's "paramount" and immediate goal (http://www.nih.gov/news/pr/sep2003/od-30.htm). And, as mentioned above, the 2010 committee convened by the Institute of Medicine and chaired by John Mendelsohn, the soft-spoken former president of the MD Anderson Cancer Center, arrived at an equally harsh conclusion: "The system for conducting cancer clinical trials in the United States is approaching a state of crisis. Changes are urgently needed if we are to continue to make progress against the second leading cause of death in this country. If the clinical trials system does not improve its efficiency and effectiveness, the introduction of new treatments for cancer will be delayed and patient lives will be lost unnecessarily." Nearly everyone involved in the clinical-trials process knows the system is broken—and nearly everyone has known it for a long, long time.

Chapter 12: Zero to Ninety

229 Epigraph: Farber et al. 1956, 6.

230 *Over six feet tall:* Information about Farber draws from a number of sources. See Bailey 1974; Mukherjee 2010, 18–36 in particular; D. Nathan 2007, 38–44; Miller 2006; D'Angio 1975; and Dana-Farber Cancer Institute, "Who Was Sidney Farber?" See also original Farber papers cited below. For a wonderful photograph of Farber as a young pathologist, see Chabner and Roberts 2005, Figure 1, 66.

230 *The ravages of the disease:* Hersh et al. 1965, 105. "Major causes of death in acute leukemia," the oncologists had measured, "were infection in 70 percent of patients and hemorrhage in 52 percent. In 38 percent of the patients there was more than one cause of death."

231 *By the late 1940s:* Lucia 1941, 120ff gives an exhaustive list of the treatments used—or at least tried—during the day across the range of leukemias. Beyond radiation, antibiotics, and transfusion, a host of chemical agents were given to patients. They included arsenic and related substances such as antimony, bismuth, and phosphorus. Many doctors had tried benzol, a highly toxic chemical, mixed with olive oil. Natural substances—colloidal gold, silver, sulfur, and lead—killed white blood cells but came with their own dangers, including an apparent acceleration of the leukemia and internal bleeding. Equally toxic was the alkaloid *Colchicum autumnale,* the meadow saffron or autumn crocus, which at doses of just four milligrams could induce vomiting, gastric pain, diarrhea and weakness. Biological treatments were plied as well. Some tried inoculating patients with the malaria plasmodium, which, though it produced fever, killed white blood cells, and slowed the activity of the bone marrow, did not cure leukemia. See also F. Smith 1914, 921.

231 *In 1926, another:* See Minot's Nobel Prize lecture, Minot 1934.

231 *As Farber would later:* See his dedication to Minot in Farber 1949, 160n.

231 *In January of 1945:* Leuchtenberger et al. 1945, 46.

231 *Within weeks:* David G. Nathan, a leading pediatric hematologist and former president of Dana-Farber Cancer Institute, frames how remarkable such an action was—and particularly in the context of the current ethical framework for human experimentation. As he writes in his book *The Cancer Treatment Revolution* (2007, 46), "In 1946, these children were treated with an entirely experimental drug, a class of drug that had never before been given to humans. The children were too young to give informed consent. In fact, there was no formal consent process at all. The parents of the children seized the opportunity because they trusted their physician. . . . The 'informed' consent was obtained orally based on the parents' understanding that their children were going to die; that these trusted doctors were trying to save them. Today, such a process would be totally unacceptable and might even lead to prosecution. It would certainly cause the removal of all National Institutes of Health (NIH) grants, vilification in the medical literature, and, in some cases, in the public media."

232 *Farber observed what:* Farber 1949, 160.

232 *At first, he wondered:* Gilman 1963, 576–77, recalls the first clinical trial with nitrogen mustard in this compelling essay: "The results of the experiments in mice were sufficiently encouraging to consider a therapeutic trial in man. Consequently, the animal data were presented to Gustav E. Lindskog, who was then Assistant Professor of Surgery. Lindskog agreed to supervise the clinical trial and not many days thereafter, early in December 1942, an X-ray resistant patient in the terminal stages of lymphosarcoma was selected as a suitable subject. The tumor masses involved the axilla, mediastinum, face and

submental regions, with a resulting cyanosis, venous dilatation and edema of the face and the upper part of the chest. Chewing and swallowing had become almost impossible and a tracheotomy set was kept close at hand for immediate use. The blood picture was within normal limits. The selection of a proper dose of a highly toxic chemical warfare agent for administration to man for the first time was made with unwarranted confidence. We knew that the suppression of bone marrow function in animals was completely reversible. Moreover there was a fairly wide margin between the dose of a nitrogen mustard that was acutely lethal and that required to affect lymphoid tissue. Furthermore there was little species variation in susceptibility to the cytotoxic action. On this basis it was decided to administer a dose of 0.1 mg. per kilogram of tris P-chloroethylamine daily for ten days or for a shorter period if the total granulocyte count dropped below 5,000 per cu. mm. Apparently we thought it more appropriate to initiate clinical trial with a full therapeutic dose than to titrate slowly up to an effective dose in a moribund patient. The selection of the daily dose turned out to be a most fortunate guess, but our acumen on the duration of therapy left much to be desired."

232 *But then, after:* Many writers have credited the revelation to Farber alone. Nathan 2007 states that correspondence unearthed between the men reveals that the evolved thinking was a product of conversations between Farber and SubbaRow.

232 *In November of 1947:* Farber 1949, 162. See also Farber et al. 1948, which provides case reports of five of the ten responders.

233 *When the results:* Farber et al. 1948.

233 *Many simply did not:* D. Miller 2006, 22.

233 *That drug would come soon:* Li, Hertz, and Spencer 1956; Djerassi et al. 1967. See also the discussion at the New York Academy of Sciences moderated by C. Gordon Zubrod and Joseph Burchenal (Zubrod and Burchenal 1971) on the class of folate antagonists. Included in the roundtable were fifteen other leading oncologists and chemists of the day. For a contemporary assessment, see Walling 2006.

233 *(Not until 1958):* Chabner and Roberts, 66; Bertino 1963. Before a cell can divide, it needs to make a carbon copy of its DNA—enough of this winding, twisting genetic material to split evenly between two cells: mother and daughter. And before it can do that, it must create, largely from scratch, the molecule's four chemical building blocks: adenine, cytosine, guanine and thymine. To make thymine, for instance, a large cellular enzyme, dihydrofolate reductase (DHFR), converts a small molecule called dihydrofolate (DHF) into tetrahydrofolate (THF)—which is used in the synthesis of thymine. (There are quite a few more steps in this metabolic chain, but this is the idea.)

Methotrexate interferes with this chain because, molecularly speaking, it's the spitting image of DHF, and like its twin, finds its way to the active site (a molecular dock) on the enzyme where DHF normally binds. This "competitive inhibition" prevents DHFR from converting DHF into THF, and thus disrupts the production of thymine. Methotrexate also works through a separate metabolic pathway to block the synthesis of other DNA building blocks. Ultimately, however, its effectiveness in killing dividing cells depends on several factors, some of which concern the normalcy of those cells. For example, certain gene mutations can make a cell resistant to the drug or prevent it from entering, concentrating in or remaining long within. Such resistance is a major reason so many cancer treatments fail.

233   *"They were resistant"*: Donald Pinkel, "A Paediatrician's Journey," in Greaves 2008, 21–22.

234   *"The evaluation of"*: Farber et al. 1956, 3.

234   *But Farber was adamant:* Ibid., 3.

234   *For Pinkel, who would:* Pinkel in Greaves 2008, 21–22.

234   *An amazing twenty-eight major:* Krakoff 1994 (chart in unpublished manuscript, given to me by author).

234   *Clinicians were so:* Leuchtenberger et al. 1945, 46.

234   *One of the swiftest:* Elion 1988.

234   *George Hitchings:* Hitchings 1988; Hitchings et al. 1950; Hitchings and Elion 1954.

235   *After some brief:* Elion 1988.

235   *The rationale behind each:* The aim of nearly all of these therapies is to disrupt the production of DNA, which is essential to all dividing cells. This approach affects not only dividing malignant cells but also healthy ones. But the strategy has a captivating logic nonetheless. That's because cancer cells divide at a faster rate, generally, than most of their normal counterparts. "Cytotoxic" chemotherapy attempts to jam that process in a variety of ingenious ways. Some drugs kill dividing cancer cells by slamming the tiny spindle on which chromosome separation takes place. A class of antibiotics called anthracyclines (including Adriamycin and Doxil) interferes with the replication of DNA by inducing structural changes in the strands themselves—a process called intercalation.

235   *As late as 1960:* This is discussed in the notes for chapter 3, under *"And as recently."* The NCI's SEER program records five-year relative survival rates for leukemia for patients diagnosed in 1960–63 as 14 percent. But many prominent oncologists of the day estimated that a far smaller share of childhood leukemia patients survived even that long. Surveying forty-three leukemia specialists around the country, Burchenal and Murphy (1965) found evidence to support that a mere fifty-three children and eighteen adults were alive five

years after diagnosis. In most chemotherapy clinical trials undertaken through the year 1963, the share of leukemia survivors approached 10 percent or less by two years of follow-up. See patient survival graphs in Frei et al. 1958, 1130 and in sources discussed above. John Cairns, a leading physician and microbiologist who wrote much-discussed commentaries on cancer in the 1970s and 1980s, cites comparable data from the Children's Cancer Study Group (1985, 56): "Only about 10 percent of the children diagnosed in 1956 as having leukemia were still alive two years after diagnosis; by 1978 the number of two-year survivors was roughly 70 percent." Cairns includes a vivid chart that makes the turnaround evident in a few stark lines.

236 *The reason was drug resistance:* See, for example, Curt, Clendeninn, and Chabner 1984.

236 *At the start of the 1960s:* For personal background on Skipper, see Simpson–Herren and Wheeler 2006. For a description of the kinetics work, see Skipper, Schabel, and Wilcox 1964; Chabner and Roberts, 67; and DeVita, Serpick, and Carbone 1970. "If the dose of the effective drug could be increased enough or treatment begun when the cell population was small enough," explain DeVita and colleagues (892), "either the tumor population could be reduced to zero or the small residual of cells could be controlled by the host's own defense mechanism." All it took was for one malignant cell to survive the onslaught of toxic therapy and the cancer might return. The theory, christened the "cell-kill hypothesis," helped explain why even "complete remissions" were often so temporary and suggested a possible way around this dilemma. See also Mukherjee 2010, 139–41.

236 *The key revelation:* Interview with Emil J. Freireich, October 30, 2006; Frei 1997, 2554; Case 1997, 77.

237 *Jay, the son of:* Frei 1997, 2558.

237 *One summer afternoon:* See Frei et al. 1961.

237 *The thinking was not:* See DeVita and Chu 2008, 8647 in particular; Frei et al. 1965b, 650; Frei et al. 1961, 448.

237 *Less than a year:* Freireich, Karon, and Frei 1964; Frei et al. 1965b. For a discussion by Freireich, see Case 1997, 81ff. See also DeVita, Serpick, and Carbone 1970 on the use of combination chemotherapy in the cure of Hodgkin's disease. See also Ochoa 1969, 926.

238 *One group of Boston doctors, including:* Dameshek et al. 1965, 221. Likewise, as Vincent DeVita and Edward Chu report (2008, 8649), "the MOMP and MOPP protocols were met with fierce resistance both in and out of the NIH Clinical Center as they were regarded as too big a departure from the norm." Still more potent resistance met Min Chiu Li, who in 1958 led a National Cancer Institute team that cured, with methotrexate, the first solid tumor—a

rare cancer of the placenta called choriocarcinoma—and who would later win a Lasker Award for his research. DeVita and Chu report that when Li persisted "in using his radical treatment," C. Gordon Zubrod, Li's boss at the newly opened NCI clinical center, asked him to leave (ibid., 8647).

238 *Most of the drugs:* Frei 1997, 2557; Anjo J. P. Veerman, "Diagnosis, Prophylaxis, and Treatment of Central Nervous System Involvement in Acute Lymphoblastic Leukemia," in Pui 2003, 173.

238 *Donald Pinkel, then director:* Pinkel 1979, 1128 and throughout; Rubnitz and Pui 1997.

238 *By 1971 five-year:* For this and figures two paragraphs below, see Boring, Squires, and Tong 1993, 25. The five-year relative survival rate for children diagnosed with acute lymphocytic leukemia in the period 1960–63 was 14 percent; in 1970–73, 34 percent; in 1974–76, 52.5 percent; and in 1977–79, 67 percent. The data are from the National Cancer Institute, Cancer Statistics Branch, SEER program. The same data are shown in Greenlee et al. 2000, 31.

238 *Jay Freireich would:* Interview with Emil J. Freireich, October 30, 2006; Frei 1997, 2558–59.

239 *The turnaround in survival:* Boring, Squires, and Tong 1993, 25 report the five-year relative survival rate for Wilms' tumor as 79.6 percent in the period 1977–79; Greenlee et al. 2000 report it at 78 percent. For children with Hodgkin's disease in the latter period, Boring, Squires, and Tong cite an 83.2 percent survival rate; Greenlee et al., 84 percent. Such discrepancies are common in reporting NCI SEER data for a given period, though most variances tend to be within a percentage point or two.

239 *Protocols for ALL:* Pui and Evans 2006.

239 *On a trip to St. Jude:* October 18, 2004.

Chapter 13: Fossils

241 *Four stories up:* Information on the American Museum of Natural History, dinosaur hunting, and the sciences of paleontology and fossil reconstruction is drawn from the following: American Museum of Natural History 1937, 2005, and 2006; Bird 1939, 1941, and 1985; Brown 1907 and 1908; Dingus, Lowell, and Norell 2007; and Leaf 2009.

243 *A 1999 RAND Corporation study:* National Bioethics Advisory Commission 1999, 1:1. "Archives of human biological materials range in size from fewer than 200 specimens to more than 92 million," the investigators found. "Conservatively estimated, at least 282 million specimens (from more than 176 million individual cases) are stored in the United States, and the collections are growing at a rate of over 20 million cases per year."

243 *I did not comprehend:* I was a member of the External Advisory Board for the University of California, San Francisco's Prostate Cancer SPORE (NCI-designated Specialized Program of Research Excellence) in 2005 and 2006. For additional background on the NCI tissue effort, see Friede et al. 2003; Eiseman et al. 2003; NCI 2007; NIH 2008. See also Fenstermacher et al. 2005; Goodman, Thornquist, Edelstein et al. 2006; and Maschke 2010.

244 *In keeping with this:* NCI 2011, iii, 43.

244 *Doctors, as it is:* Lilja et al. 2007; Lilja, Ulmert, and Vickers 2008; Wolf et al. 2010.

246 *(Typically, about 6 percent):* Massett et al. 2011, Table 2, 10.

246 Footnote: *Nearly five years:* Paris et al. 2010, 196.

247 *Or, quite often the tissue:* NIH 2008, 2–3.

247 *Cut off from the circulation:* Blow 2007 has an extraordinary analysis of the problem. See also Hicks, Kushner, and McCarthy 2011 for a discussion of the effects of "cold ischemic time"; and Nkoy et al. 2010 for the effects on the detection of the estrogen receptor (ER) and progesterone receptor (PR) in breast cancer tissue. Nkoy and colleagues examined the records of more than five thousand women with breast cancer whose receptor "status" (positive or negative) was tested at seven Utah hospitals. The hospitals, which were run by the same company, used a single automated laboratory testing process for ER/PR. The investigators found, however, that the frequency of a "negative" status report for both receptors—meaning that they were not functioning—differed significantly on each day of the week. What's more, the later in the week the surgery was performed (and the tissue sample prepared), the more likely it was to be found negative when testing was done. The reason? Often, those samples taken on or close to the weekend were left around to be processed on the following Monday. The issue is serious—and common—for women. Patients with receptor-positive tumors typically have a better prognosis than those with receptor-negative tumors, and the treatment between the two groups generally differs as well. A false-negative ER/PR test result can, therefore, have serious real-world consequences for patients.

247 *All of this:* Friede et al. 2003, vii.

248 *(In one 2008 study):* Horning 2009. Issue discussed in FDA 2008, Oncologic Drugs Advisory Committee meeting, December 16.

248 *When the National Cancer Institute:* Massett et al. 2011, Table 4, 11.

248 *A 2010 report:* NCI 2010b, 2. See also NCI 2010a, the NCI's "Action Plan" for pancreatic cancer research for 2011, in which agency officials admit (12), "The lack of specimens from early-stage cancers is a significant impediment to both the discovery and validation of biomarkers." Moreover, "obtaining such samples is the single most expensive aspect of diagnostic test development,"

according to the institute (Cancer Center Directors Working Group 2006, 59). That cost is often so unmanageable that it drives would-be test developers away from the task.

249 *After the study on tissue:* National Bioethics Advisory Commission 1999; Friede et al. 2003.

250 *I got the chance:* National Cancer Institute Symposium, *International Harmonization of Biorepository Practices* (Washington, DC, November 10, 2005).

250 (*One key question*): Skloot 2007. Rebecca Skloot writes beautifully about the profound issues surrounding human–tissue specimens here and in *The Immortal Life of Henrietta Lacks* (2010).

250 *By 2009, the annual:* NCI/2nd Annual BRN Symposium, Office of Biorepositories and Biospecimen Research (Bethesda, MD, March 17, 2009).

251 *In 1996, two Canadian:* AbeBooks company timeline, http://www.abebooks .com/docs/CompanyInformation/Timeline/.

251 *On Labor Day weekend:* Forbes 400 entry for Pierre Omidyar, September 2012, http://www.forbes.com/profile/pierre-omidyar/. eBay company history from http://www.ebayinc.com/history.

251 *But then, it is only easy:* See Compton 2009. Compton, who was then director of the NCI's Office of Biorepositories and Biospecimen Research, showed a slide entitled "The USA Lags Behind Other National Initiatives." Among those biobanking efforts that had, by then, been successfully launched were Iceland's DeCode Biobank, the Estonian Genome Project, the UK Biobank, Finland's GenomEUtwin, the pan–European Biobanking and Biomolecular Resources Research Infrastructure, Biobank Japan, and the Singapore Tissue Network. See also Cambon–Thomsen 2004 and Zika et al. 2010.

252 *Almost from the minute:* Interviews with Kathy Giusti, January 30, 2007, as well as with Paul Giusti, September 6, 2007, and Karen Andrews, August 29, 2007. Additional information in the following pages is drawn from an earlier interview with Kathy Giusti, June 23, 2006. See also Jerome Groopman's (2008) marvelous profile of Giusti and other business-trained cancer warriors.

256 *So Kathy did an end run:* Multiple Myeloma Research Consortium. For more information, see http://www.themmrc.org/model_mmrc.php.

258 *The Internet is not, fundamentally:* For a fascinating take, see Alvestrand 2004. See also Benkler 2006 on Wikipedia and the essential role of consensus (72–73), as well as a discussion of "cooperation gain" in networks (87–89).

258 *"The great thing about":* Interview with David Agus, January 4, 2006, and follow-up conversations, April 16, 2007, and in December 2012. See also his presentation at the 2009 BRN symposium.

258 *Consider, for example, the sophisticated:* Personal communication with Francis Barany; Kononen et al. 1998. It is worth putting the amount of data these

machines produce in perspective. Simply recording which of, say, twenty thousand human genes is active (being expressed) in a hundred tumor samples yields 2 million data points. Imagine an Excel file twenty thousand rows long and a hundred rows across, and you'll get the idea. But that's just a start. Collectively, these genes may "code" for as many as one hundred thousand proteins—which means there are potentially billions of "signaling" interactions between genes and proteins and between various proteins in human cells. Many billions of data points, that is. In a single patient. Even managing this staggering amount of data, though, isn't the real problem. A fantastically larger challenge is that these fleeting biological signals are recorded in data points that are in turn created by different machines using different software, algorithms, and experimental protocols. This information is expressed in different vocabularies and values. *That* is the problem.

259 *The molecular signals:* Alvis Brazma (a bioinformatics expert at the University of Cambridge), John Quackenbush (a computational biologist at Harvard), and colleagues sounded the call to arms regarding standardization of microarrays—or ways to "normalize" their readings so that data from different systems can be compared—in several papers at the beginning of last decade; see Brazma et al. 2001 and Quackenbush 2002. See also Ashburner et al. 2000; Stoeckert, Causton, and Ball 2002; Miller and Attwood 2003; Quackenbush 2004; Brazma, Krestyaninova, and Sarkans 2006; and the commentary by the editors of *Nature Biotechnology* (Anon. 2006).

259 *Likewise, there are no standard:* See Yaziji et al. 2008. Yaziji and fellow members of the Standardization Ad-Hoc Consensus Committee point out that, despite the importance of estrogen receptor (ER) status in determining a breast cancer patient's prognosis and treatment decisions (that is, whether to use hormonal therapy), the procedures for ER testing by immunohistochemistry are not standardized across laboratories—which leads to "high rates of 'false-negative' results worldwide." Wolff et al. 2007 and Vaught 2011 discuss the same problem with relation to HER2 testing in women with breast cancer, a problem that also results in high rates of both false-positive and false-negative readings. The stakes are high: women who are treated based on a mistakenly "positive" HER2-status report are typically given expensive drugs and biological therapies (such as Herceptin), which can sometimes cause serious side effects of their own; women who receive false-negative readings may miss out on a treatment that could help them. Lane 2005, 491, and Brosh and Rotter 2009, 708, make the same complaints about the protein p53, which is implicated in a huge number of cancers. See also Bustin, Vandesompele, and Pfaffl 2009 for a similar take with respect to PCR (polymerase chain reaction), a commonly used technology for studying DNA. For sweeping assessments of

the lack of standardization in the cancer research effort, see also Poste 2011, 156–57; President's Cancer Panel 2005, 34; Nass, Moses, and Mendelsohn 2010, 82–87; and Kean 2012. Astoundingly, leading cancer researchers have complained about this issue from the outset of the cancer war (see Meinert 1980), yet cancer's Tower of Babel gets only higher and more cacophonous.

259 *The inability to establish:* The National Cancer Institute did make at least a modest effort to create a system to wrangle the immense quantity of molecular data generated in cancer studies into a resource that could be widely shared among researchers. In 2004, the institute launched a project—called the Cancer Biomedical Informatics Grid, or caBIG—that, over the next seven years, would sprawl into multiple subprojects and consume between $350 million and $500 million of taxpayer investment, by various estimates. Then, in March 2011, a board of scientific advisers convened by the NCI issued a devastating report about the project. It concluded, in essence, that the cancer agency's bioinformatics team had spent too much time and resources designing new technology and overcomplicated systems and not enough time working with the scientists who actually create the data to find a common path. Many of caBIG's six dozen "tools" were barely functional, badly buggy, or couldn't be downloaded by researchers. What's more, said the review panel, the program was littered with organizational and intellectual conflicts of interest. (See Goldberg 2011 for a thorough analysis.) By April 2012, the caBIG was dead. Harold Varmus, a Nobel Prize–winning scientist and the NCI's director, sent a four-paragraph announcement saying that after undertaking a "thorough reassessment" of the project, the institute had "begun charting a new course for the informatics infrastructure that will support the NCI's research programs" (Varmus 2012). The truly sad part—beyond even the huge waste of taxpayer money—is that the idea of creating a genuine interoperable network for cancer data has lost credibility and backers. And it remains, despite the failure of caBIG, a good, and even essential, idea.

Chapter 14: The One-Eyed Surgeon

261 *The boy's name:* The story of Denis Burkitt draws heavily from three carefully reported biographies—Glemser 1970; Kellock 1985; and Nelson 1998—as well as from the academic papers of Burkitt and those of his contemporaries. Burkitt also shares part of the tale that follows in his Charles S. Mott Prize lecture, republished in the journal *Cancer* (Burkitt 1983a). For Burkitt's first sightings of the children with the jaw tumors, see Glemser, 49–50; Kellock, 45–46; and Nelson, 72–75.

261 *The lower jaw:* Babak et al. 2011; Fanibunda and Matthews 1999, 185.

261 *Burkitt had been:* For discussion of the Buganda kingdom, see Rainer 2005, 8–9.

262 *Though he ran:* For a description of the Mulago Hospital, see Epstein and Eastwood 1993, 92; Coakley 2006, 18.

262 *He was a decent one:* Epstein and Eastwood 1993, 89.

262 *Kwashiorkor:* Glemser 1970, 6–10; and writing about Hugh Carey Trowell and kwashiorkor, 51–62.

262 *The region seemed:* Burkitt 1962, 385; Scrimshaw and Béhar 1961, 2046–47 in particular; Pialoux et al. 2007, 319–27; Coakley 2006, 20.

262 *In Burkitt's first eighteen:* Epstein and Eastwood 1993, 92.

263 *By the end:* Glemser 1970, 44–45; Kellock 1985, 37.

263 *He had three:* Nelson (1998) gives an extensive account of Burkitt's family.

263 *At the age of eleven:* Glemser 1970, 21–22, 27; Epstein and Eastwood 1993, 90.

263 It had not been easy: The Colonial Medical Service was a branch of the British Colonial Service. For background, see Crozier 2007, xi, 4–5.

264 *On the grass outside:* Burkitt (1983) recalls the child in Jinja as a boy; Glemser 1970, Nelson 1998, and Epstein and Eastwood 1993 report the same. Others who have written about the incident, including Kellock 1985, 46 and Coakley 2006, report the child as a girl. Adding to the confusion is that Kellock's biography of Burkitt was done with Burkitt's active cooperation—and, indeed, the latter shares the book's copyright. See Glemser 1970, 64, for more.

264 *Burkitt took several:* Kellock 1985, 46; Glemser 1970, 49.

264 *His daughters would:* Nelson 1998, 75.

264 *By any stretch:* Biographical details are drawn from Glemser 1970; Nelson 1998; Epstein and Eastwood 1993; and others, as well as from photographs.

266 *The pathologist in each:* Epstein and Eastwood 1993, 93.

266 *The Irish surgeon:* Ibid., 93.

266 *What's more, suggested:* O'Conor and Davies 1960, 526; O'Conor 1961, 270–72.

267 *He had even penned:* Cook, Albert R., "Notes on the Diseases Met with in Uganda, Central Africa," *Journal of Tropical Medicine* 4 (1901): 175–178. Cited in Alexander 1983, 797; Davies et al. 1964, 260; Parkin et al. 2003, 167. Glemser 1970, 65, cites the year as 1902. Anon. 1972, 345, reports it as 1904.

267 *Now, with scores of case:* Anon. 1972, 348, which reproduces one of Burkitt's age-distribution charts.

268 *Then he sent off a paper:* Burkitt 1958; Glemser 1970, 107.

268 *George Oettlé was:* Glemser 1970, 69–71; Epstein and Eastwood 1993, 94.

268 *Within months of his arrival:* Epstein and Eastwood 1993, 92; Coakley 2006, 18.

269 *He submitted his observations:* Kellock 1985, 50. Epstein and Eastwood reproduce Burkitt's own typed and handwritten list of 368 articles and five books,
which spanned fifty-five years—from a 1938 report for the *British Medical
Journal* on a saccular aneurysm in the left common iliac artery to his last publication, a brief memoir for the *Journal of the Irish Colleges of Physicians and
Surgeons.* With some irony, it was titled "Unpromising Beginnings."

269 *His plan was to send:* Burkitt 1962, 17; Coakley 2006, 19; Kellock 1985, 49.

269 *He printed up:* Glemser 1970, 71.

269 *He spent weeks:* Ibid.

269 *"We couldn't afford fourpence":* Ibid., 72.

269 *The lymphomas were occurring:* Burkitt 1962, 17.

270 *While the emerging geographic:* Burkitt 1958, 218–23; Varmus and Weinberg
1993, 168–69.

270 *Tony Epstein ran a lab:* Epstein and Eastwood 1993, 94; Glemser 1970, 159–
61, 171–72; and Coakley 2006, 20.

270 *Twelve people had shown:* Glemser 1970, 160; Epstein and Eastwood 1993, 94.

270 *Its title:* Glemser 1970, 160.

270 *The apparently rigid:* Ibid., 160–61; Epstein and Eastwood 1993, 94; de-The et
al. 1978, 756–57.

270 *In 1908:* Morange 2002, 3; Beeman 2005, 392; Moore and Chang 2010, 878.

271 *Three years later:* Rous 1911, 398–411; Thorne 1914; Rous 1966; Milt 1969,
219–20; Andrewes 1971, 644–46; Vogt 1996, 1559–62.

271 *Experiments similar to:* Two decades after Rous's 1911 report came another
important discovery from Richard Shope, an Iowa-born virologist whose laboratories were the farm and the field. In the early 1930s, Shope was studying
two curious viruses he'd found in cottontail rabbits. The first of these caused
fibromas, or seemingly benign swellings on the rabbits' skins. The second—a
papillomavirus—was more interesting. The wild cottontails Shope had seen in
the Midwest often had blackish, horny warts under their fur. When ground up
and pressed through a cell-free filter like the one Rous had used two decades
earlier, the wart extract could infect healthy rabbits, both wild and domesti-
cated. But then, in a series of tests, Shope found something strange. In the pap-
illoma tumors he generated in *tame* rabbits (who commonly weren't exposed to
the cottontail virus), the cells at the base of the warts would often evolve into
something more sinister: squamous cell carcinoma. Malignant growths under
the skin would follow months later. Just as Rous had discovered, this was a
genuine cancer—apparently caused in some way by a virus. (See Oberling and
Guérin 1954, 385–95; Andrewes 1971, 648; Andrewes 1979; Rous and Beard
1934.) As luck would have it, the cottontail-rabbit papillomavirus kicked open
the door for a slew of additional oncogenic viruses—though all, it appeared,

were limited to animals. By the late 1950s, researchers had uncovered some twenty different tumor viruses in nine species ranging from horses and squirrels to mice. One such discovery was made by Peter Nowell's mentor Balduin Lucké. In 1938, he alit upon a herpesvirus that caused a spontaneous and deadly kidney tumor in the northern leopard frog (see Oberling and Guérin 1954, 384–85). Despite the mounting evidence of a viral role in cancer, the mainstream research community continued to dismiss the connection as unsubstantiated, irrelevant, or just flatly untrue. The prejudice (and animus) ran so deep that John Bittner, a young scientist at Jackson Laboratory—a hallowed redoubt for the study of cancer genetics, in Bar Harbor, Maine—felt pressure to camouflage his own discovery of a cancer virus in vaguely worded language. (Clarence Cook Little, his boss, and a driving force behind the creation of the National Cancer Institute, was vehemently in the antivirus camp.) In a series of brilliant experiments in the late 1930s, Bittner proved that a type of mammary cancer in mice was indeed caused by a virus—this one cleverly transmitted from parent to progeny through mother's milk. Fearful of attack, however, the scientist called the causative agent Milk Factor. (In 1942, the culpable viral particle was isolated by electron microscope, and there could be no more evasion.) Bittner came clean about his weak ruse many years later: "If I had called it a virus, my grant applications would have automatically been put into the category of 'unrespectable proposals,'" he wrote in reflection. "As long as I used the word 'factor,' it was respectable genetics" (G. Klein 1990, 120–21). For more background, see Oberling and Guérin 1954, 397–405.

271 *In the mid-1970s* (footnote): See Stehelin et al. 1976; Bishop 1989; Varmus 1989; Hunter 1984; G. S. Martin 2001; Bishop 2003; and Heinrichs 2006.

272 *After the speech:* Glemser 1970, 161. For some more perspective on how remarkable this sharing of specimens was, see Klein and Klein 1989, 20–21. George Klein relates writing letters to numerous hospitals in Africa and to international organizations, requesting tumor, blood, and serum from Burkitt's lymphoma patients. Then he wrote to Peter Clifford, a surgeon at the Kenyatta National Hospital in Nairobi, and "the material started coming in a continuous flow," Klein recalls. "It arrived with chronometric precision on the single direct flight from Nairobi, late Tuesday afternoon. Large dry ice boxes carried hundreds of sera, and a special wet ice package contained fresh biopsy material. There was always a long list in Clifford's own handwriting with all the essential details and a brief 'good luck' message."

272 *Just as Burkitt:* Burkitt and O'Conor 1961.

273 *As biographer Glemser:* Glemser 1970, 65.

273 *Ted Williams:* Ibid., 74–75.

273 *In Burkitt's estimation:* Ibid., 75.

274   *As it happened:* Burkitt 1962, 380–81; Glemser 1970, 75; Epstein and Eastwood 1993, 94; Kellock 1985, 55; Coakley 2006, 20.

274   *The two left Kampala:* Burkitt kept a journal of the expedition, of which Glemser (1970, 200–236) reproduces excerpts in the biography's appendix. See also
pages 76–86 for Glemser's summary of the itinerary.

274   *In all, the team:* Burkitt 1962, 381.

274   *At each stop:* Many commentators have called attention to Burkitt's seemingly
unfailing cheerfulness and energy. See, for example, Epstein and Eastwood
1993, 100.

274   *On the shores:* Burkitt 1962, 384.

274   *Near the town of Tunduma:* Burkitt journal entry, Tuesday, October 17, in
Glemser 1970, 216.

275   *From Karonga to the town:* Burkitt journal entry, Saturday, October 21
(5:45 a.m.), ibid., 217.

275   *A pathologist at the hospital:* Nelson 1998, 106.

275   *On some stretches:* "It's incredible how much dust you pick up on a trip like
this. Everything gets impregnated with dust," Burkitt wrote on October 17, in
Glemser 1970, 216–17.

275   *To pass time:* Burkitt journal entry, Wednesday, October 11 (8:20 p.m.), ibid.,
208–9.

275   *Burkitt, reflecting upon the journey:* Ibid., 79.

275   *It was the dividend:* Ibid., 80.

276   *By the time:* Burkitt 1962, 380, 384–85.

276   *Alexander Haddow worked:* Ibid., 380; Glemser 1970, 84–86; Coakley 2006,
20; Nelson 1998, 118–19. Note this Haddow was an entomologist. A second
Alexander Haddow, a celebrated pioneer in the field of cancer chemotherapy,
also figures into the Burkitt story. The latter Haddow gave the closing remarks
at an international conference of Burkitt's lymphoma in Kampala, Uganda, in
January 1966, as noted below.

276   *Another colleague, pathologist:* Burkitt 1962, 385.

277   *The feat had been managed:* O'Brien 2001, 7656–58; Skloot 2011, 30, 35–37,
and throughout, for a remarkable discussion on the complex ethical issues surrounding human tissue in medical research. See also Leibel 1991 and Masters
2002 for how easily contamination can occur in cell lines and, as a result, how
erroneous some research findings drawn from them can be. See also Wells
2005, who discusses the "well behaved" 3T3 cell line developed by George
Todaro and Howard Green in the early 1960s, a decade after the HeLa cell
line established by George Gey (discussed in Skloot 2011).

278   *After first going:* Glemser 1970, 172; Epstein, Achong, and Barr 1964, 702;
Epstein 1979.

278 *The German–born Henles:* Glemser 1970, 175–77; Epstein et al. 1965; Henle and Henle 1966; and Burchenal 1966, 2397. For general discussion of the discovery's historical importance, see Thorley-Lawson and Allday 2008.

279 *Which brought up a nagging:* Thompson and Kurzrock 2004, 803.

279 *There were plenty of additional:* Bornkamm 2009; Rowe et al. 2009; Cardy, Sharp, and Little 2001.

279 *To begin with:* Donati 2005; van den Bosch et al. 1993.

280 *In the early nineteenth:* Rowe et al. 2009, citing Guy de-The who proposed the notion in a 1985 paper. Epstein and Eastwood 1993, in turn, credit Sir Harold Himsworth for the idea: Himsworth described Burkitt's lymphoma as "something of a Rosetta stone" for the field of human carcinogenesis in the foreword to a 1970 textbook edited by Burkitt and Dennis H. Wright. The Rosetta stone analogy is popular in cancer research. Rowley (1990b) uses the term to describe "molecular genetics" generally in her Clowes Lecture at the 1990 meeting of the American Association for Cancer Research. V. Craig Jordan (2003b, 338), likewise, asked if the drug tamoxifen was the Rosetta stone for breast cancer.

280 *After days in the operating room:* In the 1950s and 1960s, Burkitt published papers on these makeshift "artificial legs," boots, and calipers in the *East African Medical Journal.* See also Kellock 1985, 43–44.

281 *Several years earlier:* Burkitt, Oettgen, and Burchenal 1963; Burchenal 1966 and 1968; Clarkson et al. 2006. See also discussions in chapter 3 and chapter 12.

281 *Sidney Farber had used:* See chapter 12; Yarris and Hunter 2003.

281 *He begged some methotrexate:* Glemser 1970, 137–39.

282 *Soon other physicians:* Klein and Klein 1989: 20–24; Glemser 1970 141–58; Anon. 1972, 347.

282 *Then, after the lecture:* Nelson 1998, 144–46; Kellock 1985, 92–93. Burchenal 1966, 2393, and Haddow 1970, 749, present data from the conference, held in Kampala, Uganda, in January 1966 by the Union Internationale Contre le Cancer.

284 *The amount spent for Burkitt's:* Glemser 1970, 104. "I would think that at six hundred and fifty pounds," remarked Ted Williams to Glemser, "it's the cheapest piece of major research of this century." E. Nelson (1998, 108) says the trip cost £678 British pounds and included visits to fifty-seven hospitals, not fifty-six. Burkitt also frequently remarked that great discoveries could be made on the cheap. "Some lessons to be learned," he wrote (Burkitt 1983b, 155), "were: 1. Dollars cannot be turned into ideas though the reverse can occur. My total research grants for my first 18 months that delineated the lymphoma belt amounted to £75 (under $150). 2. There is still a place for

research in the absence of expensive equipment. 3. There is value in friendly cooperation with those of totally different abilities, background, and outlook."

284   *The discovery of the Philadelphia:* Nowell 1977, 53.

284   *As the US Office:* OTA 1991, 199.

284   *When Burkitt is remembered* (footnote): See Kellock 1985 and Nelson 1998.

285   *While the cure rates:* See the thoughtful discussion by Ribeiro and Sandlund 2008.

285   *(The cost of the appropriate):* Cardy, Sharp, and Little 2001, 303.

Chapter 15: Matterhorn

289   *Rising 14,692 feet:* 4,478 meters. *Encyclopaedia Brittanica,* http://www.global .britannica.com/EBchecked/topic/369684/Matterhorn.

289   *But for nearly eight decades:* The tale is drawn from Edward Whymper's 1900 memoir, *Scrambles Amongst the Alps in the Years 1860–69* (1996), throughout. For Whymper's revelation that the eastern face was not quite as steep as it looked, see ibid., 272–77; for his final approach from Zermatt on July 13, 1865, see ibid., 372–82. See also Jensen 1987, 76–79.

290   *"That awful mountain":* Jensen 1987, 78.

290   *Elwood Jensen, who would later:* The story is drawn from an interview with Jensen, August 27, 2007, as well as from Jensen 1987, 2004a, and 2005. See also Jensen 2004b; Jensen and de Sombre 1972; Jensen and Jordan 2003; Jensen and Khan 2004; and Jensen et al. 2010.

290   *The tale:* Jensen 2005, 1439–40. In 2004, Jensen won the Albert Lasker Basic Medical Research Award, a prize that is often a precursor to the Nobel.

290   *Through the late 1950s:* Ibid., 1440.

291   *With that in mind:* Ibid., and interview with Jensen.

291   *But Jensen and a postdoctoral:* Jensen 2005, 1440. For earlier use of radioactive tracers in this manner, see Yankwich 1949 and Carter 1948. The latter, written by a student at Mississippi State College for Women, won first place in a 1948 undergraduate competition for science.

291   *Estrogen did not go:* Jensen and de Sombre 1973, 126; Jensen 2004, 1019–20; Owens 2006, S10.

292   *By the 1970s:* Jensen and Jordan 2003, 1980–83; Jordan 2003a, 208; Jordan 2009, 1246–47.

295   *So does the system:* Willis 1988, 14, says the Empire State Building was "erected in eleven months from the first steel columns to the finished building," a time frame others have cited as well. A report in the *New York Times,* March 22, 1931 (Anon. 1931), the day after the last of the scaffolding was removed from a mooring mast atop the building, noted that the building had "taken only a little more than a year for construction." The steelwork began on March 17,

1930. See also reports in the *Times* for March 6 and April 1, 1930, and April 26 and May 2, 1931. The building's official opening, presided over by President Herbert Hoover, was on May 1, 1931. The Empire State stood as the tallest building in the world for some four decades, until the World Trade Center was completed in the early 1970s, followed by the Sears Tower in Chicago. On April 30, 2012, the rebuilt One World Trade Center surpassed the Empire State Building's height, though that building had yet to open as of February 2013. The organization Skyscraper.org notes that it took but twenty months for the Empire State Building to be "designed, engineered, erected, and ready for tenants" (http://www.skyscraper.org/TALLEST_TOWERS/t_empire.htm).

295 *The first Intel microprocessor:* Intel Corporation 1987; Intel 2006; and Hoffman 2010, 1. Intel introduced its programmable 4004 microprocessor with an ad in the November 15, 1971, issue of *Electronic News,* "Announcing a new era of integrated electronics." The chip was the first "general-purpose microprocessor on the market—a 'building block' that engineers could purchase and then customize with software to perform different functions in a wide variety of electronic devices" (Intel 2006). The 4004 had 2,300 transistors and a clock speed of 740 kHz, or 740,000 cycles per second. (Clock speed measures how fast a processor performs an activity.) The Intel Core i7 975 Extreme (introduced in 2010), with 781 million transistors, clocks at 3.33 GHz, or 3.33 billion cycles per second, according to some estimates. The Intel 4004 chip could perform 92 kIPS, or 92,000 instructions per second, compared with roughly 177,000 MIPS—"177 thousand million," or 177 billion—instructions per second. Intel began rolling out the Core i7 family of chips in 2008. Just two years earlier, in 2006, Intel introduced its Core 2 Duo processors, which contained fewer than 300 million transistors. See also notes for chapter 11 on "Moore's Law."

296 *The idea of the Ranger mission:* See Johnson 2002, 99ff; Hall 1977, 15–24, 54 (for planned scientific experiments); Witkin 1962; Koppes 1978.

296 *The spacecraft was less a vehicle:* Hall 1977, 54–62.

296 *The first attempt:* Johnson 2002, 100; Hall 1977, 99–101.

296 *The Atlas rocket shot:* Hall 1977, 101–2.

296 *The high point:* Ibid., 94, 103.

296 *The launch of* Ranger 2: Ibid., 105–9.

297 *Two months later:* Ibid., 143–47.

297 Ranger 4 *had a little:* Ibid., 152–55; Witkin 1962a, 1; Associated Press 1962. The AP's headline was "Idiot Ranger Fumbles Its Way to the Moon."

297 Ranger 5 *followed:* Hall 1977, 167–70. "Ranger 5 was a disaster," Hall sums up. "So, too, it seemed, was the project."

297 *There could be little doubt:* Ibid., 171–76; Johnson 2002, 101–6.

298   *As later flights:* Hall 1977, 176–80; Johnson 2002, 107–10.

298   *"Systems management":* Johnson 2002, subtitle of book and throughout; see, in particular, 7–16. See also Johnson's analysis of the differences between the American and European space programs. Johnson quotes the summation of economist Antonie Knoppers: "The technology gap 'is not so much the result of differences in technological prowess, except in some special research-intensive sectors, as [it is] of differences in management and marketing approaches and—possibly above all—in attitudes."

298   *Just after the moon shot's:* Alexander 1969, 114.

300   *Having a single:* This was one idea proposed in the "Report of the National Cancer Institute Clinical Trials Program Review Group," known as the Armitage Report (NCI 1997, 50). The President's Cancer Panel suggested this simple fix as well (President's Cancer Panel 2005, 45). In a handful of select settings, such as pediatric trials run through the NCI's Children's Oncology Group, centralized IRBs have been in place for several years and have worked well.

302   *More Americans, in fact, will die:* Death counts are the Pentagon's official figures and include deaths of US military personnel from hostile action only, except as noted below. Counts derive from Leland and Oboroceanu 2010. Official casualty data for Iraq and Afghanistan theaters, as of April 30, 2012, are drawn from iCasualties.org, http://www.icasualties.org/oef/, and include deaths from nonhostile sources as well. Vietnam War deaths derive from CACCF 2013. Mortality estimates for Indian and Barbary wars, plus Bosnian intervention, are from various sources. I have included the most established mortality figures I could find for the following conflicts: Revolutionary War, Barbary (pirate) skirmishes, War of 1812, Mexican War, Indian wars (various), Civil War (both Union and Confederate forces), Spanish-American War, World War I, World War II, Korean War, Vietnam conflict, Iranian Hostage Rescue Mission, Lebanon Peacekeeping Mission, Grenada Invasion ("Urgent Fury"), Panama Invasion ("Just Cause"), Persian Gulf War ("Desert Shield/ Desert Storm"), UNOSOM Somalia Operation ("Restore Hope"), Haiti Operation ("Uphold Democracy"), Bosnia Intervention, Operation Iraqi Freedom, and Operation Enduring Freedom (Afghanistan/Global War on Terrorism). As of April 30, 2012, 689,688 US servicemen and servicewomen had perished in action during these conflicts. In raw numbers alone, that is equivalent to the number of Americans who die from cancer in 14.3 months. The aim of the above is not to draw an equivalency between these groups of deaths or types of death. The soldiers, airmen, sailors, and marines who die in war die young and in the horror of war; there is no equivalency for that, in my view. Half of those who die of cancer, meanwhile, are over the age of seventy-three.

The aim of this comparison is merely to show the scale of cancer death in the United States.

302 *By the year 2020:* Bray 2012, 790; Boyle 2006, 629.

302 *That complexity was made:* Gerlinger et al. 2012.

303 *The finding, corroborating:* Longo 2012, 956.

304 *To accept one opinion survey:* Gallup 1972. Poll on "Scientific Progress," December 23, 1949. The poll was taken twenty-two years to the day before the National Cancer Act was signed into law.

List of References

Aapro, Matti S., et al. 2005. "Never Too Old? Age Should Not Be a Barrier to Enrollment in Cancer Clinical Trials." *Oncologist* 10 (March): 198–204.

Abelev, Garry I. 1968. "Production of Embryonal Serum ß-Globulin by Hepatomas: Review of Experimental and Clinical Data." *Cancer Research* 28 (July): 1344–50.

Abelev, Garry I., et al. 1963. "Production of Embryonal ß-Globulin by Transplantable Mouse Hepatomas." *Transplantation* 1: 174–80.

Ackerknecht, Erwin H. 1958. "Historical Notes on Cancer." *Medical History* 2: 114–19.

Ackerman, Todd. 2001. Associated Press. "FDA Says Drug for Leukemia Hits Mark: Treatment Aimed at Protein Gets OK." *Houston Chronicle*, May 11, A1.

Ackoff, Russell L. 2006. "A Major Mistake That Managers Make." Speech. Ackoff Collaboratory for the Advancement of the Systems Approach, University of Pennsylvania. http://www.acasa.upenn.edu/A_Major_Mistake.pdf.

Adami, Hans-Olov, David Hunter, and Dimitrios Trichopoulos, eds. 2002. *Textbook of Cancer Epidemiology.* Oxford: Oxford University Press.

Adams, Carsbie C. 1958. *Space Flight: Satellites, Space Ships, Space Stations, and Space Travel Explained.* New York: McGraw-Hill.

Adams, M. Jacob, et al. 2004. "Cardiovascular Status in Long-Term Survivors of Hodgkin's Disease Treated with Chest Radiotherapy." *Journal of Clinical Oncology* 22 (August 1): 3139–48.

Agency for Healthcare Research and Quality. 2002. "2002 Statistics on Stays in US Hospitals, Principal Diagnosis." *Hospitalization in the United States, 2002— HCUP Fact Book No. 6.*

Agus, David B. 2009. "The Power of the 'Right' Biospecimens in Clinical Research and Care." Presentation. 2009 Biospecimen Research Network Symposium: Advancing Cancer Research Through Biospecimen Science. March 16.

————. 2011. *The End of Illness.* New York: Free Press.

————. 2012. "The 2,000-Year-Old Wonder Drug." *New York Times,* December 9. (Disclosure: I assigned and edited this editorial.)

Aisenberg, Alan C. 2000. "Historical Review of Lymphomas." *British Journal of Haematology* 109 (June): 466–76.

Al-Ali, Haifa-Kathrin, et al. 2004. "High Incidence of BCR-ABL Kinase Domain Mutations and Absence of Mutations of the PDGFR and KIT Activation Loops in CML Patients with Secondary Resistance to Imatinib." *Hematology Journal* 5: 55–60.

Alberts, Bruce, et al. 1994. *Molecular Biology of the Cell.* 3rd ed. New York: Garland Publishing.

Alexander, George A. 1983. "Geographical Aspects of Cancer in Tanzania." *Journal of the National Medical Association* 75 (August): 797–804.

Alexander, Tom. 1969. "The Unexpected Payoff of Project Apollo." *Fortune,* July, 114.

Allan, James M., and Lois B. Travis. 2005. "Mechanisms of Therapy-Related Carcinogenesis." *Nature Reviews Cancer* 5 (December): 943–55.

Al-Marshad, A. G. DeMers, and C. Kahn. 2013. "Commentary: What a Difference a Decade Makes." *Annals of Emergency Medicine* 61 (February): 223–24.

Altman, Lawrence K. 2001. "The Doctor's World: Cancer Doctors See New Era of Optimism." *New York Times,* May 22.

————. 2005. "At the Helm: Oncologists with Cancer." *New York Times,* May 24.

Alvarez, Jorge A., et al. 2007. "Long-Term Effects of Treatments for Childhood Cancers." *Current Opinion in Pediatrics* 19: 23–31.

Alvestrand, Harald. 2004. "The Role of the Standards Process in Shaping the Internet." *Proceedings of the IEEE* 92 (September): 1371–74.

American Association for the Advancement of Science. 2012. AAAS R&D Budget and Policy Program, R&D in the FY 2013 Budget, Agency Tables. Department of Veterans Affairs. http://www.aaas.org/spp/rd/fy2013/.

American Association of University Professors. 2010. "No Refuge: The Annual Report on the Economic Status of the Profession, 2009–10." *Academe* 96 (March–April): 4–32.

American Cancer Society. 1959. Public Affairs Committee, American Cancer Society. *Public Affairs Pamphlet No. 286.* Retrieved at Neilson Library collection, Smith College.

————. 1975. "Cancer Statistics, 1975." *CA: A Cancer Journal for Clinicians* 25 (January–February): 8–21.

————. 2000. *Cancer Facts and Figures, 2000.*

————. 2003. *Cancer Facts and Figures, 2003.*

————. 2005a. "The Worldwide Fight Against Cancer." (ACS, with UICC and International Network for Cancer Treatment and Research.)

————. 2005b. *Cancer Prevention and Early Detection Facts and Figures, 2005.*

————. 2006. *Cancer Facts and Figures, 2006.*

————. 2007. *Global Cancer Facts and Figures, 2007.*

————. 2007b. *Strategic Plan Progress Report, 2007.*

————. 2008. *Global Cancer Facts and Figures.* 2nd ed.

————. 2009a. *Cancer Facts and Figures, 2009.*

————. 2009b. "New American Cancer Society Report Says 650,000 Cancer Deaths Avoided Between 1990 and 2005." Press release. May 27.

————. 2009c. *Strategic Plan Progress Report, 2009.*

————. 2010a. *Cancer Facts and Figures, 2010.*

————. 2010b. "The American Cancer Society, Inc., and Affiliated Entities, Combined Financial Statements as of and for the Year Ended August 31, 2010, with Summarized Financial Information for the Year Ended August 31, 2009, with Report of Independent Auditors."

————. 2010c. *Strategic Plan Progress Report, 2010.*

————. 2011. *Strategic Stewardship Report, 2011.*

————. 2012. *Cancer Facts and Figures, 2012.*

————. 2013. *Cancer Facts and Figures, 2013.*

American Institute for Cancer Research. IRS Form 990 (Return of Organization Exempt from Income Tax) for the 2010 calendar year.

American Museum of Natural History. 1937. "The 1937 American Museum–Sinclair Dinosaur Expedition." Press release. November 6.

————. 2005. Exhibition copy for "Dinosaurs: Ancient Fossils, New Discoveries, May 14, 2005–January 8, 2006."

————. 2006. Museum signage and exhibition copy for Fossil Halls.

American Society of Clinical Oncology. 2003. Highlights from ASCO's thirty-ninth annual meeting (including attendance figures), posted May 31. http://www.cancer.gov/asco2003/highlights.

————. 2012. *ASCO Profile.* http://www.ASCO.org.

Ames, Bruce N., and Lois Swirsky Gold. 1998. "The Causes and Prevention of Cancer: The Role of Environment." *Biotherapy* 11: 205–20.

Anderson, Garth R., et al. 2001. "Cancer: The Evolved Consequence of a Destabilized Genome." *BioEssays* 23: 1037–46.

Anderson, Robert N., and Harry M. Rosenberg. 1998. "Age Standardization of Death Rates: Implementation of the Year 2000 Standard." *National Vital Statistics Report* 47 (3) (October 7): 3.

Andrewes, Christopher H. 1971. "Francis Peyton Rous. 1879–1970." *Biographical Memoirs of Fellows of the Royal Society* 17 (November): 643–62.

————. 1979. "Richard Edwin Shope. December 25, 1901–October 2, 1966." *Biographical Memoirs* (of the National Academy of Sciences) 50 (12): 353–75.

Angell, Marcia. 2004. *The Truth About the Drug Companies: How They Deceive Us and What to Do About It.* New York: Random House.

Anon. 1914. "The Cause of Cancer." *New York Times*, January 3.

———. 1921. "Cancer Phobia." *Journal of the American Medical Association* 77 (October 29): 1427.

———. 1926. "Dr. Hoffman Tells of Negro Health." *New York Times*, February 6.

———. 1931. "Empire State Building Tower Complete." *New York Times*, March 22.

———. 1937. "Executive Director Named for National Cancer Council." *Science News Letter* 32 (October 30): 278.

———. 1956. "How Many Chromosomes?" *Science* 124 (September 28): 526.

———. 1970a. "Mr. Nixon's Home Front." *Newsweek*, May 18.

———. 1970b. "The New Burdens of War." *Time*, May 11.

———. 1971a. "Teddy: Will He or Won't He?" *Newsweek*, November 15.

———. 1971b. "How Congress Packs It In." *Newsweek*, December 20, 20–21.

———. 1972. "Denis Parsons Burkitt (1911–)." *CA: A Cancer Journal for Clinicians* 22 (November–December): 345–48.

———. 1974. "Sidney Farber (1903–1973)." *CA: A Cancer Journal for Clinicians* 24 (September–October): 294–96.

———. 1987. News Bulletin. *Oncologist* 2: 276–79.

———. 2002. "New Blood Test May Detect Ovarian Cancer Early." *CA: A Cancer Journal for Clinicians* 52 (May–June): 126–27.

———. 2004a. "Cancer: Featured Drugs." *Nature Reviews Drug Discovery* 3: S6, S8.

———. 2004b. "Confronting Important Uncertainties about the Effects of Treatments: The James Lind Alliance." *Health and Social Campaigners' News* 5 (March).

———. 2006. "Making the Most of Microarrays." Editorial. *Nature Biotechnology* 24 (September): 1039.

———. 2011a. "Fix the PhD." *Nature* 472 (April 21): 259–60.

———. 2011b. "The Costly War on Cancer." *Economist*, May 26.

———. 2011c. "Lawmakers May Tinker with FDA's Review Process, REMS in PDUFA." *Washington Drug Letter*, July 11.

Armitage, Peter, and Richard Doll. 1957. "A Two-Stage Theory of Carcinogenesis in Relation to the Age Distribution of Human Cancer." *British Journal of Cancer* 11 (June): 161–69.

Armstrong, David. 2005. "October 6, 2003: Cancer Advance." Follow-through brief. *Forbes*, January 31.

Arnason, Ulfar. 2006. "FORUM: 50 Years After—Examination of Some Circumstances Around the Establishment of the Correct Chromosome Number of Man. *Hereditas* 143: 202–11.

Arnst, Catherine. 2001. "The Birth of a Cancer Drug." *BusinessWeek*, July 9.

———. 2003a. "Finally, Some Pride for Erbitux' Father." *BusinessWeek*, June 11.

————. 2003b. "The Hype vs. the Hope." *BusinessWeek,* June 16.

Ashburner, Michael, et al. 2000. "Gene Ontology: Tool for the Unification of Biology." *Nature Genetics* 25 (May): 25–29.

Ashley, D. J. B. 1969. "The Two 'Hit' and Multiple 'Hit' Theories of Carcinogenesis." *British Journal of Cancer* 23 (June): 313–28.

Ashworth, Alan, et al. 2008. "Opportunities and Challenges in Ovarian Cancer Research: A Perspective from the 11th Ovarian Cancer Action/HHMT Forum, Lake Como, March 2007." *Gynecologic Oncology* 108 (March): 652–57.

Associated Press. 1962. "Idiot Ranger Fumbles Its Way to the Moon." April 24.

Atalay, Gül, et al. 2003. "Novel Therapeutic Strategies Targeting the Epidermal Growth Factor Receptor (EGFR) Family and Its Downstream Effectors in Breast Cancer." *Annals of Oncology* 14: 1346–63.

Aya, T., et al. 1991. "Chromosome Translocation and c-MYC Activation by Epstein–Barr Virus and *Euphorbia tirucalli* in B Lymphocytes." *Lancet* 337 (May 18): 1190.

Ayala, Francisco J. 2009. "Darwin and the Scientific Method." *Proceedings of the National Academy of Sciences* 106 (supp. 1) (June 16): 10033–39.

Azam, Mohammad, et al. 2003. "Mechanisms of Autoinhibition and STI-571/Imatinib Resistance Revealed by Mutagenesis of BCR-ABL." *Cell* 112 (March 21): 831–43.

Babak, Jahan–Parwar, et al. 2011. "Facial Bone Anatomy." *Medscape Reference* (online), updated June 24. Retrieved from http://emedicine.medscape.com/article/835401-overview#a1.

Bach, Peter B., Leonard B. Saltz, and Robert E. Wittes. 2012. "In Cancer Care, Cost Matters." Op-ed. *New York Times,* October 14.

Bailar, John C., III. 1987. "Cancer Control." Letter to the editor. *Science* 236 (May 29): 1049–50.

Bailar, John C., III, and Heather L. Gornik. 1997. "Cancer Undefeated." *New England Journal of Medicine* 336 (May 29): 1569–74.

Bailar, John C., III, and Frederick Mosteller, eds. 1992. *Medical Uses of Statistics.* 2nd ed. Boston: NEJM Books.

Bailar, John C., III, and Elaine M. Smith. 1986. "Progress Against Cancer?" *New England Journal of Medicine* 314: 1226–32.

Bailey, Orville T. 1974. "Sidney Farber, MD, 1903–1973." *American Journal of Pathology* 77 (November): 129–33.

Balmain, Allan, et al. 1993. "How Many Mutations Are Required for Tumorigenesis? Implications from Human Cancer Data." *Molecular Carcinogenesis* 7: 139–46.

Baltimore, David. 1997. "Homage to Howard Temin." In *Retroviruses,* edited by John M. Coffin, Stephen H. Hughes, and Harold E. Varmus. Cold Spring Harbor, NY: Cold Spring Harbor Laboratory Press. http://www.ncbi.nlm.nih.gov/books/NBK19376/.

Baltzer, Fritz. 1967. *Theodor Boveri: Life and Work of a Great Biologist.* Translated from the German by Dorothea Rudnick. Berkeley: University of California Press.

Banda, L. T., et al. 2001. "Cancer Incidence in Blantyre, Malawi, 1994–1998." *Tropical Medicine and International Health* 6 (April): 296–304.

Bangma, C. H., et al. 2007. "Overdiagnosis and Overtreatment of Early Detected Prostate Cancer." *World Journal of Urology* 25: 3–9.

Barabasi, Albert-Laszlo. 2003. *Linked.* New York: Plume. Originally published in 2002 by Perseus Publishing.

Baron, Jonathan, and Ilana Ritov. 1994. "Reference Points and Omission Bias." *Organizational Behavior and Human Decision Processes* 59: 475–98.

Barrett, J. Carl. 1993. "Mechanisms of Multistep Carcinogenesis and Carcinogen Risk Assessment." *Environmental Health Perspectives* 100: 9–20.

Barry, Isobel. 2009. "The Regression Question." *Nature Reviews Cancer* 9 (January): 8.

Barthe, Christophe, et al. 2001. "Roots of Clinical Resistance to STI-571 Cancer Therapy." *Science* 293 (September 21): 2163a.

Bascetta, Cynthia A. 2007. Letter, dated January 31, from Bascetta (Director, Health Care) and Robert E. Martin (Director, Financial Management and Assurance), US Government Accountability Office, to Senator Tom Coburn, Subcommittee on Federal Financial Management, Government Information, and International Security Committee on Homeland Security and Governmental Affairs, US Senate, regarding National Institutes of Health Extramural Research Grants: Oversight of Cost Reimbursements to Universities (GAO-07-294R).

Bast, Robert C., Jr. 1981. "Reactivity of a Monoclonal Antibody with Human Ovarian Carcinoma." *Journal of Clinical Investigation* 68 (November): 1331–37.

Bast, Robert C., Jr., Bryan Hennessy, and Gordon B. Mills. 2009. "The Biology of Ovarian Cancer: New Opportunities for Translation." *Nature Reviews Cancer* 9 (June): 415–28.

Bast, Robert C., Jr., and Robert C. Knapp. 1998. "CA 125: History, Current Status, and Future Prospects." *McGill Journal of Medicine* 3: 67–71.

Bast, Robert C., Jr., et al. 2005. "New Tumor Markers: CA125 and Beyond." *International Journal of Gynecological Cancer* 15 (November): 274–81.

Battat, Anna C., et al. 2004. "Institutional Commitment to Rectal Cancer Screening Results in Earlier-Stage Cancers on Diagnosis." *Annals of Surgical Oncology* 11: 970–76.

Battelle, John. 2005. *The Search: How Google and Its Rivals Rewrote the Rules of Business and Transformed Our Culture.* New York: Portfolio.

Baxter, Nancy N., et al. 2004. "Trends in the Treatment of Ductal Carcinoma In Situ of the Breast." *Journal of the National Cancer Institute* 96 (March 17): 443–48.

Bazell, Robert J. 1970. "Cancer Research: Senate Consultants Likely to Push for Planned Assault." *Science* 170 (October 16): 304–5.

———. 1971a. "Cancer Research Proposals: New Money, Old Conflicts." *Science* 171 (March 5): 877–79.

———. 1971b. "Lederberg Opposes Cancer Authority." *Science* 171 (March 26): 1220.

———. 1998. *Her-2: The Making of Herceptin, a Revolutionary Treatment for Breast Cancer.* New York: Random House.

Beatson, George Thomas. 1896. "On the Treatment of Inoperable Cases of Carcinoma of the Mamma: Suggestions for a New Method of Treatment, with Illustrative Cases." *Lancet* 2 (July 11): 104–7.

Beckman, Robert A., and Lawrence A. Loeb. 2005. "Genetic Instability in Cancer: Theory and Experiment." *Seminars in Cancer Biology* 15: 423–35.

Beeman, Edward A. 2005. *Robert J. Huebner, M.D.: A Virologist's Odyssey.* Text prepared for the Office of NIH History at the National Institutes of Health.

Beerenwinkel, Niko, et al. 2007. "Genetic Progression and the Waiting Time to Cancer." *PLOS Computational Biology* 3 (November 9): e225.

Beishon, Marc. 2008. "Clifton Leaf: Asking the Difficult Questions." *CancerWorld,* January/February.

Bellhouse, D. R. 2004. "The Reverend Thomas Bayes, FRS: A Biography to Celebrate the Tercentenary of His Birth." *Statistical Science* 19 (February): 3–43.

Benkler, Yochai. 2006. *The Wealth of Networks: How Social Production Transforms Markets and Freedom.* New Haven, CT: Yale University Press.

Bennani, Youssef L. 2011. "Drug Discovery in the Next Decade: Innovation Needed ASAP." *Drug Discovery Today* 16 (September): 779–92.

Ben–Neriah, Yinon, et al. 1986. "The Chronic Myelogenous Leukemia-Specific P210 Protein Is the Product of the bcr/abl Hybrid Gene." *Science* 223 (July 11): 212–14.

Bennett, Charles L., et al. 2008. "Venous Thromboembolism and Mortality Associated with Recombinant Erythropoietin and Darbepoetin Administration for the Treatment of Cancer-Associated Anemia." *Journal of the American Medical Association* 299 (February 27): 914–24.

Benson, A. B., III. 1991. "Oncologists' Reluctance to Accrue Patients onto Clinical Trials: An Illinois Cancer Center Study." *Journal of Clinical Oncology* 9 (November): 2067–75.

Benson, Charles D., and William B. Faherty. 2001. *Gateway to the Moon: Building the Kennedy Space Center Complex.* Gainesville: University Press of Florida. Originally published in 1978 by the National Aeronautics and Space Administration as part of *Moonport: A History of Apollo Launch Facilities and Operations.*

Benson, John R., et al. 2009. "Early Breast Cancer." *Lancet* 373 (April 25): 1463–79.

Berenson, Alex. 2005. "Cancer Drugs Offer Hope, but at a Huge Expense." *New York Times*, July 12.

———. 2006. "A Cancer Drug Shows Promise, at a Price That Many Can't Pay." *New York Times*, February 15.

Berger, Leslie. 2007. "Cancer Care Seeks to Take Patients Beyond Survival." *New York Times*, May 22.

Berman, Jules J., et al. 2006. "Precancer: A Conceptual Working Definition. Results of a Consensus Conference." *Cancer Detection and Prevention* 30 (October 31): 387–94.

Berman, Nancy G., and Robert A. Parker. 2002. "Meta-analysis: Neither Quick nor Easy." *BMC Medical Research Methodology* 2 (August 9): 10.

Berry, Donald A. 1991. "Experimental Design for Drug Development: A Bayesian Approach." *Journal of Biopharmaceutical Statistics* 1(1): 81–101.

———. 1995. "Decision Analysis and Bayesian Methods in Clinical Trials." In *Recent Advances in Clinical Trial Design and Analysis*, edited by Peter F. Thall, 125–54. Boston: Kluwer Academic Publishers.

———. 2001. "Adaptive Trials and Bayesian Statistics in Drug Development." *Biopharmaceutical Report* 9: 1–11 (with comments by George Chi, H. M. James Hung, and Robert O'Neill).

———. 2004. "Bayesian Statistics and the Efficiency and Ethics of Clinical Trials." *Statistical Science* (February) 19: 175–87.

Berry, Donald A., et al. 2005. The Cancer Intervention and Surveillance Modeling Network (CISNET) Collaborators. "Effect of Screening and Adjuvant Therapy on Mortality from Breast Cancer." *New England Journal of Medicine* 353 (October 27): 1784–92.

Bertino, Joseph R. 1963. "The Mechanism of Action of the Folate Antagonists in Man." *Cancer Research* 23 (September): 1286–306.

———. 1971. "New Approaches to Chemotherapy with Folate Antagonists: Use of Leucovorin 'Rescue' and Enzymatic Folate Depletion." *Annals of the New York Academy of Sciences* 186 (November 30): 486–95.

Beutler, E. 2000. "Introduction to Janet D. Rowley." *Leukemia* 14 (March): 511–12. Monograph from the Acute Leukemia Forum 1999 on Advances and Controversies in the Therapy of Acute Myelogenous Leukemia.

Beveridge, W. I. B. 1960. *The Art of Scientific Investigation*. Reprint, New York: Vintage Books, 1960. Originally published 1950.

Bhatia, Smita, and Petra Roberts. 2005. "What Is the Risk of Second Malignant Neoplasms After Childhood Cancer?" *Nature Clinical Practice Oncology* 2 (April): 182–83.

Bhatia, Smita, et al. 2003. "High Risk of Subsequent Neoplasms Continues with Extended Follow-Up of Childhood Hodgkin's Disease: Report from the Late Effects Study Group." *Journal of Clinical Oncology* 21 (December 1): 4386–94.

Bhatia, Smita, et al. 2006. "Medical and Psychosocial Issues in Childhood Cancer Survivors." In *Oncology: An Evidence-Based Approach,* edited by Alfred E. Chang, et al. New York: Springer.

Bignold, Leon P. 2006. "Cancer Morphology, Carcinogenesis and Genetic Instability: A Background." In *Cancer: Cell Structures, Carcinogens and Genomic Instability,* edited by Leon P. Bignold, 1–24. Basel, Switzerland: Birkhäuser Verlag.

Biographical Directory of the United States Congress, 1774–Present. http://bioguide .congress.gov/.

Bionest Partners and Exane BNP Paribas. 2006. *Oncology Pipelines: Searching Is Not Finding, Sector Review.* March.

Bird, Roland T. 1939. "Thunder in His Footsteps." *Natural History Magazine,* May. Retrieved from http://www.naturalhistorymag.com/picks-from-the-past/ 241755/thunder-in-his-footsteps.

———. 1941. "A Dinosaur Walks into the Museum," *Natural History Magazine,* February. Retrieved from http://www.naturalhistorymag.com/picks-from-the-past/ 081795/a-dinosaur-walks-into-the-museum.

———. 1985. *Bones for Barnum Brown: Adventures of a Dinosaur Hunter.* Edited by V. Theodore Schreiber. Fort Worth: Texas Christian University Press.

Birmingham, Karen. 2004. "An Inauspicious Start for the U.S. National Biospecimen Network." *Journal of Clinical Investigation* 113 (February): 320.

Bishop, J. Michael. 1989. "Retroviruses and Oncogenes II." Nobel Lecture, the Nobel Prize in Physiology or Medicine 1989 (December 8). Retrieved from http://www .nobelprize.org/nobel_prizes/medicine/laureates/1989/bishop-lecture.html.

———. 2003. *How to Win the Nobel Prize: An Unexpected Life in Science.* Cambridge, MA: Harvard University Press.

Bissell, Mina J. 2007. "Phenotype Overrides Genotype in Normal Mammary Gland and Breast Cancer." AACR-Pezcoller Award Lecture, American Association for Cancer Research 2007 Annual Meeting, Los Angeles, April 15.

Bissell, Mina J., H. Glenn Hall, and Gordon Parry. 1982. "How Does the Extracellular Matrix Direct Gene Expression?" *Journal of Theoretical Biology* 99 (November 7): 31–68.

Bissell, Mina J., and Derek Radisky. 2001. "Putting Tumors in Context." *Nature Reviews Cancer* 1 (October): 46–54.

Black, Paul H. 1980. "Shedding from the Cell Surface of Normal and Cancer Cells." *Advances in Cancer Research* 32: 75–199.

Black, William C., and H. Gilbert Welch. 1997. "Screening for Disease." *American Journal of Roentgenology* 168 (January): 3–11.

Blackburn, Elizabeth H., et al. 2011. Cancer Progress Report Writing Committee. *AACR Cancer Progress Report 2011: Transforming Patient Care Through Innovation.* American Association for Cancer Research.

Blood Pressure Lowering Treatment Trialists' Collaboration. 2003. "Effects of Different Blood-Pressure-Lowering Regimens on Major Cardiovascular Events: Results of Prospectively-Designed Overviews of Randomised Trials." *Lancet* 362 (November 8): 1527–35.

Blow, Nathan. 2007. "Tissue Issues." *Nature* 448 (August): 959–62.

Blue Ridge Institute for Medical Research. 2006–11. "Ranking Tables of National Institutes of Health (NIH) Award Data," http://www.brimr.org/NIH_Awards/. Note: BRIMR obtains the annual figures from the NIH's Research Portfolio Online Reporting Tool (RePORT), at http://report.nih.gov/award/trends/Aggregate Data.cfm, and orders the institutional recipients of funding in ranking tables, as the NIH itself did prior to 2006. The NIH stopped publishing its own lists, it said, in part because of "responses received from the grantee community suggesting that ranking tables were not necessary." Data for years prior to 2006 are drawn from the NIH's own published rankings.

Blume-Jensen, Peter, and Tony Hunter. 2001. "Oncogenic Kinase Signalling." *Nature* 411 (May 17): 355–65.

Bodey, Gerald P., et al. 1966. "Quantitative Relationships Between Circulating Leukocytes and Infection in Patients with Acute Leukemia." *Annals of Internal Medicine* 64 (February 1): 328–40.

Bogoyevitch, Marie A., and David P. Fairlie. 2007. "A New Paradigm for Protein Kinase Inhibition: Blocking Phosphorylation Without Directly Targeting ATP Binding." *Drug Discovery Today* 12 (August): 622–33.

Bohlius, Julia, et al. 2006a. "Cancer-Related Anemia and Recombinant Human Erythropoietin: An Updated Overview." *Nature Clinical Practice Oncology* 3 (March): 152–64.

———. 2006b. "Recombinant Human Erythropoietins and Cancer Patients: Updated Meta-Analysis of 57 Studies Including 9,353 Patients." *Journal of the National Cancer Institute* 98 (May 17): 708–14.

Bonadonna, Gianni, and Armando Santoro. 1982. "Evolution in the Treatment Strategy of Hodgkin's Disease." *Advances in Cancer Research* 36: 257–93.

Bonetta, Laura. 2008. "Enhancing NIH Grant Peer Review: A Broader Perspective." *Cell* 135 (October 17): 201–4.

Booth, Bruce, and Rodney Zemmel. 2003. "Quest for the Best." *Nature Reviews Drug Discovery* 2 (October): 838–41.

Boring, Catherine C., Teresa S. Squires, and Tony Tong. 1993. "Cancer Statistics, 1993." *CA: A Cancer Journal for Clinicians* 43 (January–February): 7–26.

Bouck, Noël, et al. 1996. "How Tumors Become Angiogenic." *Advances in Cancer Research* 69: 135–74.

Bouvard, Véronique, et al. 2009. "Special Report: Policy. A Review of Human Carcinogens—Part B: Biological Agents." *Lancet Oncology* 10 (April): 321–22.

Boyle, Peter. 2006. "The Globalisation of Cancer." *Lancet* 368 (August 19): 629–30.

Braakhuis, Boudewijn J. M., et al. 2003. "A Genetic Explanation of Slaughter's Concept of Field Cancerization: Evidence and Clinical Implications." *Cancer Research* 63 (April 15): 1727–30.

Brainard, Jeffrey. 2004. "What the NIH Bought with Double the Money." *Chronicle of Higher Education,* February 6.

Branford, Susan, and Timothy Hughes. 2005. "Detection of BCR-ABL Mutations and Resistance to Imatinib Mesylate." In *Methods in Molecular Medicine, Vol. 125: Myeloid Leukemia: Methods and Protocols,* edited by Harry Iland et al., 93–106. New York: Humana Press.

Branford, Susan, et al. 2003. "Detection of BCR-ABL Mutations in Patients with CML Treated with Imatinib Is Virtually Always Accompanied by Clinical Resistance, and Mutations in the ATP Phosphate-Binding Loop (P-loop) Are Associated with a Poor Prognosis." *Blood* 102 (July 1): 276–83.

Brawley, Otis W. 2002. "Some Perspective on Black-White Cancer Statistics." *CA: A Cancer Journal for Clinicians* 52 (November–December): 322–25.

Bray, Freddie, et al. 2012. "Global Cancer Transitions According to the Human Development Index (2008–2030): A Population–Based Study." *Lancet Oncology* 13 (August): 790–801.

Brazma, Alvis, et al. 2001. "Minimum Information About a Microarray Experiment (MIAME). Toward Standards for Microarray Data." *Nature Genetics* 29 (December): 365–71.

Brazma, Alvis, Maria Krestyaninova, and Ugis Sarkans. 2006. "Standards for Systems Biology." *Nature Reviews Genetics* 7 (August): 593–605.

Brennan, Donald J., et al. 2010. "Antibody-Based Proteomics: Fast-Tracking Molecular Diagnostics in Oncology." *Nature Reviews Cancer* 10 (September): 605–17.

Breuer, Roderick H., et al. 2005. "The Natural Course of Preneoplastic Lesions in Bronchial Epithelium." *Clinical Cancer Research* 11 (January 15): 537–43.

Brewster, Abenaa M., et al. 2008. "Residual Risk of Breast Cancer Recurrence 5 Years After Adjuvant Therapy." *Journal of the National Cancer Institute* 100 (August 20): 1179–83.

Brinkley, Bill R. 2003. Obituary of T. C. Hsu. *ASCB Newsletter.* Retrieved from American Society for Cell Biology's newsletter archive, May 10, 2007.

Brosh, Ran, and Varda Rotter. 2009. "When Mutants Gain New Powers: News from the Mutant p53 Field." *Nature Reviews Cancer* 9 (October): 701–13.

Brouwer, C. A. J. 2007. "Changes in Body Composition After Childhood Cancer Treatment: Impact on Future Health Status—a Review." *Critical Reviews in Oncology/Hematology* 63: 32–46.

Brown, Barnum. 1907. "Gastroliths." *Science* 25 (March 8): 392.

————. 1908. Field notebooks from the paleontologist's expedition to Montana ("Hell Creek Formation"), posted online by the American Museum of Natural History. Retrieved from http://research.amnh.org/paleontology/notebooks/brown–1908/.

Brown, Martin L., and Bruce Fireman. 1995. "Evaluation of Direct Medical Costs Related to Cancer." *Journal of the National Cancer Institute* 87 (March 15): 399–400.

Brown, Martin L., Joseph Lipscomb, and Claire Snyder. 2001. "The Burden of Illness of Cancer: Economic Cost and Quality of Life." *Annual Review of Public Health* 22 (May): 91–113.

Brown, Martin L., Gerald F. Riley, Arnold L. Potosky, and Ruth D. Etzioni. 1999. "Obtaining Long-Term Disease Specific Costs of Care: Application to Medicare Enrollees Diagnosed with Colorectal Cancer." *Medical Care* 37 (December): 1249–59.

Brown, Martin L., et al. 2001. "The Burden of Illness of Cancer: Economic Cost and Quality of Life." *Annual Review of Public Health* 22: 91–113.

Browning, E. S., and Gregory Zuckerman. 2002. "What Stock Investors Need: First, Trust in Firms' Numbers." *Wall Street Journal,* July 17.

Brownlee, Shannon. 2003. "Health, Hope and Hype: Why the Media Oversells Medical 'Breakthroughs.'" *Washington Post,* August 3.

————. 2007. *Overtreated: Why Too Much Medicine Is Making Us Sicker and Poorer.* New York: Bloomsbury USA.

Bud, R. F. 1978. "Strategy in American Cancer Research After World War II: A Case Study." *Social Studies of Science* 8 (November): 425–59.

Buescher, Paul A. 2010. *Statistical Primer No. 13.* Division of Public Health, State Center for Health Statistics, North Carolina Department of Health and Human Services. Revised May 2010, 1–8.

Buffet, C., et al. 1989. "Des-gamma-carboxyprothrombin in Hepatocellular Carcinoma After Vitamin K1 Injection." *Digestive Diseases and Sciences* 34: 963–64.

Buono, Michael J., and Fred W. Kolkhorst. 2001. "Estimating ATP Resynthesis During a Marathon Run: A Method to Introduce Metabolism." *Advances in Physiology Education* 25 (June): 70–71.

Burchenal, Joseph H. 1966. "Geographic Chemotherapy: Burkitt's Tumor as a Stalking Horse for Leukemia: Presidential Address." *Cancer Research* 26 (December): 2393–405.

————. 1968. "Long-Term Survivors in Acute Leukemia and Burkitt's Tumor." *Cancer* 21 (April): 595–99.

Burchenal, Joseph H., Warren P. L. Myers, Lloyd F. Craver, and David A. Karnofsky. 1949. "The Nitrogen Mustards in the Treatment of Leukemia." *Cancer* 2 (January): 1–17.

Burchenal, Joseph H., and M. Lois Murphy. 1965. "Long-Term Survivors in Acute Leukemia." *Cancer Research* 25 (October): 1491–94.

Burkitt, Denis P. 1951. "Primary Hydrocele and Its Treatment: Review of 200 Cases." *Lancet* 1 (1951): 1341–47.

———. 1958. "A Sarcoma Involving the Jaws in African Children." *British Journal of Surgery* 46 (November): 218–23.

———. 1962. "A 'Tumor Safari' in East and Central Africa." *British Journal of Cancer* 16 (September): 379–86.

———. 1969. "Etiology of Burkitt's Lymphoma: An Alternative Hypothesis to a Vectored Virus." *Journal of the National Cancer Institute* 42 (January): 19–28.

———. 1983a. "Charles S. Mott Award: The Discovery of Burkitt's Lymphoma." *Cancer* 51 (May 15): 1777–86.

———. 1983b. "Citation Classic—A Sarcoma Involving the Jaws in African Children." *Current Contents/Life Sciences* 21 (May 23): 155.

Burkitt, Denis P., M. S. R. Hutt, and D. H. Wright. 1965. "The African Lymphoma: Preliminary Observations on Response to Therapy." *Cancer* 18 (April): 399–410.

Burkitt, Denis P., and Greg T. O'Conor. 1961. "Malignant Lymphoma in African Children: I. A Clinical Syndrome." *Cancer* 14 (March/April): 258–69.

Burkitt, Denis P., H. F. Oettgen, and Joseph H. Burchenal. 1963. "Malignant Lymphoma Involving the Jaw in African Children: Treatment with Methotrexate." *Cancer* 16: 616–23.

Burstein, Harold J., et al. 2004. "Ductal Carcinoma In Situ of the Breast." *New England Journal of Medicine* 350 (April 1): 1430–41.

Buscher, Leo F., Jr. 2002. Chief Grants Management Officer, National Cancer Institute. *Everything You Wanted to Know About the NCI Grants Process . . . But Were Afraid to Ask*. NIH Publication No. 03-1222.

Bustin, Stephen A., Jo Vandesompele, and Michael W. Pfaffl. 2009. "Standardization of qPCR and RT-qPCR: New Guidelines Seek to Promote Accurate Interpretation of Data and Reliable Results." *Genetic Engineering and Biotechnology News* 29 (August): 1.

Butler, Thomas P., and Pietro M. Gullino. 1975. "Quantitation of Cell Shedding into Efferent Blood of Mammary Adenocarcinoma." *Cancer Research* 35 (March 1): 512–16.

Bylinsky, Gene. 1971. "Cancer Cells Begin to Yield Their Secrets." *Fortune*, November, 156–59, 223–26.

———. 1985. "Science Scores a Cancer Breakthrough." *Fortune*, November 25.

———. 1988. "Technology in the Year 2000." *Fortune*, July 18.

Byrnes, Nanette, et al. 2002. "Accounting in Crisis." *BusinessWeek*, January 28.

CACCF. 2013. Combat Area Casualties Current File for Southeast Asia, Electronic and Special Media Records Services Division Reference Report, National Archives.

http://www.archives.gov/research/military/vietnam-war/casualty-statistics .html#year. Data retrieved January 10, 2013.

Cairns, John. 1978. *Cancer: Science and Society.* San Francisco: W. H. Freeman.

———. 1985. "The Treatment of Diseases and the War Against Cancer." *Scientific American* 253 (November): 51–59.

———. 1997. *Matters of Life and Death: Perspectives on Public Health, Molecular Biology, Cancer, and the Prospects for the Human Race.* Princeton, NJ: Princeton University Press.

Calin, George A., and Carlo M. Croce. 2006. "MicroRNA Signatures in Human Cancers." *Nature Reviews Cancer* 6 (November): 857–66.

Cambon–Thomsen, Anne. 2004. "The Social and Ethical Issues of Post-Genomic Human Biobanks." *Nature Reviews Genetics* 5 (November): 866–73.

Cancer Center Directors Working Group. 2006. *Accelerating Successes Against Cancer: Recommendations from the NCI-designated Cancer Center Directors.* John Mendelsohn, chair (NIH).

Cannon, Christopher P., et al. 2004. "Intensive versus Moderate Lipid Lowering with Statins after Acute Coronary Syndromes." *New England Journal of Medicine* 350 (April 8): 1495–504.

Capell, Kerry. 2009. "Novartis: Radically Remaking Its Drug Business." *Business-Week,* June 11.

Carbone, Michele, and Harvey I. Pass. 2004. "Multistep and Multifactorial Carcinogenesis: When Does a Contributing Factor Become a Carcinogen?" *Seminars in Cancer Biology* 14 (December): 399–405.

Cardoso, Fatima, et al. 2002. "Second and Subsequent Lines of Chemotherapy for Metastatic Breast Cancer: What Did We Learn in the Last Two Decades?" *Annals of Oncology* 13: 197–207.

Cardy, Amanda H., Linda Sharp, and Julian Little. 2001. "Burkitt's Lymphoma: A Review of the Epidemiology." *Kuwait Medical Journal* 33 (December): 293–306.

Carmichael, D. Erskine. 1973. *The Pap Smear: Life of George N. Papanicolaou.* Springfield, IL: Charles C. Thomas.

Carpenter, Lucy M., et al. 2008. "Antibodies Against Malaria and Epstein–Barr Virus in Childhood Burkitt Lymphoma: A Case-Control Study in Uganda." *International Journal of Cancer* 122 (March 15): 1319–23.

Carter, Fairie Lyn. 1948. "The Use of Tracers in the Study of the Living Cell." *BIOS* 19 (May): 112–23.

Carter, Richard. 1961. *The Gentle Legions: A Probing Study of the National Voluntary Health Organizations.* Garden City, NY: Doubleday.

Case, Gretchen A. 1997. "National Cancer Institute Oral History Project: Interview with Emil J. Freireich, M.D." Conducted June 19, AR-9705-012240. Rockville, MD: History Associates.

Casey, Kevin, et al. 2007. Publication Steering Committee, representing the University of California, Columbia University, Harvard University, Johns Hopkins Medicine/Johns Hopkins University, Partners Healthcare (Brigham and Women's Hospital and Massachusetts General), University of Texas at Austin, Washington University in St. Louis, University of Wisconsin, Madison, and Yale University. "Within Our Grasp—or Slipping Away? Assuring a New Era of Scientific and Medical Progress. A Statement by a Group of Concerned Universities and Research Institutions." March.

Casey, Kevin, et al. 2008. Publication Steering Committee, representing Brown University, Duke Medicine, Harvard University, Ohio State University Medical Center, Partners Healthcare (Brigham and Women's Hospital and Massachusetts General), University of California, Los Angeles, Vanderbilt University. "A Broken Pipeline? Flat Funding of the NIH Puts a Generation of Science at Risk. A Follow-Up Statement by a Group of Concerned Universities and Research Institutions." March.

Casper, Monica J., and Adele E. Clarke. 1998. "Making the Pap Smear into the 'Right Tool' for the Job: Cervical Cancer Screening in the USA, circa 1940–95." *Social Studies of Science* 28 (April): 255–90.

Caspersson, Torbjorn, et al. 1970. "Identification of the Philadelphia Chromosome as a Number 22 by Quinacrine Mustard Fluorescence Analysis." *Experimental Cell Research* 63 (November): 238–40.

Cassileth, Barrie R. 2003. "Clinical Trials: Time for Action." Editorial. *Journal of Clinical Oncology* 21 (March 1): 765–66.

C-Change. 2005. *Cost and Functional Requirements for Cancer Clinical Trials: A Guidance Document for Implementing Effective Cancer Clinical Trials* (Version 1.2). June 7.

Cech, Thomas R., et al. 2005. National Research Council. *Bridges to Independence: Fostering the Independence of New Investigators in Biomedical Research, Report by the Committee on Bridges to Independence: Identifying Opportunities for and Challenges to Fostering the Independence of Young Investigators in the Life Sciences.* Washington, DC: National Academies Press.

———. 2008. Committee on Alternative Models for the Federal Funding of Science, American Academy of Arts and Sciences, ARISE Report. *Advancing Research in Science and Engineering: Investing in Early-Career Scientists and High-Risk, High-Reward Research.* Cambridge, MA: American Academy of Arts and Sciences.

Centers for Disease Control and Prevention. *United States Cancer Statistics (USCS): 1999–2009 Cancer Incidence and Mortality,* web-based report. Atlanta: US Department of Health and Human Services, Centers for Disease Control and Prevention and National Cancer Institute. http://apps.nccd.cdc.gov/uscs/.

Chabner, Bruce A., and Thomas G. Roberts, Jr. 2005. "Chemotherapy and the War on Cancer." *Nature Reviews Cancer* 5 (January): 65–72.

Challis, G. B., and H. J. Stam. 1990. "The Spontaneous Regression of Cancer: A Review of Cases from 1900 to 1987." *Acta Oncologica* 29: 545–50.

Chalmers, Thomas C. 1981. "The Clinical Trial." *Milbank Memorial Fund Quarterly/ Health and Society* 59: 324–39.

Cheng, Steven, et al. 2009. "A Sense of Urgency: Evaluating the Link Between Clinical Trial Development Time and the Accrual Performance of CTEP-Sponsored Studies." *Journal of Clinical Oncology* (2009 ASCO Annual Meeting Proceedings, postmeeting ed., supp.) 27 (18S) (June 20): CRA6509.

Cheok, Meyling H., and William E. Evans. 2006. "Acute Lymphoblastic Leukaemia: A Model for the Pharmacogenomics of Cancer Therapy." *Nature Reviews Cancer* 6 (February): 117–29.

Christensen, Damaris. 2002. "Tracking Tumors: Looking for Early Signs of a Therapy's Success." *Science News* 161 (March 2): 139–40.

Christie, D. A., and E. M. Tansey, eds. 2007. "The Discovery, Use and Impact of Platinum Salts as Chemotherapy Agents for Cancer. The Transcript of a Witness Seminar Held by the Wellcome Trust Centre for the History of Medicine at UCL, London, on 4 April 2006." London: Wellcome Trust Centre.

CISNET. 2006. "The Impact of Mammography and Adjuvant Therapy on US Breast Cancer Mortality (1975–2000): Collective Results from the Cancer Intervention and Surveillance Modeling Network." A 126-page monograph published by the *Journal of the National Cancer Institute*. October.

Citri, Ami, and Yosef Yarden. 2006. "EGF-ERBB Signalling: Towards the Systems Level." *Nature Reviews Molecular Cell Biology* 7 (July): 505–16.

Clark, Kim B., W. Bruce Chew, and Takahiro Fujimoto. 1987. "Product Development in the World Auto Industry." *Brookings Papers on Economic Activity* 1987 (3): 729–81.

Clark, Michael James, et al. 2010. "U87MG Decoded: The Genomic Sequence of a Cytogenetically Aberrant Human Cancer Cell Line." *PLOS Genetics* 6 (January) (e1000832): 1–16.

Clarkson, Bayard D., Margaret Foti, et al. 2006. "Joseph H. Burchenal: In Memoriam (1912–2006)." *Cancer Research* 66 (December 15): 12037–38.

Coakley, Davis. 2006. "Denis Burkitt and His Contribution to Haematology-Oncology." *British Journal of Haematology* 135 (October): 17–25.

Cobleigh, Melody A. 1999. "Multinational Study of the Efficacy and Safety of Humanized Anti-HER2 Monoclonal Antibody in Women Who Have HER2-Overexpressing Metastatic Breast Cancer That Has Progressed After Chemotherapy for Metastatic Disease." *Journal of Clinical Oncology* 17 (September): 2639–48.

Coffin, John M., Stephen M. Hughes, and Harold E. Varmus, eds. 1997. "A Brief Chronicle of Retrovirology." In *Retroviruses*. Cold Spring Harbor, NY: Cold Spring Harbor Laboratory Press. Retrieved from the National Library of Medicine's National Center for Biotechnology Information, at http://www.ncbi.nlm .nih.gov/books/bv.fcgi?rid=rv.section.18.

Cohen, Joshua, Elly Stolk, and Maartje Niezen. 2007. "The Increasingly Complex Fourth Hurdle for Pharmaceuticals." *Pharmacoeconomics* 25 (9): 727–34.

Cohen, Martin H., et al. 2002. "Report from the FDA: Approval Summary for Imatinib Mesylate Capsules in the Treatment of Chronic Myelogenous Leukemia." *Clinical Cancer Research* 8 (May): 935–42.

Cohn, Victor. 1984. Untitled news story ("Top federal health officials yesterday launched an unprecedented program to cut cancer deaths in half"). *Washington Post*, March 7.

———. 1986. "The Cancer War: Disputed Victory." *Washington Post*, September 30.

Cole, M. P., C. T. A. Jones, and I. D. H. Todd. 1971. "A New Antioestrogenic Agent in Late Breast Cancer: An Early Clinical Appraisal of ICI46474." *British Journal of Cancer* 25 (June): 270–75.

Cole, Warren H. 1981. "Efforts to Explain Spontaneous Regression of Cancer." *Journal of Surgical Oncology* 17: 201–9.

Collingwood, Harris. 2001. "The Earnings Game: Everybody Plays, Nobody Wins." *Harvard Business Review* 79 (6) (June): 65–74.

Collins, Francis. 2010a. "NIH in the 21st Century: The Director's Perspective." Statement before the Committee on Energy and Commerce, Subcommittee on Health, United States House of Representatives, June 15.

———. 2010b. "Scientists Need a Shorter Path to Research Freedom." *Nature* 467 (October 7): 635.

Collins, Francis S., Michael Morgan, and Aristides Patrinos. 2003. "The Human Genome Project: Lessons from Large-Scale Biology." *Science* 300 (April 11): 286–90.

Comis, Robert L., and John Crowley. 2006. Coalition of Cancer Cooperative Groups. *Report to Global Access Project: Baseline Study of Patient Accrual onto Publicly Sponsored US Cancer Clinical Trials*. Philadelphia. February 1.

Comis, Robert L., et al. 2000. *A Quantitative Survey of Public Attitudes Towards Cancer Clinical Trials*. Coalition of National Cancer Cooperative Groups, Cancer Research Foundation of America, Cancer Leadership Council and Oncology Nursing Society.

Compton, Carolyn C. 2009. "The Cancer Human Biobank (caHUB): Advancing the Vision of Personalized Medicine, Filling the Infrastructure Gap for Translational Research." Presentation. 2nd Annual Biospecimen Research Symposium, March 17.

Comptroller General of the United States. 1984. *Assuring Reasonableness of Rising Indirect Costs on NIH (National Institutes of Health) Research Grants: A Difficult Problem.* GAO/HRD-84-3. Washington, DC: US General Accounting Office, March 16.

Conference on Human Subject Protection and Financial Conflicts of Interest. 2000. National Institutes of Health, Bethesda, MD, August 15–16. http://www.hhs.gov/ohrp/archive/coi/8-15.htm.

Congressionally Directed Medical Research Program. Website. http://cdmrp.army.mil/about/fundinghistory.shtml.

Congressional Record. 1971. Vol. 117, Part 38, US House of Representatives, 92nd Congress, 1st sess., November 15, 1971, 41158–59.

Conley, John, and Dan Vorhaus. 2010. "Pigs Fly: Federal Court Invalidates Myriad's Patent Claims." *Genomics Law Report,* March 30. http://www.genomicslawreport.com.

Cooke, Robert. 2001. *Dr. Folkman's War: Angiogenesis and the Struggle to Defeat Cancer.* New York: Random House.

Coussens, Lisa M., and Zena Werb. 2002. "Inflammation and Cancer." *Nature* 420 (December 19–26): 860–67.

Coussens, Lisa, et al. 1985. "Tyrosine Kinase Receptor with Extensive Homology to EGF Receptor Shares Chromosomal Location with *neu* Oncogene." *Science* 230 (December 6): 1133–39.

Couzin, Jennifer, and Greg Miller. 2007. "Boom and Bust." *Science* 316 (April 20): 356–61.

Cragun, Janiel Marie. 2011. "Screening for Ovarian Cancer." *Cancer Control* 18 (January): 16–21.

Craver, Lloyd F. 1942. "Treatment of Leukemia by Radioactive Phosphorus." *Bulletin of the New York Academy of Medicine* 18 (April): 254–62.

Croce, Carlo M. 1986. "Chromosome Translocations and Human Cancer." *Cancer Research* 46: 6019–23.

Crow, James F., and William F. Dove. 1996. "Recollections of Howard Temin (1934–1994)." *Genetics* 144 (September): 1–6.

Crozier, Anna. 2007. *Practising Colonial Medicine: The Colonial Medical Service in British East Africa.* New York: I. B. Tauris.

Culliton, Barbara J. 1985a. "Who Runs NIH?" *Science* 227 (March 29): 1562–64.

———. 1985b. "NIH Bills Moving Through Congress." *Science* 229 (July 5): 3.

———. 1986. "Congress Boosts NIH Budget 17.3%." *Science* 234 (November 14): 808–9.

———. 1987. "GAO Report Angers Cancer Officials." *Science* 236 (April 24): 380–81.

———. 1988. "Hammer Seeks $1 Billion to Cure Cancer." *Science* 240 (April 1): 19.

Curt, Gregory A., Neil J. Clendeninn, and Bruce A. Chabner. 1984. "Drug Resistance in Cancer." *Cancer Treatment Reports* 68 (January): 87–99.

Curtin, Lester R. 1992. Office of Research and Methodology, National Center for Health Statistics. "A Short History of Standardization for Vital Events," edited by M. Feinleib and A. O. Zarate. In *Reconsidering Age Adjustment Procedures: Workshop Proceedings, Vital and Health Statistics* 4 (29): 11–16.

Curtin, Lester R., and Richard J. Klein. 1995. "Direct Standardization (Age-Adjusted Death Rates)." *Healthy People 2000 Statistical Notes* 6 (rev.) (March).

Cutler, David M., Allison B. Rosen, and Sandeep Vijan. 2006. "The Value of Medical Spending in the United States, 1960–2000." *New England Journal of Medicine* 355 (August 31): 920–27.

Daley, George Q., and David Baltimore. 1988. "Transformation of an Interleukin 3-Dependent Hematopoietic Cell Line by the Chronic Myelogenous Leukemia-Specific P210 bcr/abl Protein." *Proceedings of the National Academy of Sciences* 85 (December): 9312–16.

Daley, George Q., et al. 1987. "The CML-Specific P210 bcr-abl Protein, Unlike v-abl, Does Not Transform NIH/3T3 Fibroblasts." *Science* 237 (July 31): 532–35.

Daley, George Q., et al. 1990. "Induction of Chronic Myelogenous Leukemia in Mice by the P210 bcr/abl Gene of the Philadelphia Chromosome." *Science* 247 (February 16): 824–30.

Dalla-Favera, Riccardo, Marco Bregni, Jan Erikson, David Patterson, Robert C. Gallo, and Carlo Croce. 1982. "Human c-*myc onc* Gene Is Located on the Region of Chromosome 8 That Is Translocated in Burkitt Lymphoma Cells." *Proceedings of the National Academy of Sciences* 79 (December): 7824–27.

Dalla-Favera, Riccardo, et al. 1983. "Translocation and Rearrangements of the c-myc Oncogene Locus in Human Undifferentiated B-Cell Lymphomas." *Science* 219: 963–67.

Dalton, William S., and Stephen H. Friend. 2006. "Cancer Biomarkers: An Invitation to the Table." *Science* 312 (May 26): 1165–68.

Dameshek, William, et al. 1965. "Editorial: Therapy of Acute Leukemia, 1965." *Blood* 26 (August): 220–25.

Dana-Farber Cancer Institute. IRS Form 990 (Return of Organization Exempt from Income Tax) for the 2010 calendar year.

———. "Who Was Sidney Farber? Sidney Farber, MD. A Career in Cancer Research Driven by the Power of an Idea." Revised posting at http://www.dana -farber.org/About-Us/History-and-Milestones.aspx.

D'Angio, Giulio J. D. 1975. "Dr. Sidney Farber." Eulogy presented at the American Cancer Society's National Conference on Childhood Cancer, Dallas, TX, May 16–18, 1974. *Cancer* 35 (March supp.): 863–65.

Danovi, Safia Ali. 2008. "Finding the Needle in the Haystack." *Nature Reviews Cancer* 8 (September): 659.

Darlington, Cyril D. 1953. *The Facts of Life*. London: George Allen & Unwin.

Dashatwar, P. 2005. "Medical Philately: Dr. Yellapragada SubbaRow (1895–1948)." *Journal of the Association of Physicians of India* 53 (July): 652.

Dave, Sandeep S., et al. 2006. "Molecular Diagnosis of Burkitt's Lymphoma." *New England Journal of Medicine* 354 (June 8): 2431–42.

David, A. Rosalie, and Michael R. Zimmerman. 2010. "Cancer: An Old Disease, a New Disease or Something in Between?" *Nature Reviews Cancer* 10 (October): 728–33.

David, Eric, Tony Tramontin, and Rodney Zemmel. 2009. "The Road to Positive R&D Returns." *Nature Reviews Drug Discovery* 8 (August): 609–10.

Davies, J. N. P., Sally Elmes, M. S. R. Hutt, L. A. R. Mtimavalye, R. Owor, and Lorna Shaper. 1964. "Cancer in an African Community, 1897–1956. An Analysis of the Records of Mengo Hospital, Kampala, Uganda: Part I." *British Medical Journal* 1 (February 1): 259–64.

Davies, Kevin, and Michael White. 1996. *Breakthrough: The Race to Find the Breast Cancer Gene*. New York: John Wiley & Sons.

Davis, Alan C. 1996. "The Legislative Process of the National Cancer Act, 1970–71: Problems and Resolutions." *Cancer* 78 (December 15): 2585–89.

Davis, Devra. 2007a. *The Secret History of the War on Cancer*. New York: Basic Books.

———. 2007b. "Off Target in the War on Cancer." Op-ed. *Washington Post*, November 4.

Davis, Robert L., James B. Konopka, and Owen N. Witte. 1985. "Activation of the c-abl Oncogene by Viral Transduction or Chromosomal Translocation Generates Altered c-abl Proteins with Similar In Vitro Kinase Properties." *Molecular and Cellular Biology* 5 (January): 204–13.

Day, Nick E., Stephen Duffy, and Eugenio Paci, eds. 2005. "Overdiagnosis and Overtreatment of Breast Cancer." *Breast Cancer Research* (review series published online, August 25).

Dean, Michael, Tito Fojo, and Susan Bates. 2005. "Tumour Stem Cells and Drug Resistance." *Nature Reviews Cancer* 5 (April): 275–84.

de Caestecker, Mark P., et al. 2000. "Role of Transforming Growth Factor-β Signaling in Cancer." *Journal of the National Cancer Institute* 92 (September 6): 1388–1402.

de Duve, Christian. 1984. *A Guided Tour of the Living Cell*. New York: *Scientific American* in collaboration with Rockefeller University Press.

de Haen, Paul. 1976. "Compilation of New Drugs: 1940 thru 1975." *Pharmacy Times* 42 (March): 40–74.

————. 1983. *New Drug Parade: A Historical Mini-Review, 1954–1982.* Englewood, CO: Paul de Haen International. Presented as a poster exhibit at the 19th Annual Meeting of the Drug Information Association, July 28, 1983, Washington, DC.

Deininger, Michael, Elisabeth Buchdunger, and Brian J. Druker. 2005. "The Development of Imatinib as a Therapeutic Agent for Chronic Myeloid Leukemia." *Blood* 105 (April 1): 2640–53.

de Klein, Annelies, et al. 1982. "A Cellular Oncogene Is Translocated to the Philadelphia Chromosome in Chronic Myelocytic Leukaemia." *Nature* 300 (December 23): 765–67.

Del Giudice, Ilaria, et al. 2009. "Spontaneous Regression of Chronic Lymphocytic Leukemia: Clinical and Biologic Features of 9 Cases." *Blood* 114 (July 16): 638–46.

Delhalle, Sylvie, et al. 2004. "A Beginner's Guide to NF-kß Signaling Pathways." In Marc Diederich, ed., *Signal Transduction Pathways, Chromatin Structures, and Gene Expression Mechanisms as Therapeutic Target. Annals of the New York Academy of Sciences* 1030 (December): 1–13.

Denby, David. 2004. "The Life of the Party." *Fortune,* January 26.

DeRenzo, Evan G. 2000. "Coercion in the Recruitment and Retention of Human Research Subjects, Pharmaceutical Industry Payments to Physician–Investigators and the Moral Courage of the IRB." *IRB: A Review of Human Subjects Research* 22 (2) (March/April): 1–5.

Desdouits, Frédéric, et al. 2006. *Oncology Pipelines: Searching Is Not Finding.* Paris: Bionest Partners, Exane BNP Paribas, March.

de Solla Price, Derek John. 1963. *Little Science, Big Science.* New York: Columbia University Press.

————. 1975. *Science Since Babylon.* New Haven, CT: Yale University Press.

de-The, Guy, et al. 1978. "Epidemiological Evidence for Causal Relationship Between Epstein–Barr Virus and Burkitt's Lymphoma from Ugandan Prospective Study." *Nature* 274 (August 24): 756–61.

DeVita, Vincent T., Jr. 1987. "Cancer Data Defended." Letter to editor. *Science News* 131 (7) (February 14): 99, 109.

————. 1997. "The War on Cancer Has a Birthday, and a Present." *Journal of Clinical Oncology* 15 (March): 867–69.

————. 2003. "Hodgkin's Disease: Clinical Trials and Travails." *New England Journal of Medicine* 348 (June 12): 2375–76.

DeVita, Vincent T., Jr., and Edward Chu. 2008. "A History of Cancer Chemotherapy." *Cancer Research* 68 (November 1): 8643–53.

DeVita, Vincent T., Jr., and Susan Molloy Hubbard. 1993. "Hodgkin's Disease." *New England Journal of Medicine* 328 (February 25): 560–65.

DeVita, Vincent T., Jr., Arthur A. Serpick, and Paul P. Carbone. 1970. "Combination Chemotherapy in the Treatment of Advanced Hodgkin's Disease." *Annals of Internal Medicine* 73 (December 1): 881–95.

DeVita, Vincent T., Jr., et al. 1980. "Curability of Advanced Hodgkin's Disease with Chemotherapy: Long-Term Follow-Up of MOPP-Treated Patients at the National Cancer Institute." *Annals of Internal Medicine* 92 (May 1): 587–95.

Devitt, James E., and W. Gordon Beattie. 1964. "The Rational Treatment of Carcinoma of the Breast?" *Annals of Surgery* 160 (July): 71–80.

Diamandis, Eleftherios P. 2004. "Mass Spectrometry as a Diagnostic and a Cancer Biomarker Discovery Tool: Opportunities and Potential Limitations." *Molecular and Cellular Proteomics* 3.4 (April 1): 367–78.

Dick, John E. 2003. "Self-Renewal Writ in Blood." *Nature* 423 (May): 231–33.

Dickman, Paul W., and Hans-Olov Adami. 2006. "Interpreting Trends in Cancer Patient Survival." *Journal of Internal Medicine* 260 (August): 103–17.

Dietrich, Arne, and Narayanan Srinivasan. 2007. "The Optimal Age to Start a Revolution." *Journal of Creative Behavior* 41 (March): 54–74.

Dignam, James J. 2000. "Differences in Breast Cancer Prognosis Among African–American and Caucasian Women." *CA: A Cancer Journal for Clinicians* 50 (January–February): 50–64.

DiKötter, Frank. 1998. "Race Culture: Recent Perspectives on the History of Eugenics." *American Historical Review* 103 (April): 467–78.

Dilts, David M., Neil P. Boyd, and H. H. Whorms. 1991. "The Evolution of Control Architectures for Automated Manufacturing Systems." *Journal of Manufacturing Systems* 10: 79–93.

Dilts, David M., Alan B. Sandler, et al. 2006. "Processes to Activate Phase III Clinical Trials in a Cooperative Oncology Group: The Case of Cancer and Leukemia Group B." *Journal of Clinical Oncology* 24 (October 1): 4553–57.

Dilts, David M., Alan B. Sandler, et al. 2008. "Development of Clinical Trials in a Cooperative Group Setting: The Eastern Cooperative Oncology Group." *Clinical Cancer Research* 14 (June 1): 3427–33.

Dilts, David M., Alan B. Sandler, et al. 2009. "Steps and Time to Process Clinical Trials at the Cancer Therapy Evaluation Program." *Journal of Clinical Oncology* 27 (April 10): 1761–66.

Dilts, David M., et al. 2010. "Phase III Clinical Trial Development: A Process of Chutes and Ladders." *Clinical Cancer Research* 16 (November 15): 5381–89.

DiMasi, Joseph A. 2001. "New Drug Development in the United States from 1963 to 1999." *Clinical Pharmacology and Therapeutics* 69 (May): 286–96.

DiMasi, Joseph A., and Henry G. Grabowski. 2007. "Economics of New Oncology Drug Development." *Journal of Clinical Oncology* 25 (January 10): 209–16.

DiMasi, Joseph A., Ronald W. Hansen, and Henry G. Grabowski. 2003. "The Price of Innovation: New Estimates of Drug Development Costs." *Journal of Health Economics* 22 (March): 151–85.

Dingus, Lowell, and Mark A. Norell. 2007. "The Bone Collector." *Discover,* March.

Djerassi, Isaac, Sidney Farber, Esshagh Abir, and William Neikirk. 1967. "Continuous Infusion of Methotrexate in Children with Acute Leukemia." *Cancer* 20 (February): 233–42.

Dolberg, David S., and Mina J. Bissell. 1984. "Inability of Rous Sarcoma Virus to Cause Sarcomas in the Avian Embryo." *Nature* 309 (June 7): 552–56.

Dolberg, David S., et al. 1985. "Wounding and Its Role in RSV-Mediated Tumor Formation." *Science* 230 (November 8): 676–78.

Donati, Daria. 2005. "Malaria, B Lymphocytes and Epstein–Barr Virus: Emerging Concepts on Burkitt's Lymphoma Pathogenesis." Author's manuscript, from the Center for Infectious Medicine, Karolinska Institutet, Stockholm, Sweden (September).

Donegan, William L. 2006. "History of Breast Cancer." In *Breast Cancer,* 2nd ed., edited by David J. Winchester, et al., 1–14. Hamilton, ON, Canada: BC Decker.

Dores, Graca, et al. 2005. "Long-Term Cause-Specific Mortality Among 41,146 One-Year Survivors of Hodgkin Lymphoma (HL)." 2005 ASCO Annual Meeting, Abstract 6511. *Journal of Clinical Oncology* 23 (June 1 supp.): 6511.

Downs, Anthony. 1964. "Inside Bureaucracy." Essay. Retrieved from www.rand.org/pubs/papers/2008/P2963.pdf.

Dranoff, Glenn. 2004. "Cytokines in Cancer Pathogenesis and Cancer Therapy." *Nature Reviews Cancer* 4 (January): 11–22.

Druker, Brian J., and Nicholas B. Lydon. 2000. "Lessons Learned from the Development of an Abl Tyrosine Kinase Inhibitor for Chronic Myelogenous Leukemia." *Journal of Clinical Investigation* 105 (January): 3–7.

Druker, Brian J., et al. 2001a. "Activity of a Specific Inhibitor of the BCR-ABL Tyrosine Kinase in the Blast Crisis of Chronic Myeloid Leukemia and Acute Lymphoblastic Leukemia with the Philadelphia Chromosome." *New England Journal of Medicine* 344 (April 5): 1038–42.

Druker, Brian J., et al. 2001b. "Efficacy and Safety of a Specific Inhibitor of the BCR-ABL Tyrosine Kinase in Chronic Myeloid Leukemia." *New England Journal of Medicine* 344 (April 5): 1031–37.

Du Bois, W. E. Burghardt. 1897. "Race Traits and Tendencies of the American Negro. By Frederick L. Hoffman, F.S.S." Review. *Annals of the American Academy of Political and Social Science* 9: 127–33. Available online at Google Books.

Du Bois, W. E. Burghardt, ed. 1906. *The Health and Physique of the Negro American.* Atlanta, GA: Atlanta University Press. Excerpted in *American Journal of Public Health* 93 (2) (February 2003): 272–76.

Dueñas-González, Alfonso, et al. 2005. "Epigenetics of Cervical Cancer. An Overview and Therapeutic Perspectives." *Molecular Cancer* 4 (October 25): 38.

Duenwald, Mary, and Denise Grady. 2003. "Young Survivors of Cancer Battle Effects of Treatment." *New York Times,* January 8.

Dupree, A. Hunter. 1986. *Science in the Federal Government: A History of Policies and Activities.* Baltimore: Johns Hopkins University Press. Originally published in 1957 by Harvard University Press.

Dvorak, Harold F. 1986. "Tumors: Wounds That Do Not Heal." *New England Journal of Medicine (Seminars in Medicine of the Beth Israel Hospital, Boston)* 315 (December 25): 1650–59.

Dvorak, Harold F., et al. 1995. "Vascular Permeability Factor, Vascular Endothelial Growth Factor, Microvascular Hyperpermeability, and Angiogenesis." *American Journal of Pathology* 146 (May): 1029–39.

Dy, Grace K., and Alex A. Adjei. 2008. "Systemic Cancer Therapy: Evolution over the Last 60 Years." *Cancer* 113 (supp. 7): 1857–87.

Eastman, Peggy. 2004. "Health Officials Defend Ambitious New US Cancer-Reduction Goals." *Oncology Times,* March 25.

Editors. 2004. "Pazdur's Revenge." Editorial. *Wall Street Journal,* December 20.

———. 2005a. "How About a 'Kianna's Legacy'?" Editorial. *Wall Street Journal,* March 24.

———. 2005b. "Kianna's Legacy—II." Editorial. *Wall Street Journal,* December 23.

———. 2007. "Cancer on the Run." *New York Daily News,* January 18.

Editors of *Fortune.* 1962. *The Space Industry: America's Newest Giant.* Englewood Cliffs, NJ: Prentice-Hall.

Edwards, Brenda K., et al. 2010. "Annual Report to the Nation on the Status of Cancer, 1975–2006." *Cancer* 116 (February 1): 544–73.

Eichenwald, Kurt, and Gina Kolata. 1999. "Drug Trials Hide Conflicts for Doctors." *New York Times,* May 16.

Einhorn, Nina, et al. 1992. "Prospective Evaluation of Serum CA 125 Levels for Early Detection of Ovarian Cancer." *Obstetrics and Gynecology* 80 (July): 14–18.

Eiseman, Elisa, Gabrielle Bloom, Jennifer Brower, Noreen Clancy, and Stuart S. Olmsted. 2003. *Case Studies of Existing Human Tissue Repositories: "Best Practices" for a Biospecimen Resource for the Genomic and Proteomic Era.* Prepared for the National Cancer Institute and the National Dialogue on Cancer. Santa Monica, CA: RAND Science and Technology.

Eisen, Andrea, and Barbara L. Weber. 1999. "Prophylactic Mastectomy—the Price of Fear." *New England Journal of Medicine* 340 (January 14): 137–38.

Ekena, Kirk, John A. Katzenellenbogen, and Benita S. Katzenellenbogen. 1998. "Determinants of Ligand Specificity of Estrogen Receptor-α: Estrogen Versus Androgen Discrimination." *Journal of Biological Chemistry* 273 (January 9): 693–99.

Elandt-Johnson, Regina C. 1975. "Definition of Rates: Some Remarks on Their Use and Misuse." *American Journal of Epidemiology* 102 (4) (October): 267–71.

El-Deiry, Wafik S., ed. 2005. "Tumor Progression and Therapeutic Resistance." *Annals of the New York Academy of Sciences* 1059 (November): 1–195.

Eli Lilly Prevention Task Force. 2005. Indianapolis, IN. January 10–11.

Elion, Gertrude B. 1988. "The Purine Path to Chemotherapy." Nobel Lecture, the Nobel Prize in Physiology or Medicine, 1988 (December 8). Retrieved from http://www.nobelprize.org/nobel_prizes/medicine/laureates/1988/elion–lecture.html.

Elkin, Elena B., et al. 2005. "The Effect of Changes in Tumor Size on Breast Carcinoma Survival in the United States: 1975–1999." *Cancer* 104 (September 15): 1149–57.

Emanuel, Ezekiel J., et al. 2013. "A Plan to Fix Cancer Care." *New York Times,* March 24.

Endicott, Kenneth M. 1957. "The Chemotherapy Program." *Journal of the National Cancer Institute* 19 (August 2): 283.

English, Rebecca, Yeonwoo Lebovitz, and Robert Giffin. 2010. Institute of Medicine. *Transforming Clinical Research in the United States: Challenges and Opportunities, Workshop Summary.* Washington, DC: National Academies Press.

Epstein, M. A. 1956. "The Identification of the Rous Virus; A Morphological and Biological Study." *British Journal of Cancer* 10 (March): 33–48.

———. 1957. "Observations on the Rous Virus; Fine Structure and Relation to Cytoplasmic Vacuoles." *British Journal of Cancer* 11 (June): 268–73.

———. 1964. "Cultivation In Vitro of Human Lymphoblasts from Burkitt's Malignant Lymphoma." *Lancet* 283 (February 1): 252–53.

———. 1979. "Citation Classic: Virus Particles in Cultured Lymphoblasts from Burkitt's Lymphoma." *Current Contents/Life Sciences* 14 (April 2): 156.

Epstein, M. A., Bert G. Achong, and Yvonne M. Barr. 1964. "Virus Particles in Cultured Lymphoblasts from Burkitt's Lymphoma." *Lancet* 283 (March 28): 702–3.

Epstein, Sir Anthony, and M. A. Eastwood. 1995. "Denis Parsons Burkitt. 28 February 1911–23 March 1993." *Biographical Memoirs of Fellows of the Royal Society* 41 (November): 88–102.

Epstein, M. A., et al. 1965. "Morphological and Biological Studies on a Virus in Cultured Lymphoblasts from Burkitt's Lymphoma." *Journal of Experimental Medicine* 121 (May 1): 761–70.

Epstein, M. A. et al. 1985. "Historical Background: Burkitt's Lymphoma and Epstein–Barr Virus." In *Burkitt's Lymphoma: A Human Cancer Model,* edited by G. Lenoir, G. O'Conor, and C. L. Olweny, 17–27. International Agency for Research on Cancer (IARC) Scientific Publications 60.

Erikson, Jan, et al. 1986. "Heterogeneity of Chromosome 22 Breakpoint in Philadelphia-Positive (Ph¹) Acute Lymphocytic Leukemia." *Proceedings of the National Academy of Sciences* 83 (March): 1807–11.

Ernster, Virginia L., et al. 2002. "Detection of Ductal Carcinoma In Situ in Women Undergoing Screening Mammography." *Journal of the National Cancer Institute* 94 (October 16): 1546–54.

Escalon, Enrique A. 1999. "Acute Lymphocytic Leukemia in Childhood." *International Pediatrics* 14: 83–89.

Espey, David K., et al. 2007. "Annual Report to the Nation on the Status of Cancer, 1975–2004, Featuring Cancer in American Indians and Alaska Natives." *Cancer* 110 (November 15): 2120.

Etzioni, Ruth, et al. 2003. "The Case for Early Detection." *Nature Reviews Cancer* 3 (April): 1–10.

Faça, Vitor M., and Samir M. Hanash. 2009. "In–Depth Proteomics to Define the Cell Surface and Secretome of Ovarian Cancer Cells and Processes of Protein Shedding." *Cancer Research* 69 (February 1): 728–30.

Faça, Vitor M., et al. 2008. "Proteomic Analysis of Ovarian Cancer Cells Reveals Dynamic Processes of Protein Secretion and Shedding of Extra-Cellular Domains." *PLOS ONE* 3 (June 18): e2425.

Faguet, Guy B. 2005. *The War on Cancer: An Anatomy of Failure, a Blueprint for the Future.* Dordrecht, The Netherlands: Springer.

Fairchild, A. L., and G. M. Oppenheimer. 1998. "Public Health Nihilism vs. Pragmatism: History, Politics, and the Control of Tuberculosis." *American Journal of Public Health* 88 (July): 1105–17.

Fanibunda, K., and J. N. S. Matthews. 1999. "Relationship Between Accessory Foramina and Tumour Spread in the Lateral Mandibular Surface." *Journal of Anatomy* 195 (August): 185–90.

Farber, Emmanuel. 1984. "Cellular Biochemistry of the Stepwise Development of Cancer with Chemicals: G. H. A. Clowes Memorial Lecture." *Cancer Research* 44 (December): 5463–74.

Farber, Emmanuel, and Ross Cameron. 1980. "The Sequential Analysis of Cancer Development." *Advances in Cancer Research* 31: 125–26.

Farber, Sidney. 1949. "Some Observations on the Effect of Folic Acid Antagonists on Acute Leukemia and Other Forms of Incurable Cancer." *Blood* 4 (February 1): 160–67.

Farber, Sidney, Louis K. Diamond, Robert D. Mercer, Robert F. Sylvester, Jr., and James A. Wolff. 1948. "Temporary Remissions in Acute Leukemia in Children Produced by Folic Acid Antagonist, 4-Aminoptenyl-Glutamic Acid (Aminopterin)." *New England Journal of Medicine* 238 (June 3): 787–93.

Farber, Sidney, Rudolf Toch, Edward Manning Sears, and Donald Pinkel. 1956. "Advances in Chemotherapy of Cancer in Man." *Advances in Cancer Research* 4: 1–71.

Faust, Halley S., and Paul T. Menzel. 2012. *Prevention vs. Treatment: What's the Right Balance?* Oxford: Oxford University Press.

Fearon, Eric, and Bert Vogelstein. 1990. "A Genetic Model for Colorectal Tumorigenesis." *Cell* 61 (June 1): 759–67.

Federal Interagency Forum on Aging-Related Statistics. 2011. *Older Americans 2010: Key Indicators of Well-Being.* Revised January 2011. http://www.agingstats .gov/Agingstatsdotnet/Main_Site/Default.aspx.

Feinstein, Alvan R., et al. 1985. "The Will Rogers Phenomenon: Stage Migration and New Diagnostic Techniques as a Source of Misleading Statistics for Survival in Cancer." *New England Journal of Medicine* 312 (June 20): 1604–8.

Fenstermacher, David, et al. 2005. The Cancer Biomedical Informatics Grid (caBIG™), Engineering in Medicine and Biology 27th Annual Conference, Shanghai, China, September 1–4, 2005. Published in *Proceedings of the 2005 IEEE,* 743–46.

Ferrara, Napoleone, Kenneth J.Hillan, Hans-Peter Gerber, and William Novotny. 2004. "Discovery and Development of Bevacizumab, an Anti-VEGF Antibody for Treating Cancer." *Nature Reviews Drug Discovery* 3 (May): 391–400.

Ferris, Lorraine E., and C. David Naylor. 2004. "Physician Remuneration in Industry-Sponsored Clinical Trials: The Case for Standardized Clinical Trial Budgets." *Canadian Medical Association Journal* 171 (October 12): 883–86.

Feyerabend, Paul. 2010. *Against Method.* 4th ed. Introduced by Ian Hacking. London: Verso. Originally published in 1975 by New Left Books.

Fidler, Isaiah J., 1990. "Critical Factors in the Biology of Human Cancer Metastasis: Twenty-Eighth G. H. A. Clowes Memorial Award Lecture." *Cancer Research* 50 (October 1): 6130–38.

———. 2003. "The Pathogenesis of Cancer Metastasis: The 'Seed and Soil' Hypothesis Revisited." *Nature Reviews Cancer* 3 (June): 453–548.

Fidler, Isaiah J., Douglas M. Gersten, and Ian R. Hart. 1978. "The Biology of Cancer Invasion and Metastasis." *Advances in Cancer Research* 28: 149–250.

Fildes, Paul. 1940. "A Rational Approach to Research in Chemotherapy." *Lancet* 235 (May 25): 955–57.

Finch, Clement A., et al. 1977. "Kinetics of the Formed Elements of Human Blood." *Blood* (October 1) 50: 699–707.

Fireman, Bruce H., et al. 1997. "Cost of Care for Cancer in a Health Maintenance Organization." *Health Care Financing Review* 18 (Summer): 51–76.

Fisk, Nicholas M., and Rifat Atun. 2008. "Market Failure and the Poverty of New Drugs in Maternal Health." *PLOS Medicine* 5 (1) (January): e22–e28.

Fleskens, Stijn, and Piet Slootweg. 2009. "Grading Systems in Head and Neck Dysplasia: Their Prognostic Value, Weaknesses and Utility." *Head and Neck Oncology* 1 (May 11): 11.

Fletcher, Jamie I., et al. 2010. "ABC Transporters in Cancer: More Than Just Drug Efflux Pumps." *Nature Reviews Cancer* 10 (February): 147–56.

Flintoft, Louisa. 2009. "Putting Epigenetic Variation on the Map." *Nature Reviews Genetics* 10 (October): 663.

Fliss, Makiko S., et al. 2000. "Facile Detection of Mitochondrial DNA Mutations in Tumors and Bodily Fluids." *Science* 287 (March 17): 2017–19.

Flook, Bill. 2012. "Food and Drug Administration Chief Margaret Hamburg Touts Changes to Speed Up Drug Reviews." *Washington Business Journal,* February 17.

Föller, Michael. 2008. "Erythrocyte Programmed Cell Death." *IUBMB Life* 60 (October): 661–68.

Food and Drug Administration. 2001. Approval letter (NDA 21-335), dated May 10, to Robert A. Miranda, Novartis Pharmaceuticals Corporation, from Robert Temple, Office of Drug Evaluation.

———. 2004a. "FDA Approves First Angiogenesis Inhibitor to Treat Colorectal Cancer." FDA news release. February 26.

———. 2004b. US Department of Health and Human Services. "Innovation or Stagnation? Challenge and Opportunity on the Critical Path to New Medical Products." March.

———. 2007. "Warnings for Sleeping Pills." *FDA Patient Safety News,* Show #63. May.

———. 2008. Oncologic Drugs Advisory Committee (ODAC), December 16 meeting. Transcript available at http://www.fda.gov/ohrms/dockets/ac/cder08 .html.

———. 2011a. "FDA Commissioner Removes Breast Cancer Indication from Avastin Label." FDA news release. November 18. http://www.fda.gov/NewsEvents/ Newsroom/ucm279485.htm.

———. 2011b. "Questions and Answers: Removing Metastatic Breast Cancer as an Indication from Avastin's Product Labeling." http://www.fda.gov/NewsEvents/ Newsroom/ucm280533.htm.

———. Drugs@FDA. http://www.accessdata.fda.gov/scripts/cder/drugsatfda/index .cfm.

———. "List of Approved Oncology Drugs with Approved Indications." http:// www.accessdata.fda.gov/scripts/cder/onctools/druglist.cfm.

———. "NME Drug and New Biologic Approvals." Retrieved from FDA website for each year. http://www.fda.gov/Drugs/DevelopmentApprovalProcess/HowDrugs areDevelopedandApproved/DrugandBiologicApprovalReports/ucm121136.htm.

————. "Summary of NDA Approvals and Receipts, 1938 to the Present." Retrieved March 9, 2012. http://www.fda.gov/AboutFDA/WhatWeDo/History/Product Regulation/SummaryofNDAApprovalsReceipts1938tothepresent/default.htm.

Foti, Margaret. 2005. American Association for Cancer Research. Written Testimony Submitted to US House and Senate Appropriations Committees. April 15.

————. 2011. Written testimony from the American Association for Cancer Research (AACR) submitted to US House and Senate Appropriations Committees. April 15 (regarding fiscal year 2012 federal budget).

Foulds, Leslie. 1969. *Neoplastic Development.* Vol. 1. London: Academic Press, 266–72.

Franco, Rodrigo, et al. 2008. "Oxidative Stress, DNA Methylation and Carcinogenesis." *Cancer Letters* 266 (July): 6–11.

Franko, Maryrose, and Martin Ionescu-Pioggia. 2006. *Making the Right Moves: A Practical Guide to Scientific Management for Postdocs and New Faculty* (Based on the BWF-HHMI Course in Scientific Management for the Beginning Academic Investigator). 2nd ed. Research Triangle Park, NC: Burroughs Wellcome Fund; and Chevy Chase, MD: Howard Hughes Medical Institute.

Frasor, Jonna, et al. 2003. "Profiling of Estrogen Up- and Down–Regulated Gene Expression in Human Breast Cancer Cells: Insights into Gene Networks and Pathways Underlying Estrogenic Control of Proliferation and Cell Phenotype." *Endocrinology* 144 (October): 4562–74.

Fredrickson, Donald S. 1993. "Biomedical Science and the Culture Warp." In *Emerging Policies for Biomedical Research,* edited by William N. Kelley, Marian Osterweis, and Elaine Rhea Rubin, 1–42. Washington, DC: Association of Academic Health Centers.

Freeman, Chris, and Luc Soete. 1999. *The Economics of Industrial Innovation.* 3rd ed. Cambridge, MA: MIT Press.

Freemantle, Nick, and Thomas Strack. 2010. "Real-World Effectiveness of New Medicines Should Be Evaluated by Appropriately Designed Clinical Trials." *Journal of Clinical Epidemiology* 63 (October): 1053–58.

Frei, Emil, III. 1972. "Combination Cancer Therapy: Presidential Address." *Cancer Research* 32 (December): 2593–607.

————. 1997. "Confrontation, Passion, and Personalization: Emil J. Freireich." *Clinical Cancer Research* 3 (December): 2554–62.

Frei, Emil, III, and Emil J. Freireich. 1965. "Progress and Perspectives in the Chemotherapy of Acute Leukemia." *Advances in Chemotherapy* 2: 269–98.

Frei, Emil, III, Emil J. Freireich, Edmund Gehan, Donald Pinkel, James F. Holland, et al. 1961. "Studies of Sequential and Combination Antimetabolite Therapy in Acute Leukemia: 6-Mercaptopurine and Methotrexate: From the Acute Leukemia Group." *Blood* 18 (October 1): 431–54.

Frei, Emil, III, and Stephen E. Sallan. 1978. "Acute Lymphoblastic Leukemia: Treatment." *Cancer* 42 (S2) (August): 828–38.

Frei, Emil, III, et al. 1958. "A Comparative Study of Two Regimens of Combination." *Blood* 13 (December 1): 1126–48.

Frei, Emil, III, et al. 1965a. "The Nature and Control of Infections in Patients with Acute Leukemia." *Cancer Research* 25 (October): 1511–15.

Frei, Emil, III, et al. 1965b. "The Effectiveness of Combinations of Antileukemic Agents in Inducing and Maintaining Remission in Children with Acute Leukemia." *Blood* 26 (November 1): 642–56.

Freireich, Emil J., and Emil Frei III. 1964. "Recent Advances in Acute Leukemia." In *Progress in Hematology,* vol. 4, edited by Carl V. Moore and Elmer B. Brown, 187–202. New York: Grune and Stratton.

Freireich, Emil J., Myron Karon, and Emil Frei III. 1964. "Quadruple Combination Therapy (VAMP) for Acute Lymphocytic Leukemia of Childhood." *Proceedings of the American Association for Cancer Research* 5: 20.

Freireich, Emil J., Paul J. Schmidt, Marvin A. Schneiderman, and Emil Frei. 1959. "A Comparative Study of the Effect of Transfusion of Fresh and Preserved Whole Blood on Bleeding in Patients with Acute Leukemia." *New England Journal of Medicine* 260 (January 1): 6–11.

Friede, Andrew, Ruth Grossman, Rachel Hunt, Rose Maria Li, and Susan Stern, eds. 2003. National Biospecimen Network Blueprint (Constella Group).

Friedman, Herman P., and Judith D. Goldberg. 1996. "Meta-analysis: An Introduction and Point of View." *Hepatology* 23 (April): 917–28.

Friend, Tim. 2003. "Cancer Deaths Decline." *USA Today,* September 3.

Friendly, Jock. 1996. "Judge Dismisses Suit Against Stanford." *Science* 273 (September 13): 1488.

Friends of Cancer Research. 2004. "From Bench to Bedside: Defeating Cancer Through Prevention and Early Detection." FOCR Congressional briefing, Russell Senate Office Building, July 13.

Galli-Stampino, Luisa, et al. 1997. "T-Cell Recognition of Tumor-Associated Carbohydrates: The Nature of the Glycan Moiety Plays a Decisive Role in Determining Glycopeptide Immunogenicity." *Cancer Research* 57 (August 1): 3214–22.

Gallup, George H. 1972. Gallup Poll on "Scientific Progress," December 23, 1949. In *The Gallup Poll, Public Opinion 1935–1971, Volume III, 1959–1971,* edited by George H. Gallup, American Institute of Public Opinion. New York: Random House.

Galper, Shira L., et al. 2006. "Evidence to Support a Continued Stage Migration and Decrease in Prostate Cancer Specific Mortality." *Journal of Urology* 175 (March): 907–12.

Galton, D. A. G., et al. 1961. "The Use of Chlorambucil and Steroids in the Treatment of Chronic Lymphocytic Leukaemia." *British Journal of Haematology* 7: 73–98.

Gal-Yam, Einav Nili, et al. 2008. "Cancer Epigenetics: Modifications, Screening, and Therapy." *Annual Review of Medicine* 59: 267–80.

Garber, Ken. 2007. "The Fragile Tumor: New Insights into Oncogene Addiction Found." *Journal of the National Cancer Institute* 99 (February 21): 264–69.

Garfield, Eugene. 2005. "The Agony and the Ecstasy: The History and Meaning of the Journal Impact Factor." Presentation at International Congress on Peer Review and Biomedical Publication, Chicago, September 16. http://garfield.library .upenn.edu/papers/jifchicago2005.pdf.

Garg, Ravin J., et al. 2009. "The Use of Nilotinib or Dasatinib After Failure to 2 Prior Tyrosine Kinase Inhibitors: Long-Term Follow-Up." *Blood* 114 (November 12): 4361–68.

Garrett, Laurie. 2000. *Betrayal of Trust: The Collapse of Global Public Health.* New York: Hyperion.

Garrett, Reginald H., and Charles M. Grisham, eds. 2012. *Biochemistry.* 5th ed. Boston: Brooks/Cole, Cengage Learning.

Gartler, Stanley M. 2006. "The Chromosome Number in Humans: A Brief History." *Nature Reviews Genetics* 7: 655–60.

Gaydos, Lawrence A., Emil J. Freireich, and Nathan Mantel. 1962. "The Quantitative Relation Between Platelet Count and Hemorrhage in Patients with Acute Leukemia." *New England Journal of Medicine* 266 (May 3): 905–9.

Gaynon, Paul S., Michael E. Trigg, and Faith M. Uckun. 2000. "Childhood Acute Lymphoblastic Leukemia." In *Holland-Frei Cancer Medicine*, 5th ed., edited by Robert C. Bast Jr., et al., 2140–50. Hamilton, ON, Canada: BC Decker.

Geenen, Maud M., et al. 2007. "Medical Assessment of Adverse Health Outcomes in Long-Term Survivors of Childhood Cancer." *Journal of the American Medical Association* 297 (June 27): 2705–15.

Gehan, Edmund A., and Emil J. Freireich. 1974. "Non–randomized Controls in Cancer Clinical Trials." *New England Journal of Medicine* 290 (January 24): 198–203.

Genestra, Marcelo. 2007. "Oxyl Radicals, Redox-Sensitive Signalling Cascades and Antioxidants." *Cellular Signalling* 19: 1807–19.

Gennaioli, Nicola, and Ilia Rainer. 2005. "The Modern Impact of Precolonial Centralization in Africa" (November). Retrieved from Social Science Research Network (SSRN): http://ssrn.com/abstract=848164.

Gerlinger, Marco, et al. 2012. "Intratumor Heterogeneity and Branched Evolution Revealed by Multiregion Sequencing." *New England Journal of Medicine* 366 (March 8): 883–92.

German, James. 2004. "Constitutional Hyperrecombinability and Its Consequences." *Genetics* 168 (September): 1–8.

Getz, Kenneth A. 2012. "Clinical Trial Complexity." Presentation at 48th Annual Meeting of the Drug Information Association in Philadelphia, June 26 (posted online, November).

Getz, Kenneth A., Rafael A. Campo, and Kenneth I. Kaitin. 2011. "Variability in Protocol Design Complexity by Phase and Therapeutic Area." *Drug Information Journal* 45: 413–20.

Getz, Kenneth A., and John R. Vogel. 2009. "Successful Outsourcing: Tracking Global CRO Usage." *Applied Clinical Trials Online,* August 17.

Getz, Kenneth A., et al. 2008. "Assessing the Impact of Protocol Design Changes on Clinical Trial Performance." *American Journal of Therapeutics* 15 (September/October): 450–57.

Giaccone, Giuseppe, and Jose Antonio Rodriguez. 2005. "EGFR Inhibitors: What Have We Learned from the Treatment of Lung Cancer?" *Nature Clinical Practice Oncology* 2 (11): 554–61.

Gibbs, W. Wayt. 2003. "Untangling the Roots of Cancer." *Scientific American* (July).

Gilchrist, Harry L., ed. 1940. *Military Surgeon: Journal of the Association of Military Surgeons of the United States.* Vols. 86–87. Carlisle, PA: The Association.

Gillies, Robert J., Daniel Verduzco, and Robert A. Gatenby. 2012. "Evolutionary Dynamics of Carcinogenesis and Why Targeted Therapy Does Not Work." *Nature Reviews Cancer* 12 (July): 487–93.

Gilman, Alfred. 1963. "The Initial Clinical Trial of Nitrogen Mustard." *American Journal of Surgery* 105 (May): 574–78.

Gilman, Alfred, and Frederick S. Philips. 1946. "The Biological Actions and Therapeutic Applications of the B-Chloroethyl Amines and Sulfides." *Science* 103 (April 5): 409–15.

Giordano, Sharon H., et al. 2004. "Is Breast Cancer Survival Improving? Trends in Survival for Patients with Recurrent Breast Cancer Diagnosed from 1974 Through 2000." *Cancer* 100 (January 1): 44–52.

Glaspy, John A., et al. 2009. "Erythropoietin in Cancer Patients." *Annual Review of Medicine* 60: 181–92.

Glaspy, John A., et al. 2010. "Erythropoiesis-Stimulating Agents in Oncology: A Study-Level Meta-analysis of Survival and Other Safety Outcomes." *British Journal of Cancer* 102: 301–15.

Glassberg, Helene, and Daniel J. Rader. 2008. "Management of Lipids in the Prevention of Cardiovascular Events." *Annual Review of Medicine* 59 (February): 79–94.

Glassman, Cynthia A. 2003. SEC Commissioner. "Financial Reform: Relevance and Reality in Financial Reporting." Speech delivered at National Association for Business Economics, Atlanta, September 16.

Gleick, James. 1993. "The Telephone Transformed—Into Almost Everything." *New York Times Magazine,* May 16.

Glemser, Bernard. 1970. *Mr. Burkitt and Africa.* Cleveland: World Publishing Company.

Glickman, Seth W., et al. 2009. "Ethical and Scientific Implications of the Globalization of Clinical Research." *New England Journal of Medicine* 360 (February 19): 816–23.

Goetz, Mario E., and Andreas Luch. 2008. "Reactive Species: A Cell-Damaging Rout Assisting to Chemical Carcinogens." *Cancer Letters* 266 (July): 73–83.

Goetz, Thomas. 2009. "Cancer and the New Science of Early Detection." *Wired,* January, 80ff.

Goff, Stephen P., et al. 1980. "Structure of the Abelson Murine Leukemia Virus Genome and the Homologous Cellular Gene: Studies with Cloned Viral DNA." *Cell* 22 (December): 777–85.

Goldberg, Kirsten Boyd. 2006. *Cancer Letter* (April 7): 2.

———. 2009. "NCI Raises R01 Payline to 16th Percentile for Fiscal 2009, up from 12th Last Year." *Cancer Letter* 35 (12) (March 27): 1–2.

Goldberg, Paul. 2002. *Cancer Letter,* see January 4 issue and related coverage in subsequent issues.

———. 2011. "Eight Years Too Late? Scrutiny of caBIG Exposes Conflicts, Bonanza for Contractors." *Cancer Letter* 37 (March 18): 1–7.

Goldman, Charles A., et al. 2000. *Paying for University Research Facilities and Administration.* Santa Monica: RAND Corporation.

Goodman, Alice. 2006. "Sky-High Costs for New Drugs: Weighing Enormous Expenses Against Tiny Extensions of Life." *Oncology Times,* June 10.

Goodman, Gary E., Mark D. Thornquist, Cim Edelstein, et al. 2006. "Biorepositories: Let's Not Lose What We Have So Carefully Gathered!" *Cancer Epidemiology, Biomarkers, and Prevention* 15 (April): 599–601.

Goodsell, David S. 1998. *The Machinery of Life.* New York: Springer-Verlag.

Gordian, Maria A., Navjot Singh, and Rodney W. Zemmel. 2006. "Why Drugs Fall Short in Late-Stage Trials." *McKinsey Quarterly,* November.

Gorlick, Richard, et al. 1996. "Intrinsic and Acquired Resistance to Methotrexate in Acute Leukemia." *New England Journal of Medicine* 335 (October 3): 1041–48.

Gormally, Emmanuelle, et al. 2007. "Circulating Free DNA in Plasma or Serum as Biomarker of Carcinogenesis: Practical Aspects and Biological Significance." *Mutation Research* 635 (May–June): 105–17.

Gorre, Mercedes E., et al. 2001. "Clinical Resistance to STI-571 Cancer Therapy Caused by BCR-ABL Gene Mutation or Amplification." *Science* 293 (August 3): 876–80.

Gortzak-Uzan, Limor, et al. 2008. "A Proteome Resource of Ovarian Cancer Ascites: Integrated Proteomic and Bioinformatic Analyses to Identify Putative Biomarkers." *Journal of Proteome Research* 7 (January): 339–51.

Gould, Stephen Jay. 2002. *The Structure of Evolutionary Theory.* Cambridge, MA: Belknap Press of the Harvard University Press.

Gould, Stephen Jay, and Niles Eldredge. 1986. "Punctuated Equilibrium at the Third Stage." *Systematic Zoology* 35 (1) (March): 143–48.

Govindan, Ramaswamy. 2007. "Phase III Failure Rates in Oncology Drugs Unacceptable." *Oncology News International* 16 (August 1).

Grabowski, Henry G., and Jeffrey L. Moe. 2008. "Impact of Economic, Regulatory and Patent Policies on Innovation in Cancer Chemoprevention." *Cancer Prevention Research* 1 (July): 84–90.

Grady, Denise. 2003. "A Conversation With: Elias Zerhouni; Learning the Science of Leading." *New York Times,* July 15.

Gratzer, Walter. 2002. *Eurekas and Euphorias: The Oxford Book of Scientific Anecdotes.* Oxford: Oxford University Press.

Graves, Theresa A., and Kirby I. Bland. 2009. "Carcinoma In Situ of the Breast: Ductal and Lobular Origin." In *General Surgery: Principles and International Practice,* 2nd ed., edited by Kirby I. Bland et al., 1509–21. New York: Springer.

Gray, Richard, et al. 2000. Correspondence related to the QUASAR Collaborative Group. *Lancet* 356 (October): 1276.

Greaves, Mel. 2007. "Darwinian Medicine: A Case for Cancer." *Nature Reviews Cancer* 7 (March): 213–21.

Greaves, Mel F., ed. 2008. *White Blood: Personal Journeys with Childhood Leukaemia.* Singapore: World Scientific.

Green, Lee A., et al. 2006. "Impact of Institutional Review Board Practice Variation on Observational Health Services Research." *Health Services Research* 41 (February): 214–30.

Green, Mark R. 2004. "Editorial: Targeting Targeted Therapy." *New England Journal of Medicine* 350 (May 20): 2191–93.

Greenfield, D. M., et al. 2006. "High Incidence of Late Effects Found in Hodgkin's Lymphoma Survivors, Following Recall for Breast Cancer Screening." *British Journal of Cancer* 94 (February 27): 469–72.

Greenlee, Robert T., et al. 2000. "Cancer Statistics, 2000" *CA: A Cancer Journal for Clinicians* 50 (January–February): 7–33.

Greenwald, Peter, and E. J. Sondik. 1986. *Cancer Control Objectives for the Nation: 1985–2000.* NCI Monographs No. 2, US Department of Health and Human Services.

Greenwood, Addison. 2007. "CA125: Biography of an Ovarian Biomarker." *NCI Cancer Bulletin* 4 (January 30): 5.

Groffen, John, et al. 1984. "Philadelphia Chromosomal Breakpoints Are Clustered Within a Limited Region, bcr, on Chromosome 22." *Cell* 36 (January): 93–99.

Groopman, Jerome. 2001. "The Thirty Years' War." *New Yorker,* June 4, 52–63.

———. 2008. "Buying a Cure: What Business Know-How Can Do for Disease." *New Yorker,* January 28, 38–43.

Gross, Ludwik. 1974a. "The Role of Viruses in the Etiology of Cancer and Leukemia in Animals and in Humans." *Proceedings of the National Academy of Sciences* 94 (April): 4237–38.

———. 1974b. "Facts and Theories on Viruses Causing Cancer and Leukemia." *Proceedings of the National Academy of Sciences* 71 (May): 2013–17.

Grosse, Yann, et al. 2009. "Special Report: Policy. A Review of Human Carcinogens— Part A: Pharmaceuticals." *Lancet Oncology* 10 (January): 13–14.

Grove, Andrew S. 1996. "Taking on Prostate Cancer." *Fortune,* May 13.

———. 1999. *Only the Paranoid Survive.* New York: Doubleday. Originally published in 1996.

Gupta, Udayan, ed. 2000. *Done Deals: Venture Capitalists Tell Their Stories.* Cambridge, MA: Harvard Business School Press, 95–100.

Haddow, Alexander. 1970. "David A. Karnofsky Memorial Lecture: Thoughts on Chemical Therapy." *Cancer* 26 (October): 737–54.

———. 1973. "Molecular Repair, Wound Healing, and Carcinogenesis: Tumor Production a Possible Overhealing?" *Advances in Cancer Research* 16: 181–234.

———. 1974. "Addendum to 'Molecular Repair, Wound Healing, and Carcinogenesis: Tumor Production a Possible Overhealing?'" *Advances in Cancer Research* 20: 343–66.

Hahn, William C., and Robert A. Weinberg. 2002. "Modeling the Molecular Circuitry of Cancer." *Nature Reviews Cancer* 2 (May): 331–41. Accompanying the paper was a poster designed by artist Claudia Bentley, "A Subway Map of Cancer Pathways." The poster, now interactive, can be retrieved at the *Nature* website, http://www.nature.com/nrc/journal/v2/n5/weinberg_poster/index.html.

Hall, Joseph Lorenzo. 2003. "Columbia and Challenger: Organizational Failure at NASA." *Space Policy* 19 (November): 239–47.

Hall, R. Cargill. 1977. *Lunar Impact: A History of Project Ranger.* NASA SP-4210. Retrieved from National Aeronautics and Space Administrations' History Office, http://history.nasa.gov/SP-4210/pages/Cover.htm.

Halliday, Gary M., et al. 1995. "Spontaneous Regression of Human Melanoma/ Nonmelanoma Skin Cancer: Association with Infiltrating CD4+ T Cells." *World Journal of Surgery* 19: 352–58.

Halperin, Morton H. 1974. *Bureaucratic Politics and Foreign Policy.* Washington, DC: Brookings Institution.

Hanahan, Douglas, and Robert A. Weinberg. 2000. "The Hallmarks of Cancer." *Cell* 100 (January 7): 57–70.

————. 2011. "Hallmarks of Cancer: The Next Generation." *Cell* 144 (March 4): 646–74.

Hand, Eric, with Meredith Wadman. 2008. "222 NIH Grants: 22 Researchers." *Nature* 452 (March 20): 258.

Haney, Daniel Q. 1986. Associated Press. "Study Says Americans Are Losing the War Against Cancer." May 7.

Harari, Daniel, and Yosef Yarden. 2000. "Molecular Mechanisms Underlying ErbB2/HER2 Action in Breast Cancer." *Oncogene* 19 (December 9): 6102–14.

Harper, Michael J. K., and Arthur L. Walpole (Imperial Chemical Industries). 1966. "Contrasting Endocrine Activities of cis and trans Isomers in a Series of Substituted Triphenylethylenes." *Nature* 212 (October 1): 87.

Harper, Peter S. 2006. "The Discovery of the Human Chromosome Number in Lund, 1955–1956." *Human Genetics* 119: 226–32.

Harrell, Joshua Chuck, Wendy W. Dye, D. Craig Allred, et al. 2006. "Estrogen Receptor Positive Breast Cancer Metastasis: Altered Hormonal Sensitivity and Tumor Aggressiveness in Lymphatic Vessels and Lymph Nodes." *Cancer Research* 66 (September 15): 9308–15.

Harries, M., and I. Smith. 2002. "The Development and Clinical Use of Trastuzumab (Herceptin)." *Endocrine-Related Cancer* 9: 75–85.

Harrington, David P. 1999. "The Tea Leaves of Small Trials." *Journal of Clinical Oncology* 17 (May): 1336–38.

Harvard School of Public Health. 2011. Office of Research Strategy and Development. "NIH Payline Updates as of October 25, 2011." Retrieved April 14, 2012. http//www.hsph.harvard.edu/research/research-strategy-and-development/ (under "Identifying Funding Opportunities").

Hawthorne, Fran. 2005. *Inside the FDA: The Business and Politics Behind the Drugs We Take and the Food We Eat.* Hoboken, NJ: John Wiley & Sons.

Health, United States (HUS). See under "National Center for Health Statistics."

Heath, Erin. 2012. "National Institutes of Health." In *AAAS Report XXXVII: Research and Development FY 2013.* Intersociety Working Group. Washington, DC: American Association for the Advancement of Science.

Hecht, Jonathan L., and Jon C. Aster. 2000. "Molecular Biology of Burkitt's Lymphoma." *Journal of Clinical Oncology* 18 (November 1): 3707–21.

Hede, Karyn. 2005. "NCI's National Biospecimen Network: Too Early or Too Late?" *Journal of the National Cancer Institute* 97 (February 16): 247–48.

Hedley, David W. 1993. "Flow Cytometric Assays of Anticancer Drug Resistance." *Annals of the New York Academy of Sciences* 677 (March): 341–53.

Heinrichs, Arianne. 2006. "Bad Seeds" (Milestone 15). In *Nature Milestones in Cancer* (April 1): S16–S17.

Heisterkamp, Nora, and John Groffen. 2002. "Philadelphia-Positive Leukemia: A Personal Perspective." *Oncogene* 21: 8536–40.

Hellquist, H., et al. 1999. "Criteria for Grading in the Ljubljana Classification of Epithelial Hyperplastic Laryngeal Lesions. A Study by Members of the Working Group on Epithelial Hyperplastic Laryngeal Lesions of the European Society of Pathology." *Histopathology* 34: 226–33.

Henderson, Brian E., Ronald K. Ross, and Leslie Bernstein. 1988. "Estrogens as a Cause of Human Cancer: The Richard and Hinda Rosenthal Foundation Award Lecture." *Cancer Research* 48 (January 15): 246–53.

Heng, Henry H. Q., et al. 2009. "Genetic and Epigenetic Heterogeneity in Cancer: A Genome-Centric Perspective." *Journal of Cellular Physiology* 220 (May 13): 538–47.

Henle, Gertrude, and Werner Henle. 1966. "Immunofluorescence in Cells Derived from Burkitt's Lymphoma." *Journal of Bacteriology* 91 (March): 1248–56.

Henry, David. 2004. "Fuzzy Numbers." *BusinessWeek,* October 4.

Heppner, Gloria H. 1984. "Tumor Heterogeneity." *Cancer Research* 44 (June): 2259–65.

Herberman, Ronald B., and Donald W. Mercer. 1990. *Immunodiagnosis of Cancer.* 2nd ed. New York: Marcel Dekker.

Herberman, Ronald B., et al. 2006. "Cancer Chemoprevention and Cancer Preventive Vaccines—a Call to Action: Leaders of Diverse Stakeholder Groups Present Strategies for Overcoming Multiple Barriers to Meet an Urgent Need." *Cancer Research* 66 (December 15): 11540–49.

Herbst, Roy S., Amir Onn, and John Mendelsohn. 2003. "The Role of Growth Factor Signaling in Malignancy." In *Signal Transduction in Cancer,* edited by David A. Frank, 19–72. Boston: Kluwer Academic Publishers.

Hersh, Evan M., Gerald P. Bodey, Boyd A. Nies, and Emil J. Freireich. 1965. "Causes of Death in Acute Leukemia: A Ten–Year Study of 414 Patients from 1954–1963." *Journal of the American Medical Association* 193 (July 12): 105–9.

Hewitt, Sylvia C., Joshua C. Harrell, and Kenneth S. Korach. 2005. "Lessons in Estrogen Biology from Knockout and Transgenic Animals." *Annual Review of Physiology* 67: 285–308.

Hicks, David G., LeeAnn Kushner, and Kristin McCarthy. 2011. "Breast Cancer Predictive Factor Testing: The Challenges and Importance of Standardizing Tissue Handling." *Journal of the National Cancer Institute Monograph* 42: 43–45.

Higgins, Brian. 2010. Representative Brian Higgins, Meeting of House Ways and Means Committee, February 3. In "Higgins Recognizes World Cancer Day." Official website of Congressman Brian Higgins (NY-27). http://higgins.house .gov/2010/02/020410-WorldCancerDay.shtml.

Higgins, Julian P. T. 2003. "Measuring Inconsistency in Meta-analyses." *British Medical Journal* 327 (September 6): 557–60.

Hill, R. P., et al. 1984. "Dynamic Heterogeneity: Rapid Generation of Metastatic Variants in Mouse B16 Melanoma Cells." *Science* 224 (June 1): 998–1000.

Hilts, Philip J. 1995. "FDA Becomes Target of Empowered Groups." Op-ed. *New York Times,* February 12.

Himmelstein, David U., et al. 2009. "Medical Bankruptcy in the United States, 2007: Results of a National Study." *American Journal of Medicine* 122 (August): 741–46. (This widely cited study of some twenty-three hundred US bankruptcy filers in 2007 found that more than 62 percent were driven primarily by medical debts.)

Hitchings, George H., Jr. 1988. "Selective Inhibitors of Dihydrofolate Reductase." Nobel Lecture, the Nobel Prize in Physiology or Medicine, 1988 (December 8). Retrieved from http://www.nobelprize.org/nobel_prizes/medicine/laureates/1988/hitchings-lecture.html.

Hitchings, George H., and Gertrude B. Elion. 1954. "The Chemistry and Biochemistry of Purine Analogs." *Annals of the New York Academy of Sciences* 60 (December): 195–99.

Hitchings, George H., Gertrude B. Elion, Elvira A. Falco, Peter B. Russell, and Henry VanderWerff. 1950. "Studies on Analogs of Purines and Pyrimidines." *Annals of the New York Academy of Sciences* 52 (July): 1318–35.

Hixson, Joe. 1967. "60,000 Miles of Blood Vessels." *Science News* 92 (December 2): 546–47.

Hochhaus, Andreas, et al. 2002. "Molecular and Chromosomal Mechanisms of Resistance to Imatinib (STI571) Therapy." *Leukemia* 16: 2190–96.

Hodges, V. M., et al. 2007. "Pathophysiology of Anemia and Erythrocytosis." *Critical Reviews in Oncology/Hematology* 64 (November): 139–58.

Hoeschele, James D. 2009. "In Remembrance of Barnett Rosenberg." *Dalton Transactions* 48: 10648–50.

Hoffbrand, A. V., and D. G. Weir. 2001. "The History of Folic Acid." *British Journal of Haematology* 113 (June): 579–89.

Hoffman, Beatrix R. 2003. "Scientific Racism, Insurance, and Opposition to the Welfare State: Frederick L. Hoffman's Transatlantic Journey." *Journal of the Gilded Age and Progressive Era* 2 (April): 150–90.

Hoffman, David A. 2010. "The Best Practices Act of 2010." Prepared Statement of Intel Corporation (by Intel's director of Security Policy and Global Privacy Officer) before the Committee on Energy and Commerce, Subcommittee on Commerce, Trade and Consumer Protection, U.S. House of Representatives, July 22.

Hoffman, Frederick L. 1896. "Race Traits and Tendencies of the American Negro." *Publications of the American Economic Association* (Macmillan Company) 11: 1–3.

————. 1913. "The Menace of Cancer." Paper first delivered at New Jersey Academy of Medicine, March 26, 1913; later presented at a meeting of the American Gynecological Society, Washington, DC, May 7. The speech was expanded and published in *Transactions of the American Gynecological Society* 38 (1913): 397–452.

————. 1915. *The Mortality from Cancer Throughout the World.* Newark, NJ: Prudential Press.

————. 1931. "Cancer and Smoking Habits." *Annals of Surgery* 93: 50–67.

Holbro, Thomas, and Nancy E. Hynes. 2004. "ErbB Receptors: Directing Key Signaling Networks Throughout Life." *Annual Review of Pharmacology and Toxicology* 44 (February): 195–217.

Holzman, Thomas F., and Eric J. Hebert. 2005. "Transforming the Work of Early-Stage Drug Discovery Through Bioprocess Informatics." *Drug Discovery Today* 10 (January): 61–67.

Hong, Waun Ki, and Scott M. Lippman, et al. 1990. "Prevention of Second Primary Tumors with Isotretinoin in Squamous-Cell Carcinoma of the Head and Neck." *New England Journal of Medicine* 323 (September 20): 795–801.

Horning, Sandra J. 2009. "Cancer Research and Privacy: The Problem with Being Joined at the Hip." *Journal of Clinical Oncology* 27 (August 20): 3879–80.

Howlader N., et al., eds. 2012. *SEER Cancer Statistics Review, 1975–2009 (Vintage 2009 Populations),* updated April 2012. National Cancer Institute. http://seer .cancer.gov/csr/1975_2009_pops09/.

Hsu, T. C. 1952. "Mammalian Chromosomes In Vitro: I. The Karyotype of Man." *Journal of Heredity* 43: 167–72.

Hsu, T. C., and Paul S. Moorhead. 1953. "Chromosome Anomalies in Human Neoplasms with Special Reference to the Mechanisms of Polyploidization and Aneuploidization in the Hela Strain." *Annals of the New York Academy of Sciences* 63 (March): 1083–94.

Huber, Peter. 1998. "FDA Caution Can Be Deadly, Too." Op-ed. *Wall Street Journal,* July 24.

Hudis, Clifford A. 2007. "Trastuzumab—Mechanism of Action and Use in Clinical Practice." *New England Journal of Medicine* 357 (July 5): 39–51.

Hughes, R. E. 1975. "James Lind and the Cure of Scurvy: An Experimental Approach." *Medical History* 19 (October): 342–51.

Hultén, Maj A. 2002. "Numbers, Bands and Recombination of Human Chromosomes: Historical Anecdotes from a Swedish Student." *Cytogenetic and Genome Research* 96: 14–19.

Humphries, Keith, Jodie Trafton, and Todd H. Wagner. 2003. "The Cost of Institutional Review Board Procedures in Multicenter Observational Research." *Annals of Internal Medicine* 139 (July 1): 77.

Hunter, Tony. 1984. "The Proteins of Oncogenes." *Scientific American* 251 (August): 70–79.

———. 1998. "The Croonian Lecture 1997. The Phosphorylation of Proteins on Tyrosine: Its Role in Cell Growth and Disease." *Philosophical Transactions of the Royal Society B (Biological Sciences)* 353 (April 29): 583–605.

———. 2007. "Treatment for Chronic Myelogenous Leukemia: The Long Road to Imatinib." *Journal of Clinical Investigation* 117 (August 8): 2036–43.

Huntly, Brian J. P., and D. Gary Gilliland. 2005. "Leukaemia Stem Cells and the Evolution of Cancer-Stem-Cell Research." *Nature Reviews Cancer* 5 (April): 311–21.

Hurwitz, Herbert, et al. 2004. "Bevacizumab plus Irinotecan, Fluorouracil, and Leucovorin for Metastatic Colorectal Cancer." *New England Journal of Medicine* 350 (June 3): 2335–42.

Hutchins, Laura F., et al. 1999. "Underrepresentation of Patients 65 Years of Age or Older in Cancer-Treatment Trials." *New England Journal of Medicine* 341 (December 30): 2061–67.

Hutchinson, Ezzie. 2007. "Blast It Away!" *Nature Reviews Cancer* 7 (October): 730–31.

Hutt, M. S. R., and Denis P. Burkitt. 1965. "Geographical Distribution of Cancer in East Africa: A New Clinicopathological Approach." *British Medical Journal* 2 (September 25): 719–22.

Hynes, Nancy E., and Heidi A. Lane. 2005. "ERBB Receptors and Cancer: The Complexity of Targeted Inhibitors." *Nature Reviews Cancer* 5 (May): 342–54.

Iatropoulos, Michael J. 1983. "Pathologist's Responsibility in the Diagnosis of Oncogenesis." *Toxicologic Pathology* 11: 132–42.

Iihara, Kuniko, et al. 2004. "Spontaneous Regression of Malignant Lymphoma of the Breast." *Pathology International* 54: 537–42.

IMPACT B2. 1999. International Multicentre Pooled Analysis of B2 Colon Cancer Trials (IMPACT B2) Investigators. "Efficacy of Adjuvant Fluorouracil and Folinic Acid in B2 Colon Cancer." *Journal of Clinical Oncology* 17 (May): 1356–63.

IMS Health. 2012. "IMS National Sales Perspectives, Antineoplastic Monoclonal Antibody Market, Top 5 Products." Yearly data 2006 to 2011 (provided by company in February 2012).

IMS Institute for Healthcare Informatics. 2011. "The Use of Medicines in the United States: Review of 2010." April.

Inskip, Peter D., and Rochelle E. Curtis. 2007. "New Malignancies Following Childhood Cancer in the United States, 1973–2002." *International Journal of Cancer* 121: 2233–40.

Intel Corporation. 1987. Datasheet for Intel 4004 Single Chip 4-Bit P-Channel Microprocessor. Order Number 231982 (March).

————. 2006. "Intel's First Microprocessor—the Intel 4004." Retrieved on October 15, 2009 from http://www.intel.com/museum/archives/4004.htm.

Internal Revenue Service. 2010. "Online Version of Publication 78" (now called "Exempt Organizations Select Check"). Accessed October 1, 2010. IRS.gov.

Ioannidis, John P. A. 2005. "Contradicted and Initially Stronger Effects in Highly Cited Clinical Research." *Journal of the American Medical Association* 294 (July 13): 218–28.

————. 2011. "Fund People Not Projects." *Nature* 477 (September 29): 529–31.

Irish, Jonathan M., Nikesh Kotecha, and Garry P. Nolan. 2006. "Mapping Normal and Cancer Cell Signalling Networks: Towards Single-Cell Proteomics." *Nature Reviews Cancer* 6 (February): 146–55.

Issa, Ala Y., et al. 2006. "The Role of Phytochemicals in Inhibition of Cancer and Inflammation: New Directions and Perspectives." *Journal of Food Composition and Analysis* 19: 405–19.

Jackman, Roger J., et al. 1999. "Stereotactic, Automated, Large-Core Needle Biopsy of Nonpalpable Breast Lesions: False-Negative and Histologic Underestimation Rates after Long-Term Follow-Up." *Radiology* 210 (March): 789–805.

Jackson, Malcolm J., et al. 2002. "Chapter 4: Antioxidants, Reactive Oxygen and Nitrogen Species, Gene Induction and Mitochondrial Function." *Molecular Aspects of Medicine* 23: 209–85.

Jacobs, Ian J., and Usha Menon. 2004. "Progress and Challenges in Screening for Early Detection of Ovarian Cancer." *Molecular and Cellular Proteomics* 3.4 (April 1): 355–66.

Jaffe, Elaine S., Nancy Lee Harris, Harald Stein, and James W. Vardiman, eds. 2001. *World Health Organization Classification of Tumors: Pathology and Genetics of Tumors of Haematopoietic and Lymphoid Tissues.* Lyon, France: IARC Press.

Jain, Meenakshi, et al. 2002. "Sustained Loss of a Neoplastic Phenotype by Brief Inactivation of MYC." *Science* 297 (July 5): 102–4.

Jain, Rakesh K. 2008. "Taming Vessels to Treat Cancer." *Scientific American* (January): 56–63.

James Lind Library. An online resource curated by Iain Chalmers, James Lind Initiative, Oxford, UK. http://www.jameslindlibrary.org/.

Jansen, Maurice P. H. M., et al. 2007. "HOXB13-to-IL17BR Expression Ratio Is Related with Tumor Aggressiveness and Response to Tamoxifen of Recurrent Breast Cancer: A Retrospective Study." *Journal of Clinical Oncology* 25 (February 20): 662–68.

Jasen, Patricia. 2002. "Breast Cancer and the Language of Risk, 1750–1950." *Social History of Medicine* 15: 17–43.

Jefferson, Tom, et al. 2008. "Vaccines for Preventing Influenza in Healthy Children." *Cochrane Database of Systematic Reviews,* Issue 2: CD004879.

Jemal, Ahmedin, et al. 2003. "Cancer Statistics, 2003." *CA: A Cancer Journal for Clinicians* 53 (January–February): 5–26.

Jemal, Ahmedin, et al. 2009. "Cancer Statistics, 2009." *CA: A Cancer Journal for Clinicians* 59 (July–August): 225–49.

Jemal, Ahmedin, et al. 2010. "Cancer Statistics, 2010." *CA: A Cancer Journal for Clinicians* 60 (September–October): 277–300.

Jenkinson, Helen C., et al. 2004. "Long-Term Population–Based Risks of Second Malignant Neoplasms After Childhood Cancer in Britain." *British Journal of Cancer* 91: 1905–10.

Jensen, Elwood V. 1987. "High Point." *Breast Cancer Research and Treatment* 9: 77–86. Originally presented before the Chicago Literary Club, April 12, 1965.

———. 2004a. "From Chemical Warfare to Breast Cancer Management." *Nature Medicine* 10 (October): v–viii.

———. 2004b. Acceptance Remarks, Albert Lasker Basic Medical Research Award, the Lasker Foundation. Retrieved from http://www.laskerfoundation.org/awards/2004_b_accept_jensen.htm.

———. 2005. "The Contribution of 'Alternative Approaches' to Understanding Steroid Hormone Action." *Molecular Endocrinology* 19 (June): 1439–42.

Jensen, Elwood V., and Eugene R. de Sombre. 1972. "Mechanism of Action of the Female Sex Hormones." *Annual Review of Biochemistry* 41: 203–30.

———. 1973. "Estrogen–Receptor Interaction." *Science* 182 (October 12): 126–34.

Jensen, Elwood V., Herbert I. Jacobson, Alicia A. Walf, and Cheryl A. Frye. 2010. "Estrogen Action: A Historic Perspective on the Implications of Considering Alternative Approaches." *Physiology and Behavior* 99 (February 9): 151–62.

Jensen, Elwood V., and V. Craig Jordan. 2003. "The Estrogen Receptor: A Model for Molecular Medicine." *Clinical Cancer Research* 9 (June): 1980–89.

Jensen, Elwood V., and Sohaib A. Khan. 2004. "A Two-Site Model for Antiestrogen Action." *Mechanisms of Ageing and Development* 125 (October–November): 679–82.

Jinks, Beth, and Carey Sargent. 2008. "Genentech, Roche Shares Gain on Avastin Use Approval." Bloomberg.com, February 25.

Johns Hopkins University. 2010. "Facilities and Administrative Costs." Rate agreement, with US Department of Heath and Human Services, dated May 5. Pertains to federally sponsored research conducted on campus between July 1, 2009, and June 30, 2010.

Johnson, Avery. 2009. "Cost-Effectiveness of Cancer Drugs Is Questioned." *Wall Street Journal*, June 30.

Johnson, John R., Grant Williams, and Richard Pazdur. 2003. "End Points and United States Food and Drug Administration Approval of Oncology Drugs." *Journal of Clinical Oncology* 21 (April 1): 1404–11.

Johnson, Stephen B. 2002. *The Secret of Apollo: Systems Management in American and European Space Programs*. Baltimore: Johns Hopkins University Press.

Johnston, Stephen R. D., and Mitch Dowsett. 2003. "Aromatase Inhibitors for Breast Cancer: Lesson from the Laboratory." *Nature Reviews Cancer* 3 (November): 821–31.

Jones, J. Louise. 2006. "Overdiagnosis and Overtreatment of Breast Cancer, Progression of Ductal Carcinoma In Situ: The Pathological Perspective." *Breast Cancer Research* 8 (April): 204–8.

Jordan, V. Craig. 2003a. "Tamoxifen: A Most Unlikely Pioneering Medicine." *Nature Reviews Drug Discovery* 2 (March): 205–13.

———. 2003b. "Is Tamoxifen the Rosetta Stone for Breast Cancer?" *Journal of the National Cancer Institute* 95 (March 5): 338–40.

———. 2006. "Tamoxifen (ICI46,474) as a Targeted Therapy to Treat and Prevent Breast Cancer." *British Journal of Pharmacology* 147 (supp. 1) (January): S269–S76.

———. 2008. "2008 David A. Karnofsky Memorial Award Lecture." ASCO Annual Meeting, June 1.

———. 2009. "A Century of Deciphering the Control Mechanisms of Sex Steroid Action in Breast and Prostate Cancer: The Origins of Targeted Therapy and Chemoprevention." *Cancer Research* 69 (February 15): 1243–54.

Jorgenson, Dale W. 2001. "Information Technology and the US Economy: Presidential Address Delivered at the 113th Meeting of the American Economic Association, January 6, New Orleans." *Information Technology and the US Economy* 91 (1): 1–32.

Joyce, Johanna A., and Jeffrey W. Pollard. 2009. "Microenvironmental Regulation of Metastasis." *Nature Reviews Cancer* 9 (April): 239–52.

Judson, Horace Freeland. 1979. *The Eighth Day of Creation: The Makers of the Revolution in Biology*. New York: Simon & Schuster.

Jukes, T. H., A. L. Franklin, and L. R. Stokstad. 1950. "Pteroylglutamic Acid Antagonists." *Annals of the New York Academy of Sciences* 52 (July): 1336–41.

Kaiser, Joceyln. 2008. "The Graying of NIH Research." *Science* 322 (November 7): 848–49.

Kalberer, John T., Jr. 1975. "Impact of the National Cancer Act on Grant Support." *Cancer Research* 35 (March): 473–81.

Kamb, Alexander, Susan Wee, and Christoph Lengauer. 2007. "Why Is Cancer Drug Discovery So Difficult?" *Nature Reviews Drug Discovery* 6 (February): 115–20.

Kambic, Vinko. 1997. "Epithelial Hyperplastic Lesions: A Challenging Topic in Laryngology." *Acta Oto-Laryngologica* 527 (supp.): 7–11.

Kanavos, Panos. 2006. "The Rising Burden of Cancer in the Developing World." *Annals of Oncology* 17 (supp. 8) (June): 15–23.

Kantarjian, Hagop, et al. 2002. "Hematologic and Cytogenetic Responses to Imatinib Mesylate in Chronic Myelogenous Leukemia." *New England Journal of Medicine* 346 (February 28): 645–52.

Katzenellenbogen, Benita S. 1996. "Estrogen Receptors: Bioactivities and Interactions with Cell Signaling Pathways." *Biology of Reproduction* 54 (February): 287–93.

Kean, Marcia A., ed. 2012. "Sustaining Progress Against Cancer in an Era of Cost Containment." Discussion paper for "Turning the Tide Against Cancer Through Sustained Medical Innovation" conference, June 12, 2012, Washington, DC.

Keen, Judith Clancy, and Nancy E. Davidson. 2003. "The Biology of Breast Carcinoma." *Cancer* 97 (3 supp.) (February 1): 825–33.

Kell, Douglas B., and Stephen G. Oliver. 2004. "Here Is the Evidence, Now What Is the Hypothesis? The Complementary Roles of Inductive and Hypothesis-Driven Science in the Post-Genomic Era." *BioEssays* 26 (1) (January): 99–105.

Kelland, Kate. 2011. "Cancer Cost 'Becoming Unsustainable' in Rich Nations." Reuters, September 26.

Kellock, Brian. 1985. *The Fiber Man: The Life Story of Dr. Denis Burkitt.* Belleville, MI: Lion Publishing.

Kelloff, Gary J., Scott M. Lippman, Andrew J. Dannenberg, et al. 2006. AACR Task Force on Cancer Prevention. "Progress in Chemoprevention Drug Development: The Promise of Molecular Biomarkers for Prevention of Intraepithelial Neoplasia and Cancer—a Plan to Move Forward." *Clinical Cancer Research* 12 (June): 3661–97.

Kelly, Judith P., et al. 1996. "Risk of Aspirin–Associated Major Upper-Gastrointestinal Bleeding with Enteric-Coated or Buffered Product." *Lancet* 348 (November 23): 1413–16.

Kennedy, John F. 1962. Text of President Kennedy's "Moon Speech" at Rice Stadium, Houston, Texas, September 12. Retrieved from http://er.jsc.nasa.gov/seh/ricetalk.htm.

Khakh, Baljit S., and Geoffrey Burnstock. 2009. "The Double Life of ATP in Humans." *Scientific American* 301 (December): 84–92.

Kher, Unmesh, and Odette Frey. 2007. "Drug Lord." *Time,* November 13.

Klein, Christoph A., et al. 2002. "Genetic Heterogeneity of Single Disseminated Tumour Cells in Minimal Residual Cancer." *Lancet* 360 (August): 683–89.

Klein, George, 1990. *The Atheist and the Holy City: Encounters and Reflections.* Translated by Theodore and Ingrid Friedmann. Cambridge, MA: MIT Press.

Klein, George, and Eva Klein. 1989. "How One Thing Has Led to Another." *Annual Review of Immunology* 7: 1–33.

Kliman, Allan, Lawrence A. Gaydos, Leslie R. Schroeder, and Emil J. Freireich. 1961. "Repeated Plasmapheresis of Blood Donors as a Source of Platelets." *Blood* 18 (September): 303–9.

Kluger, Jeffrey. 2007. "Space Brains." *Time,* October 8.

Knudson, Alfred G., Jr. 1971. "Mutation and Cancer: Statistical Study of Retino-blastoma." *Proceedings of the National Academy of Sciences* 68: 820–23.

Kobel, Martin, et al. 2008. "Ovarian Carcinoma Subtypes Are Different Diseases: Implications for Biomarker Studies." *PLOS Medicine* 5 (December): e232.

Kodani, Masuo. 1958. "Three Chromosome Numbers in Whites and Japanese." *Science* 127 (June 6): 1339–40.

Kola, Ismail, and John Landis. 2004. "Can the Pharmaceutical Industry Reduce Attrition Rates?" *Nature Reviews Drug Discovery* 3 (August): 711–15.

Kolata, Gina. 1986. "Cancer Progress Data Challenged." *Science* 232 (May 23): 932–33.

———. 2009. "Forty Years' War: Grant System Leads Cancer Researchers to Play It Safe." *New York Times,* June 27.

Konenen, Juha. 1998. "Tissue Microarrays for High-Throughput Molecular Profiling of Tumor Specimens." *Nature Medicine* 4 (July): 844–47.

Konopka, James B., Susan M. Watanabe, and Owen N. Witte. 1984. "An Alteration of the Human c-abl Protein in K562 Leukemia Cells Unmasks Associated Tyrosine Kinase Activity." *Cell* 37 (July): 1035–42.

Koppes, Clayton R. 1978. "JPL's Faltering Start in the Prestige Race: Rangers and Mariners, 1961–1962" Typed manuscript. Humanities Working Paper 12, California Institute of Technology (July). Retrieved from http://authors.library.caltech.edu/14514/1/HumsWP-0012.pdf

Kornberg, Arthur. 1991. *For the Love of Enzymes: The Odyssey of a Biochemist.* Cambridge, MA: Harvard University Press.

Krakoff, Irwin H. 1977. "Cancer Chemotherapeutic Agents." *CA: A Cancer Journal for Clinicians* 27 (May/June): 130–43.

———. 1994. "Progress and Prospects in Cancer Treatment: The Karnofsky Legacy (The 24th Annual David H. Karnofsky Memorial Lecture)." *Journal of Clinical Oncology* 12 (February): 432–38, and the author's manuscript for the same.

Krehl, Willard A. 1953. "James Lind, MD (October 4, 1716–July 18, 1794)." *Journal of Nutrition* 50: 1–11.

Krieger, Nancy. 2001. "The Ostrich, the Albatross, and Public Health: An Ecosocial Perspective—or Why an Explicit Focus on Health Consequences of Discrimination and Deprivation Is Vital for Good Science and Public Health Practice." *Public Health Reports* 116 (September–October): 419–23.

Krikorian, John G., et al. 1980. "Spontaneous Regression of Non–Hodgkin's Lymphoma: A Report of Nine Cases." *Cancer* 46 (November 1): 2093–99.

Kuhn, Thomas S. 1970. *The Structure of Scientific Revolutions.* 2nd ed. Chicago: University of Chicago Press. Originally published in 1962.

Kuipers, Benjamin J. 1974. "Working Paper 63: A Hypothesis-Driven Recognition System for the Blocks World." Cambridge: Massachusetts Institute of Technology, Artificial Intelligence Laboratory. March.

Kumar, Anjali S. 2005. "Overdiagnosis and Overtreatment of Breast Cancer, Rates of Ductal Carcinoma In Situ: A US Perspective." *Breast Cancer Research* 7 (December): 271–75.

Kushmerick, Martin J. 1995. "Bioenergetics and Muscle Cell Types." In *Fatigue: Neural and Muscular Mechanisms. Advances in Experimental Medicine and Biology* 384, edited by Simon C. Gandevia, et al. New York: Plenum Press/Springer.

Kutok, L., and F. Wang. 2006. "Spectrum of Epstein–Barr Virus-Associated Diseases." *Annual Review of Pathology: Mechanisms of Disease* 1: 375–404.

Lacher, Mortimer J. 1985. "Hodgkin's Disease: Historical Perspective, Current Status, and Future Directions." *CA: A Cancer Journal for Clinicians* 35 (March/April): 88–94.

Landers, Ann. 1971. "Ask Ann Landers." Syndicated newspaper columns for April 1, April 3, April 8, and April 14, in *Hartford Courant* and elsewhere.

Lane, David P. 2005. "Exploiting the p53 Pathway for the Diagnosis and Therapy of Human Cancer." *Cold Spring Harbor Symposia on Quantitative Biology.* Vol. 70. Cold Spring Harbor, NY: Cold Spring Harbor Laboratory Press.

Larson, Anne M., et al. 2005. Acute Liver Failure Study Group. "Acetaminophen–Induced Acute Liver Failure: Results of a United States Multicenter, Prospective Study." *Hepatology* 42 (December): 1364–72.

Laszlo, John. 1995. *The Cure of Childhood Leukemia: Into the Age of Miracles.* New Brunswick, NJ: Rutgers University Press.

Lau, Gloria. 2002. "AstraZeneca Tumbles After Cancer Pill Fails in Late-Stage Studies." *Investor's Business Daily,* August 20.

Lawler, Sylvia D., and B. R. Reeves. 1976. "Chromosome Studies in Man: Past Achievements and Recent Advances." *Journal of Clinical Pathology* 29: 569–82.

Leaf, Clifton. 2003. "Feed Your Head." *Fortune,* May 12.

———. 2004. "Why We're Losing the War on Cancer (and How to Win It)." *Fortune,* March 22, 76–97.

———. 2005. "The Law of Unintended Consequences." *Fortune,* September 19, 250–68.

———. 2006. "Deadly Caution." *Fortune,* February 20, 106–20.

———. 2009. "Oncology Recapitulates Phylogeny." Presentation, Advancing Cancer Research Through Biospecimen Science, 2nd Annual Biospecimen Research Network (BRN) Symposium, National Cancer Institute, March 17.

le Coutre, Philipp, et al. 2000. "Induction of Resistance to the Abelson Inhibitor STI571 in Human Leukemic Cells Through Gene Amplification." *Blood* 95 (March 1): 1758–66.

Lee, Christopher. 2007. "Slump in NIH Funding Is Taking Toll on Research." *Washington Post,* May 28.

Lee, Raphael C., Florin Despa, and Kimm J. Hamann, eds. 2005. *Cell Injury: Mechanisms, Responses, and Repair. Annals of the New York Academy of Sciences* 1066.

Le Fanu, James. 2012. *The Rise and Fall of Modern Medicine.* Rev. ed. New York: Basic Books. Originally published in 1999.

Lehninger, Albert L. 1960. "Energy Transformation in the Cell." *Scientific American* 202 (May): 102–14.

Leibel, Wayne. 1991. "When Scientists Are Wrong: Admitting Inadvertent Error in Research." *Journal of Business Ethics* 10 (August): 601–4.

Leibfarth, Linda Katherine. 2008. "Giving the Terminally Ill Their Due (Process): A Case for Expanded Access to Experimental Drugs Through the Political Process." *Vanderbilt Law Review* 61: 1281–317.

Leland, Anne, and Mari-Jana Oboroceanu. 2010. *American War and Military Operations Casualties: Lists and Statistics.* CRS Report for Congress RL32492. Washington, DC: Congressional Research Service, February 26.

LeLorier, Jacques, et al. 1997. "Discrepancies Between Meta-analyses and Subsequent Large Randomized, Controlled Trials." *New England Journal of Medicine* 337 (August 21): 536–42.

Lemmon, Mark A., and Joseph Schlessinger. 2010. "Cell Signaling by Receptor Tyrosine Kinases." *Cell* 141 (June 25): 1117–34.

Lemonick, Michael D., and Alice Park. 2001. "New Hope for Cancer." *Time,* May 28.

Lengauer, Christoph, Kenneth W. Kinzler, and Bert Vogelstein. 1997. "Genetic Instability in Colorectal Cancers." *Nature* 386 (April 10): 623–27.

Leonard, Gregory D., and Sandra M. Swain. 2004. "Ductal Carcinoma In Situ, Complexities and Challenges." *Journal of the National Cancer Institute* 96 (June 16): 906–20.

Lerner, Barron H. 1998. "Fighting the War on Breast Cancer: Debates over Early Detection, 1945 to the Present." *Annals of Internal Medicine* 129 (July): 74–78.

Letters to the Editor. 1986. "Progress Against Cancer?" *New England Journal of Medicine* 315 (October 9): 963–968; and 316 (March 19): 752–53.

Leuchtenberger, R., C. Leuchtenberger, D. Laszlo, and R. Lewisohn. 1945. "The Influence of 'Folic Acid' on Spontaneous Breast Cancers in Mice." *Science* 101 (January 12): 46.

Leukemia and Lymphoma Society. IRS Form 990 (Return of Organization Exempt from Income Tax) for the 2010 calendar year.

Levan, Albert (1956). "Chromosome Studies on Some Human Tumors and Tissues of Normal Origin, Grown In Vitro at the Sloan–Kettering Institute." *Cancer* 4 (July–August): 648–63.

Levine, Arnold S. 1982. *Managing NASA in the Apollo Era.* NASA SP-4102. Retrieved from National Aeronautics and Space Administrations' History Office, http://history.nasa.gov/SP-4102/sp4102.htm.

le Viseur, Christoph, et al. 2008. "In Childhood Acute Lymphoblastic Leukemia, Blasts at Different Stages of Immunophenotypic Maturation Have Stem Cell Properties." *Cancer Cell* 14 (July): 47–58.

Lewis, Joy H., et al. 2003. "Participation of Patients 65 Years of Age or Older in Cancer Clinical Trials." *Journal of Clinical Oncology* 21 (April 1): 1383–89.

Lewtas, Joellen. 2007. "Air Pollution Combustion Emissions: Characterization of Causative Agents and Mechanisms Associated with Cancer, Reproductive, and Cardiovascular Effects." *Mutation Research* 636: 95–133.

Li, Christopher I., et al. 2005. "Age-Specific Incidence Rates of In Situ Breast Carcinomas by Histologic Type, 1980 to 2001." *Cancer Epidemiology, Biomarkers, and Prevention* 14: 1008–11.

Li, Frederick P., et al. 1983. "Breast Carcinoma After Cancer Therapy in Childhood." *Cancer* 51 (February 1): 521–23.

Li, Min Chiu, Roy Hertz, and Donald B. Spencer. 1956. "Effect of Methotrexate Therapy upon Choriocarcinoma and Chorioadenoma." *Experimental Biology and Medicine* 93 (November): 361–66.

Library of Congress. 2013. The Vietnam-Era Prisoner-of-War/Missing-in–Action Database. As of February, 2013, an additional 1,910 US servicemen and 38 civilians are still unaccounted for. http://lcweb2.loc.gov/frd/pow/.

Light, Donald W., and Rebecca Warburton. 2011. "Demythologizing the High Costs of Pharmaceutical Research." *BioSocieties* 6: 34–50.

Lilja, Hans, et al. 2007. "Measurements of Proteases or Protease System Components in Blood to Enhance Prediction of Disease Risk or Outcome in Possible Cancer." *Journal of Clinical Oncology* 25 (February 1): 347–48.

Lind, James. 1772. *A Treatise on the Scurvy: In Three Parts, Containing an Inquiry into the Nature, Causes and Cure of That Disease, Together with a Critical and Chronological View of What Has Been Published on the Subject.* 3rd ed. London: S. Crowder, D. Wilson, et al.; 1st ed., 1753. Retrieved from Google Books.

Linde, Nancy. 2001. Writer, director, and producer, "Cancer Warrior." A *NOVA* production for WGBH/Boston television, aired February 27.

Lingle, Wilma L., et al. 1998. "Centrosome Hypertrophy in Human Breast Tumors: Implications for Genomic Stability and Cell Polarity." *Proceedings of the National Academy of Sciences* 95 (March): 2950–55.

Liotta, Lance Allen, Jerome Kleinerman, and Gerald M. Saidel. 1974. "Quantitative Relationships of Intravascular Tumor Cells, Tumor Vessels, and Pulmonary Metastases following Tumor Implantation." *Cancer Research* 34 (May): 997–1004.

Lipmann, Fritz. 1941. "Metabolic Generation and Utilization of Phosphate Bond Energy." In *Advances in Enzymology and Related Areas of Molecular Biology*, vol. 1, edited by F. F. Nord and C. H. Werkman, 100–162. New York: Interscience Publishers.

Lippman, Scott M., and Waun Ki Hong. 2002. "Cancer Prevention by Delay." *Clinical Cancer Research* 8 (February): 305–13.

Littlewood, Timothy J., Brad Schenkel, and Martin Liss. 2005. "Effect of Patient Exclusion Criteria on the Efficacy of Erythropoiesis-Stimulating Agents in Patients with Cancer-Related Anemia." *Oncologist* 10 (May): 357–60.

Loeb, Lawrence A. 2011. "Human Cancers Express Mutator Phenotypes: Origin, Consequences and Targeting." *Nature Reviews Cancer* 11 (June): 450–57.

Loeb, Lawrence A., Jason H. Bielas, and Robert A. Beckman. 2008. "Cancers Exhibit a Mutator Phenotype: Clinical Implications." *Cancer Research* 68 (May 15): 3551–57.

Loeb, Lawrence A., Keith R. Loeb, and Jon P. Anderson. 2003. "Multiple Mutations and Cancer." *Proceedings of the National Academy of Sciences* 100 (February 4): 776–81.

Lombard, David B., et al. 2005. "DNA Repair, Genome Review Stability, and Aging." *Cell* 120 (February 25): 497–512.

Longo, Dan L. 2012. "Tumor Heterogeneity and Personalized Medicine." *New England Journal of Medicine* 366 (March 8): 956–57.

Longthorne, Anders, et al. 2010. "An Analysis of the Significant Decline in Motor Vehicle Traffic Crashes in 2008." National Highway Traffic Safety Administration, Technical Report DOT HS 811 346. http://www-nrd.nhtsa.dot.gov/Pubs/811346.pdf. (Note: NHTSA and NCHS offer differing fatality figures for certain years.)

Löwy, Ilana. 1996. *Between Bench and Bedside: Science, Healing, and Interleukin–2 in a Cancer Ward*. Cambridge, MA: Harvard University Press.

Luch, Andreas. 2005. "Nature and Nurture: Lessons from Chemical Carcinogenesis." *Nature Reviews Cancer* 5 (February): 113–25.

Lucia, S. P. 1941. "Leukemia: Evaluation of the Therapy." *California and Western Medicine* 55 (September): 119–23.

Ludwig, Joseph A., and John N. Weinstein. 2005. "Biomarkers in Cancer Staging, Prognosis and Treatment Selection." *Nature Reviews Cancer* 5 (November): 845–56.

Lugo, Tracy G., et al. 1990. "Tyrosine Kinase Activity and Transformation Potency of bcr-abl Oncogene Products." *Science* 247 (March 2): 1079–82.

Lumachi, Franco, Stefano M. M. Basso, and Umberto Basso. 2008. "Breast Cancer Recurrence: Role of Serum Tumor Markers CEA and CA 15-3." In *Methods of Cancer Diagnosis, Therapy and Prognosis, Vol. 1, Breast Carcinoma*, edited by M. A. Hayat, 109–15. New York: Springer.

Lutz, Amelie M., et al. 2008. "Cancer Screening: A Mathematical Model Relating Secreted Blood Biomarker Levels to Tumor Sizes." *PLOS Medicine* 5 (August 19): e170.

Lynch, Richard G., ed. 2009. *Milestones in Investigative Pathology*. Bethesda, MD: American Society for Investigative Pathology.

Macdonald, Elizabeth, with Daniel Kruger. 2002. "Is Accounting Dead?" *Forbes*, March 4.

Magness, Ronald R., and Charles R. Rosenfeld. 1989. "Local and Systemic Estradiol-17ß: Effects on Uterine and Systemic Vasodilation." *American Journal of Physiology* 256: E536–E42.

Magrath, Ian. 1990. "The Pathogenesis of Burkitt's Lymphoma." *Advances in Cancer Research* 55: 133–270.

Malakoff, David. 2001. "NIH Prays for a Soft Landing After Its Doubling Ride Ends." *Science* 292 (June 15): 1992–95.

Mamounas, Eleftherios, et al. 1999. "Comparative Efficacy of Adjuvant Chemotherapy in Patients with Dukes' B Versus Dukes' C Colon Cancer: Results from Four National Surgical Adjuvant Breast and Bowel Project Adjuvant Studies (C-01, C-02, C-03, and C-04)." *Journal of Clinical Oncology* 17 (May): 1349–55.

Mandel, H. George, and Elliot S. Vesell. 2001. "NIH Budget Grows, but Not R01 Success Rates." *Science* 294 (October 5): 54–57.

Mandel, Michael J. 2002. "Restating the '90s." *BusinessWeek*, April 1.

Mandel, Richard. 2003. *Beacon of Hope: The Clinical Center Through Forty Years of Growth and Change in Biomedicine, 1953–1993*. Office of the NIH History, April 3. http://www.ors.od.nih.gov/medart/stetten/becon_of_hope/homepage.html.

Mansell, Peter. 2012. "'Unnecessary' Trial Procedures Cost up to US$5 Billion a Year." *PharmaTimes* online, July 3.

Marcus, Amy Docker. 2004. "Burden of Proof. At 32, a Decision: Is Cancer Small Enough to Ignore?" *Wall Street Journal*, December 20.

Marincola, Elizabeth, ed. 2004. *Career Advice for Life Scientists II*. Bethesda, MD: American Society for Cell Biology.

Mariotto, Angela B., et al. 2011. "Projections of the Cost of Cancer Care in the United States: 2010–2020." *Journal of the National Cancer Institute* 103: 117–28.

Marks, Harry M. 2000. *The Progress of Experiment: Science and Therapeutic Reform in the United States, 1900–1990*. Cambridge: Cambridge University Press. Originally published in 1997.

Martin, Aryn. 2004. "Can't Anybody Count? Counting as an Epistemic Theme in the History of Human Chromosomes." *Social Studies of Science* 34: 923–48.

Martin, G. Steven. 2001. "The Hunting of the Src." *Nature Reviews Molecular Cell Biology* 2 (June): 467–75.

Martin, Michael R., Andrea Kopstein, and Joy M. Janice. 2010. "An Analysis of Preliminary and Post-Discussion Priority Scores for Grant Applications Peer Reviewed by the Center for Scientific Review at the NIH." *PLOS ONE* 5 (11): e13526.

Martin, Robert G., et al. 1971. Letter to the editor. *New York Times,* August 9.

Martins-Green, Manuela, Nancy Boudreau, and Mina J. Bissell. 1994. "Inflammation Is Responsible for the Development of Wound-Induced Tumors in Chickens Infected with Rous Sarcoma Virus." *Cancer Research* 54 (August 15): 4334–41.

Maschke, Karen J. 2010. "Wanted: Human Biospecimens." *Hastings Center Report* 40 (September–October): 21–23.

Massagué, Joan. 2006. "HHMI's Joan Massagué on TGF-ß and Metastasis." Interview. *ScienceWatch* 17 (January/February).

Massett, Holly A., et al. 2011. "Assessing the Need for a Standardized Cancer HUman Biobank (caHUB): Findings from a National Survey with Cancer Researchers." *Journal of the National Cancer Institute Monograph* 42: 8–15.

Masters, John R. 2002. "HeLa Cells 50 Years On: The Good, the Bad and the Ugly." *Nature Reviews Cancer* 2 (April): 315–19.

Matthews, Kirstin R. W., et al. 2011. "The Aging of Biomedical Research in the United States." *PLOS ONE* 6 (12) (December 28): e29738.

Maugh, Thomas H., II. 1974. "Cancer Chemotherapy: Now a Promising Weapon." *Science* 184 (May 31): 970–74.

Maxmen, Amy. 2009. "Taking Risks to Transform Science." *Cell* 139 (October 2): 13–15.

Mayer, Robert J., Lowell E. Schnipper, and other correspondents. 1997. Letters to the editor. "Winning the War on Cancer." *New England Journal of Medicine* 337 (September 25): 931–38.

McCarthy, Nicola. 2004. "Multiple Opponents." *Nature Reviews Cancer* 4 (December): 924–25.

McCurdy, Howard E. 1991. "Organizational Decline: NASA and the Life Cycle of Bureaus." *Public Administration Review* 51 (July–August): 308–15.

McGeary, Michael, and Michael Burstein. 1999. "Report on Sources of Cancer Research Funding in the United States." Prepared for National Cancer Policy Board, Institute of Medicine. June, 1–20.

McKeown, Thomas. 1979. *The Role of Medicine: Dream, Mirage or Nemesis?* Princeton, NJ: Princeton University Press.

McKeown, Thomas, and R. G. Record. 1962. "Reasons for the Decline in Mortality in England and Wales in the Nineteenth Century." *Population Studies* 16 (2): 94–122.

McKnight, Steven L. 2009. "Unconventional Wisdom." *Cell* 138 (September 4): 817–19.

McManus, Rich. 1997. "NIDDK's Tjio Ends Distinguished Scientific Career." *NIH Record,* February 11.

McWhinney, Bruce D. 2000. "Reducing the Human and Economic Costs of Drug Therapy Complications: Responding to the Medication Safety Issue." Cardinal Health white paper. May.

MD Anderson Cancer Center. 2010. University of Texas System, Annual Financial Report, Primary Financial Statements, Fiscal Year 2010: University of Texas MD Anderson Cancer Center. "Exhibit B Statement of Revenues, Expenses, and Changes in Net Assets for the Year Ended August 31, 2010, Unaudited."

Meinert, Curtis L. 1980. "Terminology: A Plea for Standardization." Editorial. *Controlled Clinical Trials* 1 (September): 97–99.

Memorial Sloan–Kettering Cancer Center. 2011. Combined Financial Statements for Memorial Sloan–Kettering Cancer Center and Affiliated Corporations Years Ended December 31, 2011 and 2010 with Report of Independent Auditors.

Mendelsohn, Michael E., and Richard H. Karas. 1999. "The Protective Effects of Estrogen on the Cardiovascular System." *New England Journal of Medicine* 340 (June 10): 1801–11.

Mera, Robertino, et al. 2005. "Long-Term Follow-Up of Patients Treated for *Helicobacter pylori* Infection." *Gut* 54 (November): 1536–40.

Merlo, Lauren M. F., et al. 2006. "Cancer as an Evolutionary and Ecological Process." *Nature Reviews Cancer* 6 (December): 924–35.

Meropol, Neal J., and Kevin A. Schulman. 2007. "Perspectives on the Cost of Cancer Care." *Journal of Clinical Oncology* 25 (January 10): 169–70. (The essay is an overview of a special *JCO* issue focused on the cost of cancer care.)

Meropol, Neal J., et al. 2009. "American Society of Clinical Oncology Guidance Statement: The Cost of Cancer Care." *Journal of Clinical Oncology* 27: 3868–74.

Merton, Robert K. 1993. *On the Shoulders of Giants: A Shandean Postscript.* Chicago: University of Chicago Press. Originally published by the Free Press in 1965.

Merton, Robert K., and Elinor Barber. 2004. *The Travels and Adventures of Serendipity: A Study in Sociological Semantics and the Sociology of Science.* Princeton, NJ: Princeton University Press. Originally published in 1958.

Merz, Beverly. 1987. "General Accounting Office Report on Cancer Survival Statistics Raises NCI Hackles." *Journal of the American Medical Association* 257 (May 22): 20.

Metcalfe, Robert M. 2007. "It's All in Your Head." *Forbes,* May 7. Lead essay in *Forbes'* 90th Anniversary issue, "The Power of Networks."

Meyer, Jerome S. 1967. *Great Accidents in Science That Changed the World.* New York: Arco Publishing.

Michor, Franziska, et al. 2005. "Dynamics of Colorectal Cancer." *Seminars in Cancer Biology* (December 15): 484–93.

Midgley, Rachel, and David J. Kerr. 2005. "Adjuvant Chemotherapy for Stage II Colorectal Cancer: The Time Is Right!" *Nature Clinical Practice Oncology* 2 (July): 364–69.

Mijuk, Goran. 2011. "Roche's Avastin Rejected for Breast Cancer by UK Cost Body." *Wall Street Journal*, February 22.

Milken Institute Global Conference. 2005. "Starting Over with the FDA." Session at Milken Institute Global Conference, Los Angeles, April 18.

Miller, A. B., B. Hoogstraten, M. Staquet, and A. Winkler. 1981. "Reporting Results of Cancer Treatment." *Cancer* 47 (January 1): 207–14.

Miller, Crispin J., and Teresa K. Attwood. 2003. "Bioinformatics Goes Back to the Future." *Nature Reviews Molecular Cell Biology* 4 (February): 157–62.

Miller, Denis R. 2006. "A Tribute to Sidney Farber: The Father of Modern Chemotherapy." *British Journal of Haematology* 134: 20–26.

Miller, Edward D. 2005. "NIH Medical School Rankings." Editorial. *Johns Hopkins Medicine Web Notes*, July. Retrieved on January 14, 2011. http://www.hopkins medicine.org/webnotes/newsletter_draft/editorials/0507.cfm.

Miller, Henry I. 2008. "Drug Innovation Has Fallen Victim to Risk-Averse, Anti-Industry Government." Op-ed. *Investor's Business Daily*, August 7.

Miller, Kathy D., et al. 2005. "Randomized Phase III Trial of Capecitabine Compared with Bevacizumab plus Capecitabine in Patients with Previously Treated Metastatic Breast Cancer." *Journal of Clinical Oncology* 23 (February 1): 792–99.

Mills, Gordon B., Robert C. Bast, Jr., and Sudhir Srivastava. 2001. "Future for Ovarian Cancer Screening: Novel Markers from Emerging Technologies of Transcriptional Profiling and Proteomics." *Journal of the National Cancer Institute* 93 (October 3): 1437–39.

Milo, George E., et al. 1996. "Malignant Conversion of Chemically Transformed Normal Human Cells." *Proceedings of the National Academy of Sciences* 93 (May): 5229–34.

Milt, Harry. 1969. "Viruses and Cancer." *CA: A Cancer Journal for Clinicians* 19 (July/August): 219–27.

Miniño, Arialdi M., et al. 2011. "Deaths: Final Data for 2008." *National Vital Statistics Reports* 59 (December 7).

Minot, George R. 1934. "The Development of Liver Therapy in Pernicious Anemia." Nobel Lecture, the Nobel Prize in Physiology or Medicine 1934 (December 12). Retrieved from http://www.nobelprize.org/nobel_prizes/medicine/laureates/1934/minot-lecture.html.

Mintz, Beatrice, and Karl Illmensee. 1975. "Normal Genetically Mosaic Mice Produced from Malignant Teratocarcinoma Cells." *Proceedings of the National Academy of Sciences* 72 (September 1): 3585–89.

Mirand, Edwin A., and Albert S. Gordon. 1966. "Mechanism of Estrogen Action in Erythropoiesis." *Endocrinology* 78 (February 1): 325–32.

Mitelman, Felix. 1974. "Heterogeneity of Ph[1] in Chronic Myeloid Leukaemia." *Hereditas* 76: 315.

Mitka, Mike. 2007. "Scientists Warn NIH Funding Squeeze Hampering Biomedical Research." *Journal of the American Medical Association* 297 (May 2): 1867–68.

Moasser, Mark M. 2007. "Targeting the Function of the HER2 Oncogene in Human Cancer Therapeutics." *Oncogene* 26 (October 11): 6577–92.

Moed, H. F., and Th. N. Van Leeuwen. 1995. "Improving the Accuracy of Institute for Scientific Information's Journal Impact Factors." *Journal of the American Society for Information Science* 46 (6) (July): 461–67.

Moloney, William Curry. 1978. "Chronic Myelogenous Leukemia." *Cancer* 42 (August): 865–73.

Monastersky, Richard. 2007. "The Real Science Crisis: Bleak Prospects for Young Researchers." *Chronicle of Higher Education,* September 21.

Monthly Vital Statistics Report (MVSR). See under "National Center for Health Statistics."

Moore, Patrick S., and Yuan Chang. 2010. "Why Do Viruses Cause Cancer? Highlights of the First Century of Human Tumour Virology." *Nature Reviews Cancer* 10 (December): 878–89.

Moorhead, Paul S., et al. 1960. "Chromosome Preparations of Leukocytes Cultured from Human Peripheral Blood." *Experimental Cell Research* 20 (September): 613–16.

Morange, Michel. 2002. "History of Cancer Research." *Encyclopedia of Life Sciences.* Online edition. John Wiley & Sons.

Morgan Stanley Dean Witter. 2001. Equity research report on ImClone Systems: "C225 Data Expected: Framing the Issues." April 5, as well as reports throughout 2001 (June 28, November 16, December 31) and 2002 (January 8, January 22, January 24, January 25, and February 6).

Morgenson, Gretchen. 2002. "Wait a Second: What Devils Lurk in the Details?" *New York Times,* April 14.

Mosca, Lori, et al. 2004. "Evidence-Based Guidelines for Cardiovascular Disease Prevention in Women." *Journal of the American College of Cardiology* 43 (March 3): 900–921.

Moses, Harold L., and Anita B. Roberts. 2008. "The Discovery of TGF-Beta: A Historical Perspective." In *The TGF-ß Family,* edited by Rik Derynck and Kohei Miyazono, 1–28. Cold Spring Harbor, NY: Cold Spring Harbor Laboratory Press.

Moses, Harold L., et al. 1981. "Transforming Growth Factor Production by Chemically Transformed Cells." *Cancer Research* 41 (July): 2842–48.

Moss, Lenny. 2003. *What Genes Can't Do.* Cambridge, MA: MIT Press.

Mukherjee, Siddhartha. 2010. *The Emperor of All Maladies.* New York: Scribner.

Mundy, Alicia. 2011. "Resistance to FDA on Avastin Limits." *Wall Street Journal,* April 8.

Murphy, Kevin, and Robert Topel. 2003. "Diminishing Returns? The Costs and Benefits of Improving Health." *Perspectives in Biology and Medicine* 46 (Summer): S108–28.

Murray, Todd H., et al. 2010. "Costs and Benefits of the National Cancer Institute Central Institutional Review Board." *Journal of Clinical Oncology* 28 (February 1): 662–66.

Muzykantov, Vladimir R. 2010. "Drug Delivery by Red Blood Cells: Vascular Carriers Designed by Mother Nature." *Expert Opinion on Drug Delivery* 7 (April): 403–27.

Myles, Renate et al. 2011. "Stakeholder Research on Biospecimen Needs and Reactions to the Development of a National Cancer Human Biobank by the National Cancer Institute." *Journal of the National Cancer Institute Monograph* 42: 16–23.

Nandi, Satyabrata, Raphael C. Guzman, and Jason Yang. 1995. "Hormones and Mammary Carcinogenesis in Mice, Rats, and Humans: A Unifying Hypothesis." *Proceedings of the National Academy of Sciences* 92 (April): 3650–57.

Naora, Honami, and Denise J. Montell. 2005. "Ovarian Cancer Metastasis: Integrating Insights from Disparate Model Organisms." *Nature Reviews Cancer* 5 (May): 355–66.

Nass, Sharyl J., and Harold L. Moses, eds. 2007. *Cancer Biomarkers: The Promises and Challenges of Improving Detection and Treatment.* Washington, DC: Institute of Medicine, National Academies Press.

Nass, Sharyl J., Harold L. Moses, and John Mendelsohn, eds. 2010. Committee on Cancer Clinical Trials and the NCI Cooperative Group Program, Institute of Medicine. *A National Cancer Clinical Trials System for the 21st Century: Reinvigorating the NCI Cooperative Group Program.* Washington, DC: National Academies Press.

Nathan, Carl. 2007. "Aligning Pharmaceutical Innovation with Medical Need." *Nature Medicine* 13 (March): 304.

Nathan, David G. 2001. "The Relevant Biomedical Research." *Harvard Magazine,* January/February.

———. 2007. *The Cancer Treatment Revolution: How Smart Drugs and Other New Therapies Are Renewing Our Hope and Changing the Face of Medicine.* Hoboken, NJ: John Wiley & Sons.

National Aeronautics and Space Administration, NASA History Division. 1998. "Chronology of Defining Events in NASA History, 1958–1998." Retrieved from http://www.hq.nasa.gov/office/pao/History/40thann/define.htm.

National Archives. Military Records, Southeast Asia Combat Area Casualties Current File (CACCF), Record Counts by Year of Death or Declaration of Death (as of December 1998). http://www.archives.gov/research/military/vietnam-war/casualty-statistics.html#year.

National Bioethics Advisory Commission. 1999. *Research Involving Human Biological Materials: Ethical Issues and Policy Guidance.* Rockville, MD: NBAC.

National Cancer Act of 1971. 1971. Public Law 92-218, 92nd Congress, S. 1828, December 23. The complete text of the law can be found at http://legislative.cancer.gov/history/phsa/1971.

National Cancer Institute. 1971–2011. Annual NCI *Fact Books.* NCI Office of Budget and Finance. http://obf.cancer.gov/financial/factbook.htm.

———. 1997. *Report of the National Cancer Institute Clinical Trials Program Review Group* (Armitage Report). August 26.

———. 1998. "Report of the National Cancer Institute Clinical Trials Implementation Committee." Presented to the NCI Board of Scientific Advisors. September 23.

———. 2000. Division of Cancer Prevention. *The Early Detection Research Network: Translational Research to Identify Early Cancer and Cancer Risk. Initial Report.* NIH, October.

———. 2004. *NCI Cancer Bulletin.* January 20.

———. 2005. "Report of the Clinical Trials Working Group: Restructuring the National Cancer Clinical Trials Enterprise." June.

———. 2007a. *National Cancer Institute Best Practices for Biospecimen Resources.* US Department of Health and Human Services. June, 1–43.

———. 2007b. National Cancer Institute press release, "Annual Report to the Nation Finds Cancer Death Rate Decline Doubling." October 15. http://www.cancer.gov/newscenter/pressreleases/2007/reportnation2007release.

———. 2010. *Office of Biorepositories and Biospecimen Research: Setting the Standards and Creating the Infrastructure for High Quality Biospecimens* (NIH Publication No. 10-7684). October.

———. 2011. "Guidelines for Specialized Programs of Research Excellence (SPOREs)." Translational Research Program, Division of Cancer Treatment and Diagnosis, National Cancer Institute. Posted August 2011.

———. "The Childhood Cancer Survivor Study." http://www.cancer.gov/cancertopics/coping/ccss.

———. Discussion of bevacizumab. Retrieved November 18, 2011. http://www.cancer.gov/cancertopics/druginfo/fda-bevacizumab.

———. Division of Extramural Activities. "NIH Grant Review Process." http://www.deainfo.nci.nih.gov/extra/extdocs/grantrevprocess.htm.

———. Fact sheet on childhood ALL. http://www.cancer.gov/cancertopics/pdq/treatment/childALL/Patient.

———. "NCI's Clinical Trials Cooperative Group Program" (fact sheet). http://www.cancer.gov/cancertopics/factsheet/NCI/clinical-trials-cooperative-group.

National Cancer Institute Clinical Trials Program Review Group. 1997. Division of Extramural Activities report. August 26.

National Cancer Institute SEER. For SEER *Cancer Statistics Review (CSR)* 1973–1993, see Ries et al. 1996; for *CSR* 1975–2005, see Ries et al. 2005; for *CSR* 1975–2009, see Howlader et al. 2012.

———. 2013a. SEER data sets, "Standard Populations—19 Age Groups." US Standard Population, 1940–2000. http://seer.cancer.gov/stdpopulations/stdpop.19ages .html.

———. 2013b. "Glossary of Statistical Terms." http://seer.cancer.gov/cgi-bin/glossary/ glossary.pl.

National Center for Health Statistics. 1974a. "Summary Report, Final Mortality Statistics, 1970. Part II. Cause of Death." *Monthly Vital Statistics Report* 22 (11 supp.). HRA 74-1120. February 22.

———. 1974b. "Summary Report, Final Mortality Statistics, 1971. Part II. Cause of Death." *Monthly Vital Statistics Report* 23 (3 supp.). HRA 74-1120. May 24.

———. 1975. *Vital Statistics of the United States 1970, Vol. II—Mortality.* Rockville, MD.

———. 1977. National Vital Statistics System. Unpublished trend table 290A, "Deaths for 60 Selected Causes, by 10-Year Age Groups, Race, and Sex: United States, 1960–67," and separate unpublished mortality tables for the black population and accidents.

———. 1982. National Vital Statistics System. Unpublished trend table 290A, "Deaths for 69 Selected Causes, by 10-Year Age Groups, Race, and Sex: United States, 1968–78."

———. 1993. "Advance Report of Final Mortality Statistics, 1990." *Monthly Vital Statistics Report* 41 (7 supp.). PHS 93-1120. January 7.

———. 2011a. "Deaths: Final Data for 2009." *National Vital Statistics Report* 59 (10). PHS 2011-1120. December 7.

———. 2011b. "Deaths: Final Data for 2009." *National Vital Statistics Report* 60 (3). PHS 2012-1120. December 29.

———. 2012. "Deaths: Preliminary Data for 2011." *National Vital Statistics Report* 61 (6). PHS 2013-1120. October 10. (Includes some final data for 2010.)

———. *Health, United States, 1998. With Socioeconomic Status and Health Chartbook.* Hyattsville, MD.

———. *Health, United States, 2000. With Adolescent Health Chartbook.* Hyattsville, MD.

———. *Health, United States, 2002: With Chartbook on Trends in the Health of Americans.* Hyattsville, MD.

———. *Health, United States, 2007: With Chartbook on Trends in the Health of Americans.* Hyattsville, MD.

————. *Health, United States, 2009: With Special Feature on the Health of Young Adults.* Hyattsville, MD.

————. *Health, United States, 2010: With Special Feature on Medical Technology.* Hyattsville, MD.

————. *Health, United States, 2011: With Special Feature on Death and Dying.* Hyattsville, MD.

————. *Health, United States, 2012: With Special Feature on Socioeconomic Status and Health.* Hyattsville, MD.

————. *Leading Causes of Death, 1900–1998.* http://www.cdc.gov/nchs/data/dvs/lead1900_98.pdf.

National Highway Traffic Safety Administration (NHTSA). 2010. "Lives Saved in 2008 by Restraint Use and Minimum Drinking Age Laws." *Traffic Safety Facts, Crash Stats.* DOT HS 811 153. May.

————. 2012. *An Analysis of Recent Improvements to Vehicle Safety.* DOT HS 811 572. June.

National Institute on Aging, National Institutes of Health. 2012. "Blood Vessels and Aging: The Rest of the Journey." Available on NIA website.

National Institutes of Health. 2003. NIH Roadmap. NIH News, Office of the Director. September 30. http://www.nih.gov/news/pr/sep2003/od-30.htm.

————. 2008a. "Enhancing Peer Review: The NIH Announces New Scoring Procedures for Evaluation of Research Applications Received for Potential FY2010 Funding." NIH Notice Number: NOT-OD-09-024. December 2.

————. 2008b. "Summary: National Cancer Institute Biospecimen Best Practices Forum, the Conference Center at Harvard Medical, Boston, November 5, 2007." Prepared by Rose Li and Associates, Inc. for the Office of Biorepositories and Biospecimen Research, National Cancer Institute. January.

————. 2009. Statement of NIH Director, "NIH's Role in the American Recovery and Reinvestment Act (ARRA)." February 25. http://www.nih.gov/about/director/02252009statement_arra.htm.

————. 2011. Freedom of Information Request to Division of Program Coordination, Planning, and Strategic Initiatives, regarding components of Biomedical Research and Development Price Index (BRDPI). Provided in letter. February 15.

————. 2012. Peer Review Process, National Institutes of Health, Office of Extramural Research. http://grants.nih.gov/grants/peer_review_process.htm. Updated September 6.

————. Center for Scientific Review. Roster Index for Regular Standing Study Sections and Continuing Special Emphasis Panels (SEPs). http://public.csr.nih.gov/StudySections/Standing/Pages/default.aspx.

————. The NIH Almanac, Appropriations (Section 1). http://www.nih.gov/about/almanac/appropriations/index.htm.

————. Office of Extramural Research. "NIH Research Project Grant Program (R01)." Retrieved September 12, 2012. http://grants.nih.gov/grants/funding/r01.htm.

————. Office of Extramural Research, Office of Research Information Systems. "NIH R01 Equivalent and RPG Success Rates FY 1970–2009."

————. Office of Extramural Research, Office of Research Information Systems. "NIH Research Project Grant Principal Investigators and Medical School Faculty Age Distributions, 1980–2006."

————. Research Portfolio Online Reporting Tools (RePORT). Research Project Success Rates by NIH Institute for 2011.

National Panel of Consultants on the Conquest of Cancer. 1970. *National Program for the Conquest of Cancer, Report to the US Senate, Committee on Labor and Public Welfare* (Report No. 91-1402). 91st Cong., 2nd sess., November 25.

National Vital Statistics Reports (NVSR). See under "National Center for Health Statistics."

Naumov, George N., et al. 2002. "Persistence of Solitary Mammary Carcinoma Cells in a Secondary Site: A Possible Contributor to Dormancy." *Cancer Research* 62 (April 1): 2162–68.

Neergaard, Lauran. 2007. Associated Press. "Cancer Death Rates Dropping Fast." *Washington Post*, October 15. http://www.washingtonpost.com/wp-dyn/content/article/2007/10/15/AR2007101500303.html.

Neison, F. G. P. 1844. "On a Method Recently Proposed for Conducting Inquiries into the Comparative Sanatory Condition of Various Districts, with Illustrations, Derived from Numerous Places in Great Britain at the Period of the Last Census." *Quarterly Journal of the Statistical Society of London* 7 (April). London: John William Parker.

Nelson, Celeste M., and Mina J. Bissell. 2005. "Modeling Dynamic Reciprocity: Engineering Three-Dimensional Culture Models of Breast Architecture, Function, and Neoplastic Transformation." *Seminars in Cancer Biology* 15 (October): 342–52.

Nelson, Cliff L., and Norman J. Temple. 1994. "Tribute to Denis Burkitt." *Journal of Medical Biography* 2: 130–33.

Nelson, Ethel R. 1998. *Burkitt Cancer Fiber: How a Humble Surgeon Changed the World*. Brushton, NY: Teach Services.

Neubauer, Hans, et al. 2008. "Breast Cancer Proteomics Reveals Correlation Between Estrogen Receptor Status and Differential Phosphorylation of PGRMC1." *Breast Cancer Research* 10 (5) (October): R85.

New York Times Editorial Board. 2012. "Incredible Prices for Cancer Drugs." November 12.

Ng, Rick. 2004. *Drugs: From Discovery to Approval*. Hoboken, NJ: John Wiley & Sons.

Nigam, Vijai N., and Antonio Canter. 1973. "Polysaccharides in Cancer: Glycoproteins and Glycolipids." *Advances in Cancer Research* 17: 1–80.

Nishikawa, Makiya. 2008. "Reactive Oxygen Species in Tumor Metastasis." *Cancer Letters* 266 (July): 53–59.

Nissen, Steven E., et al. 2005. "Statin Therapy, LDL Cholesterol, C-Reactive Protein, and Coronary Artery Disease." *New England Journal of Medicine* 352 (January 6): 29–38.

Nkoy, Flory L., et al. 2010. "Variable Specimen Handling Affects Hormone Receptor Test Results in Women with Breast Cancer: A Large Multihospital Retrospective Study." *Archives of Pathology and Laboratory Medicine* 134 (April): 606–12.

Noble, Denis. 2006. *The Music of Life: Biology Beyond the Genome.* Oxford: Oxford University Press.

Norman, Colin. 1984. "Congress Votes NIH a Big Budget Boost." *Science* 226 (October 26): 417–18.

Norris, Floyd. 1999. "Can Regulators Keep Accountants from Writing Fiction?" *New York Times,* September 10.

Novak, Kristine. 2005. "A Healing Process." *Nature Reviews Cancer* 5 (April): 244.

Nowell, Peter C. 1960. "Phytohemagglutinin: An Initiator of Mitosis in Cultures of Normal Human Leukocytes." *Cancer Research* 20 (May): 462–66.

———. 1977. "Citation Classic." *Current Contents/Life Sciences* 42 (October 17): 53.

———. 1985. "Citation Classic." *Current Contents/Life Sciences* 8 (February 25): 19.

———. 2002. "Progress with Chronic Myelogenous Leukemia: A Personal Perspective over Four Decades." *Annual Review of Medicine* 53: 1–13.

———. 2007. "Discovery of the Philadelphia Chromosome: A Personal Perspective." *Journal of Clinical Investigation* 117 (August): 2033–35.

Nowell, Peter C., Riccardo Dalla-Favera, Janet Finan, Jan Erikson, and Carlo M. Croce. 1983. "Chromosome Translocations, Immunoglobulin Genes, and Neoplasia." In *Chromosomes and Cancer: From Molecules to Man, Bristol-Myers Cancer Symposia,* vol. 5, edited by Janet D. Rowley and John E. Ultmann, 165–82. Orlando, FL: Academic Press.

Nowell, Peter C., and David A. Hungerford. 1960. "A Minute Chromosome in Human Chronic Granulocytic Leukemia." *Science* 132 (November 18): 1497.

———. 1961. "Chromosome Studies in Human Leukemia. II. Chronic Granulocytic Leukemia." *Journal of the National Cancer Institute* 27 (November): 1013–35.

Nucifora, Giuseppina, Richard A. Larson, and Janet D. Rowley. 1993. "Persistence of the 8:21 Translocation in Patients with Acute Myeloid Leukemia Type M2 in Long-Term Remission." *Blood* 82 (August 1): 712–15.

Oatis, W. S., et al. 2009. "Interpreting Out-of-Pocket Expenditures for Cancer Patients: The Importance of Considering Baseline Household Income

Information." 2009 ASCO annual meeting. *Journal of Clinical Oncology* 27 (supp.; abstract 6541): 15s.

Oberling, C., and M. Guérin. 1954. "The Role of Viruses in the Production of Cancer." *Advances in Cancer Research* 2: 353–423.

O'Brien, Stephen J. 2001. "Cell Culture Forensics." *Proceedings of the National Academy of Sciences* 98 (July 3): 7656–58.

O'Byrne, Kenneth J., and Angus G. Dalgleish. 2001. "Chronic Immune Activation and Inflammation as the Cause of Malignancy." *British Journal of Cancer* 85 (August): 473–83.

Ochoa, Manuel, Jr. 1969. "Alkylating Agents in Clinical Cancer Chemotherapy." *Annals of the New York Academy of Sciences* 163 (October): 921–30.

O'Conor, Greg T., and J. N. P. Davies. 1960. "Malignant Tumors in African Children: With Special Reference to Malignant Lymphoma." *Journal of Pediatrics* 56 (April): 526–35.

O'Conor, Greg T. 1961. "Malignant Lymphoma in African Children: II. A Pathological Entity." *Cancer* 14 (March–April): 270–83.

Oeffinger, Kevin C., et al. 2006. "Chronic Health Conditions in Adult Survivors of Childhood Cancer." *New England Journal of Medicine* 335 (October 12): 1572–82.

Office for Human Research Protections. US Department of Health and Human Services, IRB guidebook. http://www.hhs.gov/ohrp/archive/irb/irb_guide book.htm.

Office of Management and Budget. 2010. *Budget of the US Government, Fiscal Year 2011.* Washington, DC: US Government Printing Office.

Office of Technology Assessment, US Congress. 1976. *Development of Medical Technology: Opportunities for Assessment.* NTIS order #PB-258117.

———. 1991. *Federally Funded Research: Decisions for a Decade, OTA-SET-490.* Washington, DC: US Government Printing Office. May.

———. 1993a. *Pharmaceutical R&D: Costs, Risks, and Rewards, OTA-H-522.* Washington, DC: US Government Printing Office. February.

———. 1993b. *Researching Health Risks, OTA-BBS-570.* Washington, DC: US Government Printing Office. November.

Office of the Surgeon General. 1964. *Smoking and Health: Report of the Advisory Committee to the Surgeon General of the Public Health Service.* Public Health Service Publication No. 1103.

Ogawa, Makio. 1993. "Differentiation and Proliferation of Hematopoietic Stem Cells." *Blood* 81 (June 1): 2844–53.

Ogwang, Martin D., Kishor Bhatia, Robert J. Biggar, and Sam M. Mbulaiteye. 2008. "Incidence and Geographic Distribution of Endemic Burkitt Lymphoma in Northern Uganda Revisited." *International Journal of Cancer* 123 (December 1): 2658–63.

O'Keefe, Sean. 2005. "Step by Step, NASA Is Doing What It Takes to 'Fix the Culture.'" Op-ed. *USA Today*, April 25.

O'Malley, Maureen A., Kevin C. Elliott, Chris Haufe, and Richard M. Burlan. 2009. "Philosophies of Funding." *Cell* 138 (August 21): 611–15.

Oppel, Richard A., Jr. 1999. "Benno C. Schmidt, Financier, Is Dead at 86." *New York Times*, October 22.

Ordway, Frederick I., III, and Mitchell R. Sharpe. 1979. *The Rocket Team: From the V-2 to the Saturn Moon Rocket—the Inside Story of How a Small Group of Engineers Changed World History*. New York: Thomas Y. Crowell Publishers.

Orem, Jackson, Edward Katongole Mbidde, Bo Lambert, Silvia de Sanjose, and Elisabete Weiderpass. 2007. "Burkitt's Lymphoma in Africa, a Review of the Epidemiology and Etiology." *African Health Sciences* 7 (September): 166–75.

Orkin, Stuart H., and Leonard I. Zon. 2008. "Hematopoiesis: An Evolving Paradigm for Stem Cell Biology." *Cell* 132 (February 22): 631–44.

Osborne, Cynthia, and Debu Tripathy. 2005. "Aromatase Inhibitors: Rationale and Use in Breast Cancer." *Annual Review of Medicine* 56 (February): 103–16.

Osgood, Edwin E., and Marion L. Krippaehne. 1955. "The Gradient Tissue Culture Method." *Experimental Cell Research* 9: 116–27.

O'Shaughnessy, Joyce A., et al. 2002. The American Association for Cancer Research Task Force on the Treatment and Prevention of Intraepithelial Neoplasia. "Treatment and Prevention of Intraepithelial Neoplasia: An Important Target for Accelerated New Agent Development." *Clinical Cancer Research* 8 (February): 314–46.

Otten, Alan L. 1971. "Politics and People." *Wall Street Journal*, November 18, 22.

Ottmann, Oliver G., et al. 2002. "A Phase 2 Study of Imatinib in Patients with Relapsed or Refractory Philadelphia Chromosome-Positive Acute Lymphoid Leukemias." *Blood* 100 (September 15): 1965–71.

Otto, Sarah P. 2007. "The Evolutionary Consequences of Polyploidy." *Cell* 131 (November 2): 452–62.

Owens, Albert H., Jr. 1982. "Introduction to the Symposium, Tumor Cell Heterogeneity: A Perspective." In *Tumor Cell Heterogeneity: Origins and Implications, Bristol-Myers Cancer Symposia*, vol. 4, edited by Albert H. Owens Jr., Donald S. Coffey, and Stephen B. Baylin. New York: Academic Press.

Owens, Joanna. 2006. "The Enemy Within" (Milestone 5). In *Nature Milestones in Cancer* (April 1): S10.

———. 2007. "2006 Drug Approvals: Finding the Niche." *Nature Reviews Drug Discovery* 6 (February): 99–101.

Pacey, Arnold. 1975. *The Maze of Ingenuity: Ideas and Idealism in the Development of Technology*. New York: Holmes & Meier Publishers.

———. 1990. *Technology in World Civilization: A Thousand-Year History*. Cambridge, MA: MIT Press.

————. 1994. *The Culture of Technology.* Cambridge, MA: MIT Press. Originally published in 1983.

Paget, Stephen. 1889. "The Distribution of Secondary Growths in Cancer of the Breast." *Lancet* 133 (March 23): 571–73.

Painter, Theophilus Shickel. 1923. "Studies in Mammalian Spermatogenesis: II. The Spermatogenesis of Man." *Journal of Experimental Zoology* 37: 291–336.

————. 1924. "The Sex Chromosomes of Man." *American Naturalist* 58: 506–24.

Panayiotidis, Mihalis. 2008. "Reactive Oxygen Species (ROS) in Multistage Carcinogenesis." *Cancer Letters* 266 (July): 3–5.

Papac, Rose J. 1996. "Spontaneous Regression of Cancer." *Cancer Treatment Reviews* 22: 395–423.

————. 2001. "Origins of Cancer Therapy." *Yale Journal of Biology and Medicine* 74: 391–98.

Papanicolaou, George N. 1942. "New Procedure for Staining Vaginal Smears." *Science* 95 (April 24): 438–39.

Papanicolaou, George N., and Herbert F. Traut. 1943. *Diagnosis of Uterine Cancer by the Vaginal Smear.* New York: Commonwealth Fund.

Parazzini, Fabio. 2005. "Clinical Trials in Urology: How Many Patients Are Required to Achieve Statistically Significant Results?" *BJU International* 95 (April): 717–22.

Paris, Pamela, et al. 2010. "A Group of Genome-Based Biomarkers That Add to a Kattan Nomogram for Predicting Progression in Men with High-Risk Prostate Cancer." *Clinical Cancer Research* 16 (January 1): 195–202.

Parisian, Suzanne. 2001. *FDA: Inside and Out.* Front Royal, VA: Fast Horse Press.

Parker-Pope, Tara. 2010. "The Downside of a Cancer Study Extolling CT Scans." *New York Times,* November 16.

————. 2011. "Prostate Test Finding Leaves a Swirl of Confusion." *New York Times,* October 11.

Parkin, D. M. 1998. "Epidemiology of Cancer: Global Patterns and Trends." *Toxicology Letters* 102–3 (December): 227–34.

Parkin, D. M., et al. 2003. *Cancer in Africa: Epidemiology and Prevention.* International Agency for Research on Cancer, World Health Organization, IARC Scientific Publication No. 153. Lyon, France: IARC Press.

Parran, Thomas, Jr. 1939. "Cancer and the Public Health." *Science* 90 (November 10): 427–30.

Passegué, Emmanuelle. 2006. "Cancer Biology: A Game of Subversion." *Nature* 442 (August 17): 754–55.

Pathak, S. 2004. "T. C. Hsu: In Memory of a Rare Scientist." *Cytogenetic and Genome Research* 105: 1–3.

Patlak, Margie. 2001. "Targeting Leukemia: From Bench to Bedside." *FASEB Breakthroughs in Bioscience.* Federation of American Societies for Experimental Biology, 1–12.

Patlak, Margie, Erin Balogh, and Sharyl J. Nass. 2012. National Cancer Policy Forum, Institute of Medicine. "Facilitating Collaborations to Develop Combination Investigational Cancer Therapies: Workshop Summary." Washington, DC: National Academies Press.

Patterson, James T. 1987. *The Dread Disease: Cancer and Modern American Culture* Cambridge, MA: Harvard University Press.

Patton, Stacey. 2012. "The Ph.D. Now Comes with Food Stamps." *Chronicle of Higher Education,* May 6.

Peers, Alexandra. 2006. "For Cancer Survivors, a Job Hunt Can Be the Next Big Obstacle." *New York Times,* September 17.

Peters, Christie Provost. 2004. "Fundamentals of the Prescription Drug Market, NHPF Background Paper." Washington, DC: National Health Policy Forum. August 24.

Petricoin, Emanuel F., and Lance A. Liotta. 2004. "SELDI-TOF-Based Serum Proteomic Pattern Diagnostics for Early Detection of Cancer." *Current Opinion in Biotechnology* 15 (February): 24–30.

Petricoin, Emanuel F., et al. 2006. "The Blood Peptidome: A Higher Dimension of Information Content for Cancer Biomarker Discovery." *Nature Reviews Cancer* 6 (December): 961–67.

Petryna, Adriana. 2007. "Clinical Trials Offshored: On Private Sector Science and Public Health." *BioSocieties* 2: 21–40.

Pfizer. 2004. Hank McKinnell (then CEO), meeting with Wall Street analysts, November 30. Obtained through Factiva.

Philipson, Tomas, Ernst R. Berndt, Adrian H. B. Gottschalk, and Matthew W. Strobek. 2006. "How Safe Is Too Safe? Public Safety Versus Innovation at the FDA." *Milken Institute Review* (2nd quarter): 38–45.

PhRMA. 2002. "Delivering on the Promise of Pharmaceutical Innovation: The Need to Maintain Strong and Predictable Intellectual Property Rights." White paper on the intersection of intellectual property and antitrust law in the pharmaceutical industry, submitted to the Federal Trade Commission and the Department of Justice, Antitrust Division. Washington, DC: Pharmaceutical Research and Manufacturers of America. April 22.

———. 2012. 2012 Profile of Pharmaceutical Industry, and profiles for previous years. Washington, DC: Pharmaceutical Research and Manufacturers of America.

Pinkel, Donald. 1979. "The Ninth Annual David Karnofsky Lecture. Treatment of Acute Lymphocytic Leukemia." *Cancer* 43 (March): 1128–37.

Pisano, Douglas J., and David Mantus, eds. 2004. *FDA Regulatory Affairs: A Guide for Prescription Drugs, Medical Devices, and Biologics.* Boca Raton, FL: CRC Press.

Pisu, Marie, et al. 2010. "The Out-of-Pocket Cost of Breast Cancer Survivors: A Review." *Journal of Cancer Survivorship* 4: 202–9.

Pollack, Andrew. 2002. "ImClone's Woes Cast a Broader Biotech Shadow." *New York Times,* January 21.

———. 2010. "Panel Urges FDA to Revoke Approval of Drug for Breast Cancer Treatment." *New York Times,* July 20.

———. 2012a. "Justices Send Back Gene Case." *New York Times,* March 26.

———. 2012b. "Sanofi Halves Price of Cancer Drug Zaltrap After Sloan–Kettering Rejection." *New York Times,* November 8.

Polo, Sophie E., and Stephen P. Jackson. 2011. "Dynamics of DNA Damage Response Proteins at DNA Breaks: A Focus on Protein Modifications." *Genes and Development* 25 (March 1): 409–33.

Poste, George. 2011. "Bring on the Biomarkers." *Nature* 469 (January 13): 156–57.

Poste, George, and Isaiah J. Fidler. 1980. "The Pathogenesis of Cancer Metastasis." *Nature* 283 (June 10): 139–46.

President's Cancer Panel. 2001. Harold P. Freeman, chairman, Suzanne H. Reuben, ed. *Voices of a Broken System: President's Cancer Panel Report of the Chairman, 2000–2001.* Bethesda, MD: National Cancer Institute, National Institutes of Health.

———. 2004. LaSalle D. Leffall Jr., chairman, Suzanne H. Reuben, ed. *Living Beyond Cancer: Finding a New Balance, President's Cancer Panel 2003 Annual Report.* Bethesda, MD: National Cancer Institute, National Institutes of Health.

———. 2005. LaSalle D. Leffall Jr., chairman, Suzanne H. Reuben, ed. *Translating Research into Cancer Care: Delivering on the Promise, President's Cancer Panel Report of the Chairman, 2004–2005.* Bethesda, MD: National Cancer Institute, National Institutes of Health.

———. 2008. LaSalle D. Leffall Jr., chairman, Suzanne H. Reuben, ed. *Our Nation's Investment in Cancer: Three Crucial Actions for America's Health, President's Cancer Panel 2007–2008 Annual Report.* Bethesda, MD: National Cancer Institute, National Institutes of Health.

Prestera, Tory, et al. 1993. "The Electrophile Counterattack Response: Protection Against Neoplasia and Toxicity." *Advances in Enzyme Regulation* 33: 281–96.

Price, Don K. 1965. *The Scientific Estate.* Cambridge, MA: Belknap Press of Harvard University Press.

Prochaska, Hans Joaquim, et al. 1985. "On the Mechanisms of Induction of Cancer-Protective Enzymes: A Unifying Proposal." *Proceedings of the National Academy of Sciences* 82 (December 1): 8232–36.

Prud'homme, Alex. 2004. *The Cell Game.* New York: HarperCollins.

Public Citizen. WorstPills.org website, http://www.worstpills.org/.

Public Law 75-244. 1937. The National Cancer Institute Act. Enacted August 5.

Public Law 92-218. 1971. The National Cancer Act of 1971. Enacted December 23.

Public Law 99-158. 1985. The Health Research Extension Act of 1985. Enacted November 20.

Public Papers of the Presidents of the United States. 1972. "Remarks on Signing the National Cancer Act of 1971." December 23. *Public Papers of the Presidents of the United States, Richard Nixon, 1971.* General Services Administration, National Archives and Records Service, No. 408.

Pui, Ching-Hon, ed. 2003. *Treatment of Acute Leukemias: New Directions for Clinical Research.* New York: Humana Press.

Pui, Ching-Hon, and William E. Evans. 2006. "Treatment of Acute Lymphoblastic Leukemia." *New England Journal of Medicine* 354 (January 12): 166–78.

Quackenbush, John. 2002. "Microarray Data Normalization and Transformation." *Nature Genetics* 32 (December): 496–501.

———. 2004. "Data Standards for 'omic' Science." *Nature Biotechnology* 22 (May): 613–14.

Rader, Karen. 2004. *Making Mice: Standardizing Animals for American Biomedical Research, 1900–1955.* Princeton, NJ: Princeton University Press.

Radisky, Derek C., and Mina J Bissell. 2006. "Matrix Metalloproteinase-Induced Genomic Instability." *Current Opinion in Genetics and Development* 16: 45–50.

Rak, Janusz, and Joanne L. Yu. 2004. "Oncogenes and Tumor Angiogenesis: The Question of Vascular 'Supply' and Vascular 'Demand.'" *Seminars in Cancer Biology* 14: 93–104.

Rall, David P. 1968. "Selective Aspects of Chemotherapy in Acute Leukemia and Burkitt's Tumor." *Cancer* 21 (April): 575–79.

Rapkiewicz, Amy V., et al. 2004. "Biomarkers of Ovarian Tumours." *European Journal of Cancer* 40 (November): 2604–12.

Rapoport, Alan I. 1998. "What Is the Debt Burden of New Science and Engineering PhDs?" *National Science Foundation Issue Brief.* NSF 98-318. July 18.

Rather, L. J. 1978. *The Genesis of Cancer: A Study in the History of Ideas.* Baltimore: Johns Hopkins University Press.

Re, Daniel, Roman K. Thomas, Karolin Behringer, and Volker Diehl. 2005. "From Hodgkin Disease to Hodgkin Lymphoma: Biological Insights." *Blood* 105 (June 15): 4553–60.

Real, Francisco X. 2007. "p53: It Has It All, but Will It Make It to the Clinic as a Marker in Bladder Cancer?" *Journal of Clinical Oncology* 25 (December 1): 5341–44.

Reddoch, Jim, and David Amsellem. 2006. "Cancer Chronicle: Monthly Perspectives in Oncology." Arlington, VA: FBR Research, Friedman, Billings & Ramsey & Co. January 9.

Redmond, Kathy. 2004. "The US and European Regulatory Systems: A Comparison." *Journal of Ambulatory Care Management* 27: 105–14.

Rettig, Richard A. 1977. *Cancer Crusade: The Story of the National Cancer Act of 1971.* Princeton, NJ: Princeton University Press.

———. 2000. "Are Patients a Scarce Resource for Academic Clinical Research?" *Health Affairs* 19 (November/December): 195–205.

Reya, Tannishtha, Sean J. Morrison, Michael F. Clarke, and Irving L. Weissman. 2001. "Stem Cells, Cancer, and Cancer Stem Cells." *Nature* 414 (November 1): 105–11.

Rhoads, Cornelius P. 1946. "Nitrogen Mustards in the Treatment of Neoplastic Disease: Official Statement." *Journal of the American Medical Association* 131 (June 22): 656–58.

———. 1954. "Rational Cancer Chemotherapy." *Science* 119 (January 15): 77–80.

———. 1957. "The Soluble Puzzle of Cancer Control: Imperial Cancer Research Fund Lecture delivered at the Royal College of Surgeons of England, October 9, 1956." *Annals of the Royal College of Surgeons of England* 20 (March 1957): 139–56.

Rieff, David. 2008. *Swimming in a Sea of Death: A Son's Memoir.* New York: Simon & Schuster.

Ries, Lynn A. Glockler, et al., eds. 1996. *SEER Cancer Statistics Review, 1973–1993.* National Cancer Institute. http://seer.cancer.gov/csr/1973_1993/.

Ries, Lynn A. Glockler, et al., eds. 1999. *SEER Pediatric Monograph. Cancer Incidence and Survival Among Children and Adolescents: United States SEER Program, 1975–1995.* Bethesda, MD: National Cancer Institute, NIH Pub. No. 99-4649.

Ries, Lynn A. Glockler, et al., eds. 2008. *SEER Cancer Statistics Review, 1975–2005.* Based on November 2007 *SEER* data submission. National Cancer Institute. http://seer.cancer.gov/csr/1975_2005/.

Rieselbach, Richard E., Edward E. Morse, David P. Rall, Emil Frei III, and Emil J. Freireich. 1962. "Treatment of Meningeal Leukemia with Intrathecal Aminopterin." *Cancer Chemotherapy Reports* 16 (February): 191–96.

Riley, Gerald F., et al. 1995. "Medicare Payments from Diagnosis to Death for Elderly Cancer Patients by Stage at Diagnosis." *Medical Care* 33 (August): 828–41.

Ritov, Ilana, and Jonathan Baron. 1990. "Reluctance to Vaccinate: Omission Bias and Ambiguity." *Journal of Behavioral Decision Making* 3 (October/December): 263–77.

Rivera, Gaston K., Donald Pinkel, Joseph V. Simone, Michael L. Hancock, and William M. Crist. 1993. "Treatment of Acute Lymphoblastic Leukemia: 30 Years' Experience at St. Jude Children's Research Hospital." *New England Journal of Medicine* 329 (October 28): 1289–95.

Rizzo, J. Douglas, et al. 2007. "American Society of Hematology/American Society of Clinical Oncology 2007 Clinical Practice Guideline Update on the Use of Epoetin and Darbepoetin." *Journal of Clinical Oncology* 25 (December 1): 5490–505.

Roberts, Anita B., et al. 1981. "New Class of Transforming Growth Factors Potentiated by Epidermal Growth Factor: Isolation from Non–neoplastic Tissues." *Proceedings of the National Academy of Sciences* 78 (September): 5339–43.

Roberts, Anita B., Michael B. Sporn, et al. 1986. "Transforming Growth Factor Type Beta: Rapid Induction of Fibrosis and Angiogenesis In Vivo and Stimulation of Collagen Formation In Vitro." *Proceedings of the National Academy of Sciences* 83 (June 1): 4167–71.

Roberts, Royston M. 1989. *Serendipity: Accidental Discoveries in Science.* New York: John Wiley & Sons.

Rockey, Sally. 2011. "Paylines, Percentiles and Success Rates." In "Rock Talk: Helping Connect You with the NIH Perspective." Archive of NIH Extramural Nexus. http://nexus.od.nih.gov/all/2011/02/15/paylines-percentiles-success-rates/. Posted February 15.

Rodu, Brad, and Philip Cole. 2001. "The Fifty-Year Decline of Cancer in America." *Journal of Clinical Oncology* 19 (January 1): 239–41.

Roin, Benjamin N. 2009. "Unpatentable Drugs and the Standards of Patentability." *Texas Law Review* 87 (February): 503–70.

Roller, Duane H. D., ed. 1971. *Perspectives in the History of Science and Technology.* Norman: University of Oklahoma Press.

Roodi, Nady, et al. 1995. "Estrogen Receptor Gene Analysis in Estrogen Receptor-Positive and Receptor-Negative Primary Breast Cancer." *Journal of the National Cancer Institute* 87 (March 15): 446–51.

Roos, David S. "Bioinformatics: Trying to Swim in a Sea of Data," *Science* 291 (February 16): 1260–61.

Rosato, Donna. 2002. "Worried About Corporate Numbers? How About the Charts?" *New York Times,* September 15.

Rosenberg, Barnett, Loretta Van Camp, and Thomas Krigas. 1965. "Inhibition of Cell Division in *Escherichia coli* by Electrolysis Products from a Platinum Electrode." *Nature* 205 (February 13): 698–99.

Ross, Jeffrey S., et al. 2003. "The HER-2/neu Gene and Protein in Breast Cancer 2003: Biomarker and Target of Therapy." *Oncologist* 8 (August): 307–25.

Ross, Jeffrey S., et al. 2004. "Targeted Therapy in Breast Cancer: The HER-2/neu Gene and Protein." *Molecular and Cellular Proteomics* 3 (April): 379–98.

Rothwell, P. M., et al. 2011. "Effect of Daily Aspirin on Long-Term Risk of Death due to Cancer: Analysis of Individual Patient Data from Randomised Trials." *Lancet* 377 (January 1): 31–41.

Rous, Peyton. 1911a. "Transmission of a Malignant New Growth By Means of a Cell-Free Filtrate." *Journal of the American Medical Association* 56 (January 21): 198.

————. 1911b. "A Sarcoma of the Fowl Transmissible by an Agent Separable from the Tumor Cells." *Journal of Experimental Medicine* 13 (April 1): 397–411.

————. 1966. "The Challenge to Man of the Neoplastic Cell," Nobel Lecture, the Nobel Prize in Physiology or Medicine 1966 (December 13). Retrieved from http://www.nobelprize.org/nobel_prizes/medicine/laureates/1966/rous-lecture.html.

Rowe, Martin, Gemma L. Kelly, Andrew I. Bell, and Alan B. Rickinson. 2009. "Burkitt's Lymphoma: The Rosetta Stone Deciphering Epstein–Barr Virus Biology." *Seminars in Cancer Biology* 19 (December): 377–88.

Rowley, Janet D. 1973. "Identification of a Translocation with Quinacrine Fluorescence in a Patient with Acute Leukemia." *Annales de Génétique* 16: 109–12.

————. 1973a. "A New Consistent Chromosomal Abnormality in Chronic Myelogenous Leukaemia Identified by Quinacrine Fluorescence and Giemsa Staining." *Nature* 243 (June 1): 290–93.

————. 1973b. "Chromosomal Patterns in Myelocytic Leukemia." *New England Journal of Medicine* 289 (July 26): 220–21.

————. 1975a. "Nonrandom Chromosomal Abnormalities in Hematologic Disorders of Man." *Proceedings of the National Academy of Sciences* 72 (January): 152–56.

————. 1975b. "Abnormalities of Chromsome 1 in Myeloproliferative Disorders." *Cancer* 36 (November): 1748–57.

————. 1977. "Mapping of Human Chromosomal Regions Related to Neoplasia: Evidence from Chromosomes 1 and 17." *Proceedings of the National Academy of Sciences* 74 (December): 5729–33.

————. 1980. "Chromosome Abnormalities in Cancer." *Cancer Genetics and Cytogenetics* 2: 175–98.

————. 1990a. "The Philadelphia Chromosome Translocation: A Paradigm for Understanding Leukemia." *Cancer* 65 (May 15): 2178–84.

————. 1990b. "Molecular Cytogenetics: Rosetta Stone for Understanding Cancer—Twenty-Ninth G. H. A. Clowes Memorial Award Lecture." *Cancer Research* 50 (July 1): 3816–25.

————. 2008. "Chromosomal Translocations: Revisited Yet Again." *Blood* 112 (September 15): 2183–89.

Rowley, Janet D., and Joseph R. Testa. 1982. "Chromosome Abnormalities in Malignant Hematologic Diseases." In *Advances in Cancer Research*, vol. 36, edited by George Klein and Sidney Weinhouse, 118. Waltham, MA: Academic Press.

Rowley, Janet D., and John E. Ultmann, eds. 1983. *Chromosomes and Cancer: From Molecules to Man, Bristol-Myers Cancer Symposia*, vol. 5. Orlando, FL: Academic Press.

Rubinstein, Lawrence V. 2000. "Therapeutic Studies." *Hematology/Oncology Clinics of North America* 14 (August): 849–76.

Rubnitz, Jeffrey E., and Ching-Hon Pui. 1997. "Childhood Acute Lymphoblastic Leukemia." *Oncologist* 2 (6): 374–80.

Russo, Jose, Yun–Fu Hu, Xiaoqi Yang, and Irma H. Russo. 2000. "Developmental, Cellular, and Molecular Basis of Human Breast Cancer." In *Journal of the National Cancer Institute Monographs* 27: 17–37. (The NCI also provides a straightforward explanation of estrogen's effects on breast tissue on its website.)

Rutten, Paul, Mickey Tauman, Hagai Bar-Lev, and Avner Sonnino. 2001. "Is Moore's Law Infinite? The Economics of Moore's Law." *Kellogg TechVenture 2001 Anthology.* Kellogg Institute, Northwestern University, 1–28.

Ruzek, Jennifer Y., et al. 1996. *Trends in US Funding for Biomedical Research.* San Francisco: UCSF Center for the Health Professions.

Salk, Jesse J., Edward J. Fox, and Lawrence A. Loeb. 2010. "Mutational Heterogeneity in Human Cancers: Origin and Consequences." *Annual Review of Pathology: Mechanisms of Disease* 5: 51–75.

Salomon, David S., et al. 1995. "Epidermal Growth Factor-Related Peptides and Their Receptors in Human Malignancies." *Critical Reviews in Oncology/Hematology* 19: 183–232.

Sancar, Aziz, et al. 2004. "Molecular Mechanisms of Mammalian DNA Repair and the DNA Damage Checkpoints." *Annual Review of Biochemistry* 73 (July): 39–85.

Sargent John F., Jr. 2012. *Federal Research and Development Funding: FY2012.* CRS Report for Congress R41706. Washington, DC: Congressional Research Service. January 26.

Sausville, Edward A. 2003. "Imatinib for Chronic Myelogenous Leukemia: A 9 or 24 Carat Gold Standard?" *Lancet* 361 (April 26): 1400–1401.

Savona, Michael, and Moshe Talpaz. 2008. "Getting to the Stem of Chronic Myeloid Leukaemia." *Nature Reviews Cancer* 8 (May): 341–50.

Sawyers, Charles L. 1999. "Chronic Myeloid Leukemia." *New England Journal of Medicine* 340 (April 29): 1330–40.

———. 2008. "The Cancer Biomarker Problem." *Nature* 452 (April 3): 548–52.

Sawyers, Charles L., et al. 2002. "Imatinib Induces Hematologic and Cytogenetic Responses in Patients with Chronic Myelogenous Leukemia in Myeloid Blast Crisis: Results of a Phase II Study." *Blood* 99 (May 15): 3530–39.

Scannell, Jack W., Alex Blanckley, Helen Boldon, and Brian Warrington. 2012. "Diagnosing the Decline in Pharmaceutical R&D Efficiency." *Nature Reviews Drug Discovery* 11 (March): 191–200.

Schäfer, Matthias, and Sabine Werner. 2008. "Cancer as an Overhealing Wound: An Old Hypothesis Revisited." *Nature Reviews Molecular Cell Biology* 9 (August): 628–38.

Schaller, Robert R. 1977. "Moore's Law: Past, Present, and Future." *IEEE Spectrum,* June, 53–59.

Schein, Philip S., and Barbara Scheffler. 2006. "Barriers to Efficient Development of Cancer Therapeutics." *Clinical Cancer Research* 12 (June 1): 3243–48.

Schilsky, Richard L., Ross McIntyre, James F. Holland, and Emil Frei III. 2006. "A Concise History of the Cancer and Leukemia Group B." *Clinical Cancer Research* 12 (11 supp.) (June 1): 3553s–55s.

Schlessinger, Joseph. 2000. "Cell Signaling by Receptor Tyrosine Kinases." *Cell* 103 (October 13): 211–25.

Schmeck, Harold M., Jr. 1960. "Anti-Cancer Drug Tested in Africa." *New York Times*, April 22.

———. 1971a. "Cancer: The Fight over How to Fight a Dread Disease." *New York Times*, May 16.

———. 1971b. "House Unit Votes Own Cancer Bill." *New York Times*, November 5.

———. 1971c. "Cancer Research Is Voted by House." *New York Times*, November 16.

———. 1971d. "Cancer Agency Debate: Scientific Stakes Are High." *New York Times*, December 7.

———. 1975. "Lower Survival Found for Blacks with Cancer." *New York Times*, August 28, 25.

Schwan, Severin. 2011. Roche CEO presentation of company's fiscal year 2010 results, February 2, London and New York. See the section "Projected Additional Indications Submissions of Existing Products: Projects Currently in Phase 2 and 3," 71.

Schwartz, John, Andrew C. Revkin, and Matthew L. Wald. 2005. "For NASA, Misjudgments Led to Latest Shuttle Woes." *New York Times*, July 31.

Science Careers Online. 2001–7. The GrantDoctor. "Betting on the Future." July 25, 2003; November 10, 2006. Nextwave from the journal *Science*, "Getting an NIH R01." September 28, 2001. And updated version of guide, "The NIH R01 Toolkit." July 27, 2007.

ScienceWatch. 2003. "Twenty Years of Citation Superstars." *ScienceWatch* 14 (5) (September/October): 2.

SCOTUSblog. 2012. *Association for Molecular Pathology, et al. (petitioners) v. Myriad Genetics, Inc., et al.* No. 11-725. http://www.scotusblog.com/case-files/cases/association–for-molecular-pathology-v-myriad-genetics/.

Scrimshaw, Nevin S., and Moisés Béhar. 1961. "Protein Malnutrition in Young Children." *Science* 133 (June 30): 2039–47.

Securities and Exchange Commission. 2003a. Litigation release No. 18026, *Securities and Exchange Commission v. Samuel D. Waksal*, 02-CIV-4407 (NB) (SDNY). March 11. http://www.sec.gov/litigation/litreleases/lr18026.htm.

———. 2003b. "Enforcement Proceedings: SEC Charges Martha Stewart and Her Broker Peter Bacanovic with Illegal Insider Trading." *SEC News Digest*, issue 2003-106 (June 4). http://www.sec.gov/news/digest/dig060403.txt.

Securities and Exchange Commission against Samuel D. Waksal. 2003. Amended Complaint, 02 Civ. 4407 (NRB). March 11. http://www.sec.gov/litigation/complaints/comp18026.htm.

Sell, Stewart. 1990. "Cancer-Associated Carbohydrates Identified by Monoclonal Antibodies." *Progress in Pathology* 21 (October): 1003–19.

Semple, Robert B., Jr. 1965. "Bill-Signing a Johnson Art." *New York Times,* August 15.

Senate Hearings. 1971. *Conquest of Cancer Act, 1971. Subcommittee on Health of the Committee on Labor and Public Welfare. Hearings Before the United States Senate.* 92nd Cong., 1st sess., on S. 34 . . . [and] S. 1828 . . . March 9, 10, and June 10, 1971. Washington, DC: US Government Printing Office.

———. 1997. "Winning the War on Cancer and Medicare: Physician Practice Expenses." *Hearings Before a Subcommittee of the Committee on Appropriations* (Senate Hearings 105-178). 105th Cong., 1st sess., May 7, 1997, 32.

Seruga, Bostjan, et al. 2008. "Cytokines and Their Relationship to the Symptoms and Outcome of Cancer." *Nature Reviews Cancer* 8 (November): 887–99.

Serwer, Andy. 2002a. "Dirty Rotten Numbers." *Fortune,* February 18.

———. 2002b. "The Socialite Scientist." *Fortune,* April 15.

SF424(R&R). 2011. Public Health Service, US Department of Health and Human Services. SF424 (R&R) Application Guide for NIH and Other PHS Agencies (updated July 25). http://grants.nih.gov/grants/funding/424/index.htm.

Shah, Neil P., et al. 2002. "Multiple BCR-ABL Kinase Domain Mutations Confer Polyclonal Resistance to the Tyrosine Kinase Inhibitor Imatinib (STI571) in Chronic Phase and Blast Crisis Chronic Myeloid Leukemia." *Cancer Cell* 2 (August): 117–25.

Shah, Neil P., et al. 2004. "Overriding Imatinib Resistance with a Novel ABL Kinase Inhibitor." *Science* 305 (July 16): 399–401.

Shah, Sohrab P., et al. 2009. "Mutational Evolution in a Lobular Breast Tumour Profiled at Single Nucleotide Resolution." *Nature* 461 (October 8): 809–13.

Shallit, Jeffrey. 2005. "Science, Pseudoscience, and the Three Stages of Truth." Online, University of Waterloo, Ontario, Canada, March 28.

Shannon, James A., ed. 1973. *Science and the Evolution of Public Policy.* New York: Rockefeller University Press.

Shibata, Darryl, et al. 1993. "Genetic Heterogeneity of the c-K-ras Locus in Colorectal Adenomas but not in Adenocarcinomas." *Journal of the National Cancer Institute* 85 (July 7): 1058–63.

Shojaei, Farbod, and Napoleone Ferrara. 2008. "Role of the Microenvironment in Tumor Growth and in Refractoriness/Resistance to Anti-Angiogenic Therapies." *Drug Resistance Updates* 11 (December): 219–30.

Sieber, Oliver M., Karl Heinimann, and Ian P. M. Tomlinson. 2003. "Genomic Instability—the Engine of Tumorigenesis?" *Nature Reviews Cancer* 3 (September): 701–8.

Siegel, Peter M., and Joan Massagué. 2003. "Cytostatic and Apoptotic Actions of TGF-beta in Homeostasis and Cancer." *Nature Reviews Cancer* 3 (October): 807–21.

Siegel, Rebecca, et al. 2012. "Cancer Statistics, 2012." *CA: A Cancer Journal for Clinicians* 62 (January–February): 10–29.

Siegel, Rebecca, et al. 2013. "Cancer Statistics, 2013." *CA: A Cancer Journal for Clinicians* 63 (January–February): 11–30.

Sieweke, Michael H., Nancy L. Thompson, Michael B. Sporn, and Mina J. Bissell. 1990. "Mediation of Wound-Related Rous Sarcoma Virus Tumorigenesis by TGF-ß." *Science* 248 (June 29): 1656–60.

Silverberg, Edwin, and Arthur I. Holleb. 1971. "Cancer Statistics, 1971." *CA: A Cancer Journal for Clinicians* 21: 13–31.

Silverman, Richard B. 2004. *The Organic Chemistry of Drug Design and Drug Action.* 2nd ed. Waltham, MA: Elsevier Academic Press.

Silverstein, Melvin J. 1998. "Ductal Carcinoma In Situ of the Breast: Controversial Issues." *Oncologist* 3: 94–103.

Silvestri, Gerard A., et al. 2003. "Importance of Faith on Medical Decisions Regarding Cancer Care." *Journal of Clinical Oncology* 21 (April 1): 1379–82.

Simone, Joseph V. 2004. "The Task for 2015." *Oncology Times,* March 10.

Simpson–Herren, Linda, and Glynn P. Wheeler. 2006. "Howard Earle Skipper: In Memoriam (1915–2006)" *Cancer Research* 66 (December 15): 12035–36.

Sitas, Freddy, et al. 2006. "Cancers." In *Disease and Mortality in Sub-Saharan Africa,* 2nd ed., edited by Dean T. Jamison, et al. Washington, DC: The World Bank. Retrieved online from NCBI Bookshelf.

Sjöblom, Tobias, et al. 2006. "The Consensus Coding Sequences of Human Breast and Colorectal Cancers." *Science* 314 (October 13): 268–74.

Skipper, Howard E., Frank M. Schabel, Jr., and William S. Wilcox. 1964. "Experimental Evaluation of Potential Anticancer Agents. XIII. On the Criteria and Kinetics Associated with 'Curability' of Experimental Leukemias." *Cancer Chemotherapy Reports* 35 (February): 1–111.

Skloot, Rebecca. 2006. "Taking the Least of You." *New York Times Magazine,* April 16.

———. 2011. *The Immortal Life of Henrietta Lacks.* New York: Broadway Paperbacks, Crown; originally published by Crown in 2010.

Slamon, Dennis J. 1987. "Human Breast Cancer: Correlation of Relapse and Survival with Amplification of the HER-2/neu Oncogene." *Science* 235 (January 9): 177–82.

Slamon, Dennis J., et al. 2001. "Use of Chemotherapy plus a Monoclonal Antibody Against HER2 for Metastatic Breast Cancer That Overexpresses HER2." *New England Journal of Medicine* 344 (March 15): 783–92.

Slaughter, Danely P., Harry W. Southwick, and Walter Smejkal. 1953. "'Field Cancerization' in Oral Stratified Squamous Epithelium: Clinical Implications of Multicentric Origin." *Cancer* 6 (September): 963–68.

Slavin, David. 2006. "Risk/Benefit Ratios for Pharmaceuticals: Key Factors to Consider." Presentation at "Understanding the Benefits and Risks of Pharmaceuticals" meeting at the National Academy of Sciences, Institute of Medicine, Washington, DC. May 30.

Smith, Benjamin D., Grace L. Smith, Arti Hurria, Gabriel N. Hortobagyi, and Thomas A. Buchholz. 2009. "Future of Cancer Incidence in the United States: Burdens upon an Aging, Changing Nation." *Journal of Clinical Oncology* 27 (June 10): 2758–65.

Smith, F. H. 1914. "Benzol Treatment in Two Cases of Leukemia." *Journal of the American Medical Association* 42 (March 21): 921–25.

Smith, Malcolm A., et al. 1999. "Chapter 1: Leukemia." In *Cancer Incidence and Survival Among Children and Adolescents: United States SEER Program, 1975–1995*, edited by Lynn A. G. Ries et al., 17–34. Bethesda, MD: National Cancer Institute, NIH Pub. 99-4649.

Smith, Malcolm A., et al. 2010. "Outcomes for Children and Adolescents with Cancer: Challenges for the Twenty-First Century." *Journal of Clinical Oncology* 28 (May 20): 2625–34.

Smith, Merritt Roe, and Gregory Clancey, eds. 1998. *Major Problems in the History of American Technology.* Boston: Houghton Mifflin Company.

Smithers, David W. 1962. "Cancer: An Attack on Cytologism." *Lancet* 279 (March 10): 493–99.

———. 1969. "No Cell Is an Island." *British Medical Journal* 3 (September 27): 778.

Society for Medicines Research Committee. 2004. "Successes in Drug Discovery and Design." Case Histories in Drug Discovery and Design meeting, London, December 4, 2003. *Drug News and Perspectives* 17 (April 2004): 213.

Speer, John F., et al. 1984. "A Stochastic Numerical Model of Breast Cancer Growth That Simulates Clinical Data." *Cancer Research* 44 (September): 4124–30.

Spivak, Jerry L. 2005. "The Anaemia of Cancer: Death by a Thousand Cuts." *Nature Reviews Cancer* 5 (July): 543–55.

Sporn, Michael B. 1976. "Approaches to Prevention of Epithelial Cancer During the Preneoplastic Period." *Cancer Research* 36 (July): 2699–702.

———.1978. "Chemoprevention of Cancer." *Nature* 272 (March 30): 402–3.

———. 1980. "Combination Chemoprevention of Cancer." *Nature* 287 (September 11): 107–8.

———. 1991. "Carcinogenesis and Cancer: Different Perspectives on the Same Disease." *Cancer Research* 51 (December 1): 6215–18.

———. 1996. "The War on Cancer." *Lancet* 347 (May 18): 1377–81.

———. 1999. "TGF-ß: 20 Years and Counting." *Microbes and Infection* 1 (December): 1251–53.

———. 2005. "Brinker Award Lecture: Agents That Regulate TGF-β Are Good Candidates for Prevention and Treatment of Breast Cancer." San Antonio Breast Cancer Symposium. December 8.

———. 2006. "Dichotomies in Cancer Research: Some Suggestions for a New Synthesis." *Nature Clinical Practice Oncology* 3 (July): 364–73.

———. 2011. "The Big C—for Chemoprevention." *Nature* 471 (March 20): S10–S11.

Sporn, Michael B., and Anita B. Roberts. 1992. "Transforming Growth Factor-β: Recent Progress and New Challenges." *Journal of Cell Biology* 119 (December 1): 1017–21.

Sporn, Michael B., and George J. Todaro. 1980. "Autocrine Secretion and Malignant Transformation of Cells." *New England Journal of Medicine* 303 (October 9): 878–80.

Sporn, Michael B., et al. 1976. "Prevention of Chemical Carcinogenesis by Vitamin A and Its Synthetic Analogs (Retinoids)." *Federation Proceedings* (Federation of American Societies for Experimental Biology) 35 (May 1): 1332–38.

Spranca, Mark, Elisa Minsk, and Jonathan Baron. 1991. "Omission and Commission in Judgment and Choice." *Journal of Experimental Social Psychology* 27 (January): 76–105.

Srivastava, Sudhir, et al. 2008. Cancer Biomarkers Research Group of the National Cancer Institute's Division of Cancer Prevention. *The Early Detection Research Network, Fourth Report: Investing in Translational Research on Biomarkers of Early Cancer and Cancer Risk*. NIH Publication No. 07-6135. January.

State of Florida Department of Health. 2010. *Florida Vital Statistics Annual Report, 2009*. December.

Stehelin, Dominique, Harold E. Varmus, J. Michael Bishop, and Peter K. Vogt. 1976. "DNA Related to the Transforming Gene(s) of Avian Sarcoma Viruses Is Present in Normal Avian DNA." *Nature* 260 (March 11): 170–73.

Stein, Rob. 2009. "Fierce Debate Raging over New Cancer Test Guidelines." *Washington Post*, November 22.

———. 2011. "FDA Panel Votes Against Avastin for Breast Cancer Treatment." *Washington Post*, June 29.

Stempel, Jonathan. 2012. "Myriad Wins Gene Patent Ruling from US Appeals Court." Reuters, August 16.

Stewart, David J. 2009. "Cancer: The Road to Amiens." *Journal of Clinical Oncology* 27 (January 20): 328–33.

Stewart, Sarah E. 1960. "The Polyoma Virus." *Scientific American* 203 (November): 63–71.

Stipp, David. 2000. "A New Way to Attack Cancer." *Fortune,* May 29.

Stock, C. Chester. 1954. "Experimental Cancer Chemotherapy." *Advances in Cancer Research* 2: 425–92.

Stock, C. Chester, John J. Biesele, Joseph H. Burchenal, David A. Karnofsky, Alice E. Moore, and Kanematsu Sugiura. 1950. "Folic Acid Analogs and Experimental Tumors." *Annals of the New York Academy of Sciences* 52 (July): 1360–78.

Stoeckert, Christian J., Jr., Helen C. Causton, and Catherine A. Ball. 2002. "Microarray Databases: Standards and Ontologies." *Nature Genetics* 32 (December supp.): S469–73.

Stokes, Donald E. 1977. *Pasteur's Quadrant: Basic Science and Technological Innovation.* Washington, DC: Brookings Institution Press.

Stoler, Daniel L. 1999. "The Onset and Extent of Genomic Instability in Sporadic Colorectal Tumor Progression." *Proceedings of the National Academy of Sciences* 96 (December 21): 15121–26.

Stolley, Paul D., and Tamar Lasky. 1995. *Investigating Disease Patterns: The Science of Epidemiology.* New York: Scientific American Library.

Stolowy, Hervé, and Gaétan Breton. 2004. "Accounts Manipulation: A Literature Review and Proposed Conceptual Framework." *Review of Accounting and Finance* 3 (1): 5–92.

Stossel, Thomas P. 2008. "The Discovery of Statins." *Cell* 134 (September 19): 903–5.

Strickland, Stephen P. 1971. "Integration of Medical Research and Health Policies." *Science* 173 (September 17): 1093–1103.

———. 1972. *Politics, Science, and Dread Disease: A Short History of United States Medical Research Policy.* Cambridge, MA: Harvard University Press.

Stubbe, JoAnne, and Wilfred A. van der Donk. 1998. "Protein Radicals in Enzyme Catalysis." *Chemical Reviews* 98 (April 2): 705–62.

Subcommittee on Oversight and Investigations. 2002. *An Inquiry into the ImClone Cancer Drug Story Hearings.* 107th Cong., June 13.

Sugar, Alan. 2000. "Clinical Research." *Science* 287 (March 3): 1593.

Sulston, John, and Georgina Ferry. 2002. *The Common Thread: A Story of Science, Politics, Ethics and the Human Genome.* Washington, DC: Joseph Henry Press.

Sundro, Linda G. 1991. Office of Inspector General, National Science Foundation. *Federally Sponsored Research: How Indirect Costs Are Charged by Educational and Other Research Institutions.* Washington, DC: National Science Foundation. September.

Sung, Nancy S., et al. 2003. "Central Challenges Facing the National Clinical Research Enterprise." *Journal of the American Medical Association* 289 (March 12): 1278–87.

Supreme Court of the United States. 2012. *Association for Molecular Pathology, et al. (petitioners) v. Myriad Genetics, Inc., et al.* No. 11-725, docketed December 14, 2011; judgment issued April 27, 2012. United States Court of Appeals for the Federal Circuit, Case No. 2010-1406, decision July 29, 2011. See also http://www.pubpat.org/assets/files/brca/brcacertpetitionappendix.pdf.

Surh, Young-Joon. 2003. "Cancer Chemoprevention with Dietary Phytochemicals." *Nature Reviews Cancer* 3 (October): 768–80.

Susan G. Komen Breast Cancer Foundation. 2010. IRS Form 990 (Return of Organization Exempt from Income Tax) for the 2010 calendar year.

Suzuki, Hiroyoshi, et al. 1998. "Interfocal Heterogeneity of PTEN/MMAC1 Gene Alterations in Multiple Metastatic Prostate Cancer Tissues." *Cancer Research* 58 (January 15): 204–9.

Swain, Sandra M. 2012. Letter to *New York Times* regarding Bach, Saltz, and Wittes op-ed. October 19.

Sypher, F. J. 2000. "The Rediscovered Prophet: Frederick L. Hoffman (1865–1946)." *COSMOS: The Journal of the Cosmos Club.* Retrieved at http://www.cosmos-club.org/web/journals/2000/sypher.html.

———, ed. 2002. *Frederick L. Hoffman: His Life and Works.* Philadelphia: Xlibris.

Tabarrok, Alexander T. 2000. "Assessing the FDA via the Anomaly of Off-Label Drug Prescribing." *Independent Review* 5 (Summer): 25–53.

Talalay, Paul, et al. 1988. "Identification of a Common Chemical Signal Regulating the Induction of Enzymes That Protect Against Chemical Carcinogenesis." *Proceedings of the National Academy of Sciences* (November 1) 85: 8261–65.

Talmadge, James E., and Isaiah J. Fidler. 2010. "AACR Centennial Series: The Biology of Cancer Metastasis: Historical Perspective." *Cancer Research* 70 (July 15): 5649–69.

Talpaz, Moshe, et al. 2002. "Imatinib Induces Durable Hematologic and Cytogenetic Responses in Patients with Accelerated Phase Chronic Myeloid Leukemia: Results of a Phase 2 Study." *Blood* 99 (March 15): 1928–37.

Tanford, Charles, and Jacqueline Reynolds. 2003. *Nature's Robots: A History of Proteins.* Oxford: Oxford University Press. Originally published in 2001.

Taplin, Stephen H., et al. 1995. "Stage, Age, Comorbidity, and Direct Costs of Colon, Prostate, and Breast Cancer Care." *Journal of the National Cancer Institute* 87 (March 15): 417–26.

Tapscott, Don, and Anthony D. Williams. 2006. *Wikinomics: How Mass Collaboration Changes Everything.* New York: Portfolio.

Temple, Larissa K. F., et al. 1999. "Preventive Health Care, 1999 Update: 3. Follow-Up after Breast Cancer." *Canadian Medical Association Journal* 161 (October 19): 1001–8.

Temple, Norman J., and Denis P. Burkitt. 1991. "The War on Cancer—Failure of Therapy and Research: Discussion Paper." *Journal of the Royal Society of Medicine* 84 (February): 95–98.

Texas Department of State Health Services. 2010. *Texas Vital Statistics 2009 Annual Report.*

Theisen, Christine. 2003. "Predicting the Future: Projections Help Researchers Allocate Resources." *Journal of the National Cancer Institute* 95 (June 18): 846–48.

Thiers, Fabio A., Anthony J. Sinskey, and Ernst R. Berndt. 2008. "Trends in the Globalization of Clinical Trials." *Nature Reviews Drug Discovery* 7 (January): 13–14.

Thilly, William G. 2003. "Have Environmental Mutagens Caused Oncomutations in People?" *Nature Genetics* 34 (July): 255–59.

Thomas, Duncan P. 1969. "Experiment versus Authority: James Lind and Benjamin Rush." *New England Journal of Medicine* 281 (October 23): 932–33.

Thompson, Matthew P., and Razelle Kurzrock, 2004. "Epstein–Barr Virus and Cancer." *Clinical Cancer Research* 10 (February 1): 803–21.

Thomson Reuters. 2010. ISI Web of Knowledge [v.4.7]. Web of Science, cited reference search, January 28.

Thomson Reuters. *Journal Citation Reports.* 2010.

Thorley-Lawson, David A., and Martin J. Allday. 2008. "The Curious Case of the Tumour Virus: 50 years of Burkitt's Lymphoma." *Nature Reviews Microbiology* 6 (December): 913–24.

Thornburn, Andrew. 2010. "The Need for More Cancer Research." News release. Denver: University of Colorado Newsroom, June 4.

Thorne, Van Buren. 1914. "Scientists Sure that Germs Cause Chicken Cancer: After Experimenting for Years, Dr. Peyton Rous, of the Rockefeller Institute, Makes Some Remarkable Discoveries." *New York Times,* January 11.

Thorpe, Kenneth E., and David Howard. 2003. "Health Insurance and Spending Among Cancer Patients." *Health Affairs* W3 (April 9): 183–98.

Tilghman, Shirley, et al. 1998. National Research Council. *Trends in the Early Careers of Life Scientists: Report by the Committee on Dimensions, Causes, and Implications of Recent Trends in the Careers of Life Scientists.* Washington, DC: National Academy Press.

Tjio, Joe Hin, and Albert Levan. 1956. "The Chromosome Number of Man." *Hereditas* 42 (April): 1–6.

Tobias, J. S., M. Baum, and H. Thornon. 2000. "Clinical Trials in Cancer: What Makes for a Successful Study?" *Annals of Oncology* 11 (November): 1371–73.

Tomlinson, Ian, Peter Sasieni, and Walter Bodmer. 2002. "How Many Mutations in a Cancer?" *American Journal of Pathology* 160 (March): 755–58.

Topol, Eric J. 2004. "Intensive Statin Therapy—a Sea Change in Cardiovascular Prevention." *New England Journal of Medicine* 350 (April 8): 1562–64.

Toran–Allerand, C. Dominique, Meharvan Singh, and György Sétáló, Jr. 1999. "Novel Mechanisms of Estrogen Action in the Brain: New Players in an Old Story." *Frontiers in Neuroendocrinology* 20 (April): 97–121.

Tortora, Gerard J., and Nicholas P. Anagnostakos. 1987. *Principles of Anatomy and Physiology.* 5th ed. New York: Harper & Row Publishers.

Traut, Herbert F., and George N. Papanicolaou. 1943. "Cancer of the Uterus: The Vaginal Smear in Its Diagnosis." *California and Western Medicine* 59 (2) (August): 121–22.

Trimble, Cornelia L. et al. 2005. "Spontaneous Regression of High-Grade Cervical Dysplasia: Effects of Human Papillomavirus Type and HLA Phenotype." *Clinical Cancer Research* 11 (July 1): 4717–23.

Tsiaris, Alexander, and Barry Werth. 2004. *The Architecture and Design of Man and Woman.* New York: Doubleday.

Tsimicalis, Argerie, et al. 2011. "The Cost of Childhood Cancer From the Family's Perspective: A Critical Review." *Pediatric Blood and Cancer* 56 (May): 707–17.

Tufts Center for the Study of Drug Development. 2010. "Rising Protocol Complexity, Execution Burden Varies Widely by Phase and TA." *TCSDD Impact Report* 12 (3) (May/June).

Tuttle, Todd M., et al. 2009. "Increasing Rates of Contralateral Prophylactic Mastectomy Among Patients with Ductal Carcinoma In Situ." *Journal of Clinical Oncology* 27 (March 20): 1362–67.

Tyson, John J., et al. 2011. "Dynamic Modelling of Oestrogen Signalling and Cell Fate in Breast Cancer Cells." *Nature Reviews Cancer* 11 (July): 523–32.

UBS Warburg. 2001. Global Equity Research report. Untitled. "Buy" rating on ImClone Systems, January 2.

Ugorski, Maciej, and Anna Laskowska. 2002. "Sialyl Lewis: A Tumor-Associated Carbohydrate Antigen Involved in Adhesion and Metastatic Potential of Cancer Cells." *Acta Biochimica Polonica* 49: 303–11.

Unger, Lawrence, and Robert V. Blystone. 1996. "Paradigm Lost: The Human Chromosome Story." *Bioscene* 22 (2): 3–9.

USA Today/Kaiser Family Foundation/Harvard School of Public Health. 2006. "National Survey of Households Affected by Cancer." November.

US Attorney, Southern District of New York. 2003. "Samuel Waksal Sentenced in Federal Court to 7 Years 3 Months in Prison, Fined $3 Million." Press release. June 10. http://www.usdoj.gov/usao/nys/pressreleases/June03/waksalsentencepr.pdf.

US Census Bureau. 1990. "Intercensal Estimates of the United States Resident Population by Age and Sex, 1990."

————. 2000. "All Across the USA: Population Distribution and Composition, 2000."

————. 2000. "Historical National Population Estimates, 1900 to 1999." In Web archives. Internet release date, April 11; revised June 28.

————. 2002. Current Population Reports, P25-1095.

————. 2005. "Age and Sex Distribution in 2005: Population Profile of the United States."

————. 2008a. "2008 National Population Projections." August.

————. 2008b. NP2008-T2. August 14.

————. 2010a. "Annual Estimates of the Resident Population by Sex and Five-Year Age Groups for the United States: April 1, 2000 to July 1, 2009." NC-EST2009-01. June.

————. 2010b. "Current Population Survey, Annual Social and Economic Supplement, 2009." December.

————. 2011a. "National Intercensal Estimates, 2000–2010." Census Bureau Population Estimates home page. http://www.census.gov/popest/estimates.html. September.

————. 2011b. "Resident Population by Sex and Age." http://www.census.gov/popest/archives/EST90INTERCENSAL/US-EST90INT-04.html. September 30.

————. 2011c. "2010 Census Brief: The Older Population: 2010." November.

————. 2012a. "Table 1. Annual Estimates of the Population for the United States, Regions, States, and Puerto Rico: April 1, 2010 to July 1, 2012." NST-EST2012-01. December.

————. 2012b. Table 7. Resident Population by Sex and Age: 1980 to 2010, U.S. Census Bureau, Statistical Abstract of the United States: 2012. http://www.census.gov/compendia/statab/2012/tables/12s0007.pdf.

US Court of Appeals, Second Circuit. 2006. *United States of America, Appellee, v. Martha Stewart and Peter Bacanovic, Defendants-Appellants*. 433 F.3d 273. Docket No. 04-3953(L)-CR, Docket No. 04-4081(CON)-CR. Argued March 17, 2005; decided January 6, 2006. http://bulk.resource.org/courts.gov/c/F3/433/433.F3d.273.-.04-4081.04-3953.html.

US Department of Energy. 2009. Office of Science, Office of Biological and Environmental Research. "Major Events in the U.S. Human Genome Project and Related Projects." September 11. Retrieved from http://www.ornl.gov/sci/techresources/Human_Genome/project/timeline.shtml.

————. Office of Science Genome Programs. "History of the Human Genome Project." Retrieved from http://www.ornl.gov/sci/techresources/Human_Genome/project/hgp.shtml.

US Department of Transportation. 2012a. Bureau of Transportation Statistics. National Transportation Statistics, 2010. http://www.rita.dot.gov/bts/

sites/rita.dot.gov.bts/files/publications/national_transportation_statistics/html/
table_01_11.html.

———. 2012b. *National Highway Transportation Safety Administration, Traffic Safety Facts for 2010.* Washington, DC: NHTSA publication 811659.

US General Accounting Office. 1987a. *Cancer Patient Survival: What Progress Has Been Made?* PEMD-87-13. March.

US General Accounting Office. 1987b. *University Funding: Patterns of Distribution of Federal Research Funds to Universities.* Briefing Report to the Ranking Minority Member, Committee on Appropriations, United States Senate. GAO/RCED-87-67BR. Washington, DC: United States General Accounting Office, February.

———. 1999. *NIH Clinical Trials: Various Factors Affect Patient Participation.* GAO/HEHS-99-182. September.

US Government Accountability Office. 2006a. "Drug Safety: Improvement Needed in FDA's Postmarket Decision–Making and Oversight Process." Report to Congress. GAO-06-402. March.

———. 2006b. "Science, Business, Regulatory, and Intellectual Property Issues Cited as Hampering Drug Development Efforts." Report to Congress. GAO-07-49. November.

———. 2012. *2012 Annual Report: Opportunities to Reduce Duplication, Overlap and Fragmentation, Achieve Savings, and Enhance Revenue.* Report to Congressional Addressees. February.

US House of Representatives. 1971a. *National Cancer Attack Act of 1971: Report of the Committee on Interstate and Foreign Commerce, US House of Representatives, Together with Additional Views and Minority Views, to Accompany H.R. 11302, November 10, 1971.* House Report 92-659. Washington, DC: US Government Printing Office.

———. 1971b. *National Cancer Attack Act of 1971: Hearings Before the Subcommittee on Public Health and Environment of the Committee on Interstate and Foreign Commerce, 92nd Congress, 1st Session, on H.R. 8343, H.R. 10681, S. 1828.* Washington, DC: US Government Printing Office.

———. 2004. Rep. Thomas M. Davis III (chair), House Committee on Government Reform. Hearing on Cancer Clinical Trials, Washington, DC, May 13.

———. 2006. Committee on Government Reform, Minority Staff, Special Investigations Division (prepared for Rep. Henry A. Waxman). "Medicare Drug Plans: Restrictions on Access to Formulary Drugs." March.

US National Library of Medicine. "Changing the Face of Medicine: Biography of Dr. Janet Davison Rowley." http://www.nlm.nih.gov/changingthefaceofmedicine/physicians/biography_282.html.

———. MedlinePlus service. http://www.nlm.nih.gov/medlineplus/druginformation.html.

Vallery-Radot, Rene. 1916. *Life of Pasteur.* Translated from the French by Mrs. R. L. Devonshire. New York: Doubleday, Page & Company.

van den Bosch, C. A., et al. 1993. "Are Plant Factors a Missing Link in the Evolution of Endemic Burkitt's Lymphoma?" *British Journal of Cancer* 68 (December): 1232–35.

van den Bosch, C. A., et al. 2004. "Is Endemic Burkitt's Lymphoma an Alliance Between Three Infections and a Tumour Promoter?" *Lancet Oncology* 5 (December): 738–46.

van der Merwe, Da-Elene, et al. 2006. "Mass Spectrometry: Uncovering the Cancer Proteome for Diagnostics." *Advances in Cancer Research* 96: 23–50.

van de Vijver, Marc J., et al. 2002. "A Gene-Expression Signature as a Predictor of Survival in Breast Cancer." *New England Journal of Medicine* 347 (December 19): 1999–2009.

Van Slyke, C. J. 1946. "New Horizons in Medical Research." *Science* 104 (December 13): 559–67.

Varchaver, Nicholas. 2003. "Spinning the Wheel on ImClone." *Fortune,* April 28.

Varmus, Harold E. 1989. "Retroviruses and Oncogenes I." Nobel Lecture, the Nobel Prize in Physiology or Medicine 1989 (December 8). Retrieved from http://www.nobelprize.org/nobel_prizes/medicine/laureates/1989/varmus-lecture.html.

———. 2006. "The New Era in Cancer Research." *Science* 312 (May 26): 1162–65.

———. 2012. "Announcement: New National Cancer Informatics Program (NCIP)." National Cancer Institute. Retrieved from https://cabig.nci.nih.gov/ncip_announcement/ (undated, mid-April).

Varmus, Harold, and Robert A. Weinberg. 1993. *Genes and the Biology of Cancer.* New York: Scientific American Library.

Vasella, Daniel, and Clifton Leaf. 2002. "Temptation Is All Around Us." *Fortune,* November 18.

Vasella, Daniel, with Robert Slater. 2003. *Magic Cancer Bullet: How a Tiny Orange Pill Is Rewriting Medical History.* New York: HarperBusiness.

Vastag, Brian. 2006. "Increasing R01 Competition Concerns Researchers." *Journal of the National Cancer Institute* 98 (October 18): 1436–38.

Vaught, Jim. 2011. "BioBanking and Its Role in Cancer Research and Molecular Diagnostics." Presentation, Molecular Diagnostics conference, Washington, DC. March 24.

Verma, Mukesh, and Upender Manne. 2006. "Genetic and Epigenetic Biomarkers in Cancer Diagnosis and Identifying High-Risk Populations." *Critical Reviews in Oncology/Hematology* 60 (October): 9–18.

Vogel, Charles L., et al. 2002. "Efficacy and Safety of Trastuzumab as a Single Agent in First-Line Treatment of HER2-Overexpressing Metastatic Breast Cancer." *Journal of Clinical Oncology* 20 (February 1): 719–26.

Vogt, Peter K. 1996. "Peyton Rous: Homage and Appraisal." *FASEB Journal* 10 (November): 1559–62.

von Eschenbach, Andrew. 2002. "Collaboration to Play Key Role in NCI's Future, Director Says." *Journal of the National Cancer Institute* 94 (June 5): 790–92.

———. 2004. "A Vision for the National Cancer Program in the United States." *Nature Reviews Cancer* 4 (October): 820–28.

———. 2005. "Progress with a Purpose." *Cancer* 104 (supp.) (December 15): 2903.

Waalen, Jill. 2001. "Gleevec's Glory Days." *HHMI Bulletin,* December, 10–15.

Wagner, Todd H., et al. 2003. "Cost of Operating Institutional Review Boards (IRBs)." *Academic Medicine* 78 (June): 638–44.

Wakabi, Wairagala. 2008. "Special Report: International. Kenya and Uganda Grapple with Burkitt's Lymphoma." *Lancet Oncology* 9 (April): 319.

Walker, Steven. 2005. "Making FDA Work for Patients." *Legal Backgrounder* (Washington Legal Foundation) 20 (10) (February 25).

Walling, Jackie. 2006. "From Methotrexate to Pemetrexed and Beyond: A Review of the Pharmacodynamic and Clinical Properties of Antifolates." *Investigational New Drugs* 24 (January): 37–77.

Ward, Ryan J., and Peter B. Dirks. 2007. "Cancer Stem Cells: At the Headwaters of Tumor Development." *Annual Review of Pathology: Mechanisms of Disease* 2: 175–89.

Warnakulasuriya, S., et al. 2008. "Oral Epithelial Dysplasia Classification Systems: Predictive Value, Utility, Weaknesses and Scope for Improvement." *Journal of Oral Pathology and Medicine* 37 (March): 127–33.

Warren, Joan L., et al. 2008. "Evaluation of Trends in the Cost of Initial Cancer Treatment." *Journal of the National Cancer Institute* 100 (June 18): 888–97.

Watson, James V. 1981. "What Does 'Response' in Cancer Chemotherapy Really Mean?" *British Medical Journal* 283 (July 4): 34–37.

Wattenberg, Lee W. 1966. "Chemoprophylaxis of Carcinogenesis: A Review." *Cancer Research* 26 (part 1) (July): 1520–26.

Weaver, Valerie M., et al. 1997. "Reversion of the Malignant Phenotype of Human Breast Cells in Three-Dimensional Culture and In Vivo by Integrin Blocking Antibodies." *Journal of Cell Biology* 137 (April 7): 231–45.

Weinberg, Robert A. 1996a. "How Cancer Arises." *Scientific American* (September).

———. 1996b. *Racing to the Beginning of the Road: The Search for the Origin of Cancer.* New York: Harmony Books.

———. 1998. *One Renegade Cell: How Cancer Begins.* New York: Basic Books.

———. 2006. Kirk A. Landon Prize lecture, 2006 AACR annual meeting. Published in *Cancer Letter* 32 (April 7): 5–6.

———. 2007. *The Biology of Cancer.* New York: Garland Science.

Weinberg, Robert A., and Anthony L. Komaroff. 2008. "Your Lifestyle, Your Genes and Cancer." *Newsweek,* June 14.

Weinstein, I. Bernard. 1988. "The Origins of Human Cancer: Molecular Mechanisms of Carcinogenesis and Their Implications for Cancer Prevention and Treatment—Twenty-Seventh G. H. A. Clowes Memorial Award Lecture." *Cancer Research* 48 (August 1): 4135–43.

———. 2002. "Addiction to Oncogenes: The Achilles Heal of Cancer." *Science* 297 (July 5): 63–64.

Weinstein, I. Bernard, and Andrew Joe. 2008. "Oncogene Addiction" (a "Point-Counterpoint Review") and "Response" by Dean W. Felsher. *Cancer Research* 68 (May 1): 3077–80.

Weintraub, Arlene. 2004. "Avastin's Stumble, Genentech's Tumble." *BusinessWeek,* August 16.

Weisberg, Ellen, et al. 2007. "Second Generation Inhibitors of BCR-ABL for the Treatment of Imatinib-Resistant Chronic Myeloid Leukaemia." *Nature Reviews Cancer* 7 (May): 345–56.

Weiss, Leonard. 2000a. "Observations on the Antiquity of Cancer and Metastasis." *Cancer and Metastasis Reviews* 19 (December 1): 193–204.

———. 2000b. "Early Concepts of Cancer." *Cancer and Metastasis Reviews* 19 (December 1): 205–17.

Welch, Danny Ray, and L. L. Wei. 1998. "Genetic and Epigenetic Regulation of Human Breast Cancer Progression and Metastasis." *Endocrine-Related Cancer* 5: 155–97.

Welch, H. Gilbert, and Peter C. Albertsen. 2009. "Prostate Cancer Diagnosis and Treatment After the Introduction of Prostate-Specific Antigen Screening: 1986–2005." *Journal of the National Cancer Institute* 101 (October 7): 1325–29.

Welch, H. Gilbert, and William C. Black. 2010. "Overdiagnosis in Cancer." *Journal of the National Cancer Institute* 102 (May 5): 605–13.

Welch, H. Gilbert, Lisa M. Schwartz, and Steven Woloshin. 2000. "Are Increasing 5-Year Survival Rates Evidence of Success Against Cancer?" *Journal of the American Medical Association* 283 (June 14): 2975–78.

Wells, William A. 2005. "A Cell Line That Is Under Control." *Journal of Cell Biology* 168 (March 28): 988.

Whitmore, Elaine. 2004. *Development of FDA-Regulated Medical Products: Prescription Drugs, Biologics, and Medical Devices.* Milwaukee, WI: ASQ Quality Press.

Whittemore, Alice. 1978. "Quantitative Theories of Oncogenesis." *Advances in Cancer Research* 27: 55–88.

Whymper, Edward. 1996. *Scrambles Amongst the Alps in the Years 1860–69*. Mineola, NY: Dover Publications. Originally published in London in 1900 by John Murray.

Wicha, Max S., Suling Liu, and Gabriela Dontu. 2006. "Cancer Stem Cells: An Old Idea—a Paradigm Shift." *Cancer Research* 66 (February 15): 1883–90.

Wilford, John Noble. 2005. "At NASA, Another High-Stakes Comeback Mission: For the 4th Time, Agency Starts Over." *New York Times*, July 13.

Willis, Carol, 1988. "Building the Empire State." In *Building the Empire State: A Rediscovered 1930s Notebook Charts the Construction of the Empire State Building*, edited by Carol Willis. New York: W. W. Norton & Company.

Wilson, Duff. 2010. "Risks Seen in Cholesterol Drug Use in Healthy People." *New York Times*, March 30.

Wilson, James Q. 1989. *Bureaucracy: What Government Agencies Do and Why They Do It*. New York: Basic Books.

Winchester, David J., David P. Winchester, Clifford Hudis, and Larry Norton. 2006. *Breast Cancer*. 2nd ed. Hamilton, ON, Canada: BC Decker.

Witkin, Richard. 1962a. "U.S. to Attempt Moon Shot Today. Ranger Is Designed to Take Pictures and Hit Surface." *New York Times*, April 24.

———. 1962b. "Moon Rocket Is Launched But Fails to Transmit Data; Ranger IV Is Expected to Crash on Far Side of Target Thursday." *New York Times*, April 24.

Witte, Owen N., Asim Dasgupta, and David Baltimore. 1980. "Abelson Murine Leukaemia Virus Protein Is Phosphorylated In Vitro to Form Phosphotyrosine." *Nature* 283 (February 28): 826–31.

Wolbach, S. Burt, and Percy R. Howe. 1933. "Epithelial Repair in Recovery from Vitamin A Deficiency: An Experimental Study." *Journal of Experimental Medicine* 57 (February 28): 511–26.

Wolf, Andrew, et al. 2010. "American Cancer Society Guideline for the Early Detection of Prostate Cancer: Update 2010." *CA: A Cancer Journal for Clinicians* 60 (March–April): 70–98.

Wolfe, Sidney M. 2005. Testimony, Health Subcommittee of the House Energy and Commerce Committee. "Hearing on Current Issues Related to Medical Liability Reform." February 10.

Wolff, Antonio C., et al. 2007. "American Society of Clinical Oncology/College of American Pathologists Guideline Recommendations for Human Epidermal Growth Factor Receptor 2 Testing in Breast Cancer. *Archives of Pathology and Laboratory Medicine* 131 (January): 18–43.

Wolff, Megan J. 2006. "The Myth of the Actuary: Life Insurance and Frederick L. Hoffman's Race Traits and Tendencies of the American Negro." *Public Health Reports* 121 (January–February): 84–91.

Wolff, William I., and Hiromi Shinya. 1971. "Colonofiberoscopy." *Journal of the American Medical Association* 217 (September 13): 1509–12.

———. 1973. "A New Approach to Colonic Polyps." *Annals of Surgery* 178 (September): 367–78.

———. 1974. "Earlier Diagnosis of Cancer of the Colon Through Colonic Endoscopy (Colonoscopy)." *Cancer* 34 (September supp.): 912–31.

Woloshin, Steven, Lisa Schwartz, and H. Gilbert Welch. 2005. "Warned but Worse Off." Op-ed. *New York Times,* August 22.

Wong, Stephane, and Owen N. Witte. 2004. "The BCR-ABL Story: Bench to Bedside and Back." *Annual Review of Immunology* 22: 247–306.

Wood, Laura D., et al. 2007. "The Genomic Landscapes of Human Breast and Colorectal Cancers." *Science* 318 (November 16): 1108–13.

Woodcock, Janet D. 2011. Testimony, House Committee on Energy and Commerce, Subcommittee on Health. "Hearing on Prescription Drug User Fee Act Reauthorization." July 7.

Wright, Pearce. 2001. "Joe Hin Tjio: The Man Who Cracked the Chromosome Count." *Guardian* (UK), December 11.

Xu, Yanfei, et al. 2005. "Tumor-Associated Carbohydrate Antigens: A Possible Avenue for Cancer Prevention." *Immunology and Cell Biology* 83 (August): 440–48.

Yabroff, K. Robin, et al. 2004. "Burden of Illness in Cancer Survivors: Findings from a Population–Based National Sample." *Journal of the National Cancer Institute* 96 (September 1): 1322–30.

Yabroff, K. Robin, Jennifer Lund, Deanna Kepka, et al. 2011. "Economic Burden of Cancer in the United States: Estimates, Projections, and Future Research." *Cancer Epidemiology, Biomarkers, and Prevention* 20 (October): 2006–14.

Yaffe, Michael B. 2009. "Living by the Numbers." *Science Signaling* 2 (99) (December 1): eg15.

Yager, James D., and Nancy E. Davidson. 2006. "Estrogen Carcinogenesis in Breast Cancer." *New England Journal of Medicine* 354 (January 19): 270–82.

Yale Medical School. 2012. "Yale Medical Histology." http://medcell.med.yale.edu/histology/blood.php.

Yancik, Rosemary, and Margaret E. Holmes. 2001. National Institute on Aging and National Cancer Institute. "Workshop Report: Exploring the Role of Cancer Centers for Integrating Aging and Cancer Research." Workshop. June 13–15.

Yankwich, Peter E. 1949. "Radioactive Isotopes as Tracers." Presented at the First Annual Summer Symposium on Analytical Chemistry, Northwestern University. *Analytical Chemistry* 21(3): 318–321.

Yarden, Y. 2001. "The EGFR Family and Its Ligands in Human Cancer: Signalling Mechanisms and Therapeutic Opportunities." *European Journal of Cancer* 37 (supp. 4) (September): S3–S8.

Yarris, Jonathan P., and Alan J. Hunter. 2003. "Roy Hertz, MD (1909–2002): The Cure of Choriocarcinoma and Its Impact on the Development of Chemotherapy for Cancer." *Gynecologic Oncology* 89 (May): 193–98.

Yaziji, Hadi, et al. 2008. "Consensus Recommendations on Estrogen Receptor Testing in Breast Cancer by Immunohistochemistry." *Applied Immunohistochemistry and Molecular Morphology* 16 (December): 513–20.

Yie, Shang-mian. 2008. "Prediction of Metastasis and Recurrence of Breast Carcinoma: Detection of Survivin–Expressing Circulating Cancer Cells." In *Methods of Cancer Diagnosis, Therapy and Prognosis, Vol. 1, Breast Carcinoma*, edited by M. A. Hayat, 157–74. New York: Springer.

Young, Robert C. 2010. "Cancer Clinical Trials: A Chronic but Curable Crisis." *New England Journal of Medicine* 363 (July 22): 306–9.

Young, Robert C., Vincent T. DeVita, and Ralph E. Johnson. 1973. "Hodgkin's Disease in Childhood." *Blood* 42 (August): 163–73.

Yu, Tian–Wei, and Diana Anderson. 1997. "Reactive Oxygen Species-Induced DNA Damage and Its Modification: A Chemical Investigation." *Mutation Research* 379 (October 6): 201–10.

Yunis, Jorge J. 1983. "The Chromosomal Basis of Human Neoplasia." *Science* 221 (July 15): 227–36.

Zauber, Ann G., et al. 2012. "Colonoscopic Polypectomy and Long-Term Prevention of Colorectal-Cancer Deaths." *New England Journal of Medicine* 366 (February 23): 687–96.

Zemlo, Tamara R., et al. 2000. "The Physician–Scientist: Career Issues and Challenges at the Year 2000." *FASEB Journal* 14 (February): 221–30.

Zemmel, Rodney, and Mubasher Sheikh. 2010. *Invention Reinvented: McKinsey Perspectives on Pharmaceutical R&D*. New York: McKinsey & Co.

Zerhouni, Elias A. 2006. "NIH in the Post-Doubling Era: Realities and Strategies." *Science* 314 (November 17): 1088–90.

Zhivotovsky, Boris, and Sten Orrenius. 2009. "The Warburg Effect Returns to the Cancer Stage." *Seminars in Cancer Biology* 19: 3.

Ziegler, Sandra. 2003. "Jürg Zimmermann: Extraordinary Contributions to Oncology Research" (interview with Zimmermann). Novartis Institute for Biomedical Research, internal company publication. December.

Zika, Eleni, et al. 2010. *Biobanks in Europe: Prospects for Harmonisation and Networking*. European Commission Joint Research Centre and Institute for Prospective Technological Studies. EUR 24361 EN–2010.

Zimmermann, Jürg, et al. 1997. "Potent and Selective Inhibitors of the Abl-Kinase: Phenylamino-Pyrimidine (PAP) Derivatives." *Bioorganic and Medicinal Chemistry Letters* 7 (January 21): 187–92.

Zimmerman, Rachel. 2005. "Drug Slows a Deadly Cancer, Study Finds, but Price Is Steep." *Wall Street Journal,* June 16.

Zubrod, C. Gordon. 1979. "Historic Milestones in Curative Chemotherapy." *Seminars in Oncology* 6 (4): 496–500.

———. 1984. "Origins and Development of Chemotherapy Research at the National Cancer Institute." *Cancer Treatment Reports* 68 (January): 9–19.

Zubrod, C. Gordon, and Joseph H. Burchenal. 1971. "Folate Antagonists as Chemotherapeutic Agents." *Annals of the New York Academy of Sciences* 186 (November): 516–19.

Index